REFERENCE EDITION

ENDOCRINE BOARD REVIEW 2021

Serge A. Jabbour, MD, Program Chair
Professor of Medicine
Director, Division of Endocrinology,
Diabetes & Metabolic Diseases
Sidney Kimmel Medical College
Thomas Jefferson University

Natalie E. Cusano, MD, MS
Associate Professor of Medicine
Zucker School of Medicine
at Hofstra/Northwell
Director of the Bone
Metabolism Program
Division of Endocrinology
at Lenox Hill Hospital

Tobias Else, MD
Associate Professor
Division of Metabolism,
Endocrinology, and Diabetes
University of Michigan

Frances J. Hayes, MB BCh, BAO
Associate Clinical Chief
of Endocrinology
Massachusetts General Hospital
Associate Professor of Medicine
Harvard Medical School

Jacqueline Jonklaas, MD, PhD, MPH
Professor
Division of Endocrinology
Georgetown University Medical Center

Sangeeta R. Kashyap, MD
Professor of Medicine
Cleveland Clinic Lerner
College of Medicine
Physician Scientist
Endocrinology Institute
at Cleveland Clinic

Laurence Katznelson, MD
Professor of Neurosurgery
and Medicine
Division of Endocrinology
Stanford University School of Medicine

Kathryn A. Martin, MD
Assistant Professor of Medicine
Harvard Medical School
Faculty Clinician, Reproductive
Endocrine Unit
Massachusetts General Hospital
Senior Physician Editor,
Endocrinology and Diabetes
UpToDate

Marie E. McDonnell, MD
Section Chief, Diabetes Section
Division of Endocrinology
Diabetes and Hypertension
Brigham and Women's Hospital
Harvard Medical School

Abbie L. Young, MS, CGC, ELS(D)
Medical Editor

Endocrine Society
2055 L Street NW, Suite 600, Washington, DC 20036
1-888-ENDOCRINE • www.endocrine.org

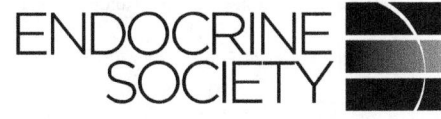
ENDOCRINE SOCIETY

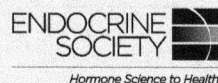

The Endocrine Society is the world's largest, oldest, and most active organization working to advance the clinical practice of endocrinology and hormone research. Founded in 1916, the Society now has more than 18,000 global members across a range of disciplines. The Society has earned an international reputation for excellence in the quality of its peer-reviewed journals, educational resources, meetings, and programs that improve public health through the practice and science of endocrinology.

For between-edition updates, visit us at:
https://www.endocrine.org/education-and-training/book-updates

Other publications:
endocrine.org/publications

ISBN: 978-1-936704-06-4
Library of Congress Control Number: 2021939128

On the Cover: © Shutterstock. (By mrmohock)

OVERVIEW

Endocrine Board Review (EBR) 13th Edition (2021) is a board examination preparation book designed for endocrine fellows who have completed or are nearing completion of their fellowship and are preparing to sit for the board certification exam, and for practicing endocrinologists in search of a comprehensive self-assessment of endocrinology, either to prepare for recertification or to update their practice. EBR consists of approximately 220 case-based, American Board of Internal Medicine (ABIM) style, multiple-choice questions. Each section follows the ABIM Endocrinology, Diabetes, and Metabolism Certification Examination blueprint, covering the breadth and depth of the certification and recertification examinations. Each case is discussed in detail with detailed answer explanations and references provided.

The EBR 13th Edition (2021) reference book is intended primarily for consultation and self-assessment of knowledge relating to endocrinology. As a reference book, educational credits are not available upon completion of the multiple-choice questions included. For information on educational products that include educational credit, please visit endocrine.org/store.

LEARNING OBJECTIVES

Upon completion of this educational activity, learners will be able to demonstrate enhanced medical knowledge and clinical skills across all major areas of endocrinology; apply knowledge and skills in diagnosing, managing, and treating a wide spectrum of endocrine disorders; and successfully complete the board examination for certification or recertification in the subspecialty of endocrinology, diabetes, and metabolism.

TARGET AUDIENCE

This activity should be of substantial interest to endocrinologists, internists, and endocrine fellows preparing for the board examination or recertification; or endocrinologists and other health care practitioners seeking a review in endocrinology.

STATEMENT OF INDEPENDENCE

The Endocrine Society has a policy of ensuring that the content and quality of this educational activity are balanced, independent, objective, and scientifically rigorous. The scientific content of this activity was developed under the supervision of the Endocrine Society's EBR faculty. There are no commercial supporters of this activity and no commercial entities have had an influence over the planning of this activity.

DISCLOSURE POLICY

The faculty, committee members, and staff who are in position to control the content of this activity are required to disclose to the Endocrine Society and to learners any relevant financial relationship(s) of the individual or spouse/partner that have occurred within the last 12 months with any commercial interest(s) whose products or services are related to the content. Financial relationships are defined by remuneration in any amount from the commercial interest(s) in the form of grants; research support; consulting fees; salary; ownership interest (eg, stocks, stock options, or ownership interest excluding diversified mutual funds); honoraria or other payments for participation in speakers' bureaus, advisory boards, or boards of directors; or other financial benefits. The intent of this disclosure is not to prevent planners with relevant financial relationships from planning or delivery of content, but rather to provide learners with information that allows them to make their own judgments of whether these financial relationships may have influenced the educational activity with regard to exposition or conclusion.

The Endocrine Society has reviewed all disclosures and resolved or managed all identified conflicts of interest, as applicable.

The faculty reported the following relevant financial relationship(s) during the content development process for this activity:

Natalie E. Cusano, MD, MS, has served as a research investigator for Shire/Takeda, a speaker for Alexion Pharmaceuticals, and DSMB member for Ascendis Pharma.

Tobias Else, MD, has served as an advisory board member to Corcept Therapeutics, HRA Pharma, and Merck, and his institution has received research support from Corcept Therapeutics, Merck, and Strongbridge Biopharma.

Sangeeta R. Kashyap, MD, has served as a consultant and coinvestigator to GI Dynamics and as a consultant to Fractyl, Inc; her institution has received research support from Fractyl, Inc, and Janssen Pharmaceuticals.

Laurence Katznelson, MD, has served as a consultant and principal investigator to Chiasma and Camarus, and he has served as an advisory board member to Novo Nordisk.

Marie E. McDonnell, MD, has served as a trial event adjudicator for a trial conducted by Eisai.

The following faculty reported no relevant financial relationships: Frances J. Hayes, MB BCh, BAO; Serge A. Jabbour, MD; Jacqueline Jonklaas, MD, PhD, MPH; and Kathryn A. Martin, MD

The medical editor for this activity reported no relevant financial relationships: Abbie L. Young, MS, CGC, ELS(D)

Endocrine Society staff associated with the development of content for this activity reported no relevant financial relationships.

DISCLAIMERS

The information presented in this activity represents the opinion of the faculty and is not necessarily the official position of the Endocrine Society.

Use of professional judgment:

The educational content in this activity relates to basic principles of diagnosis and therapy and does not substitute for individual patient assessment based on the health care provider's examination of the patient and consideration of laboratory data and other factors unique to the patient. Standards in medicine change as new data become available.

Drugs and dosages:

When prescribing medications, the physician is advised to check the product information sheet accompanying each drug to verify conditions of use and to identify any changes in drug dosage schedule or contraindications.

POLICY ON UNLABELED/OFF-LABEL USE

The Endocrine Society has determined that disclosure of unlabeled/off-label or investigational use of commercial product(s) is informative for audiences and therefore requires this information to be disclosed to the learners at the beginning of the presentation. Uses of specific therapeutic agents, devices, and other products discussed in this educational activity may not be the same as those indicated in product labeling approved by the Food and Drug Administration (FDA). The Endocrine Society requires that any discussions of such "off-label" use be based on scientific research that conforms to generally accepted standards of experimental design, data collection, and data analysis. Before recommending or prescribing any therapeutic agent or device, learners should review the complete prescribing information, including indications, contraindications, warnings, precautions, and adverse events.

ACKNOWLEDGEMENT OF COMMERCIAL SUPPORT

The activity is not supported by educational grant(s) or other funds from any commercial supporters.

Publication Date: August 2021

Contents

For between-edition updates, visit us at: https://www.endocrine.org/education-and-training/book-updates.

LABORATORY REFERENCE RANGES

Reference ranges vary among laboratories. Conventional units are listed first with SI units in parentheses.

Lipid Values

High-density lipoprotein (HDL) cholesterol

    Optimal ------------------------- >60 mg/dL (SI: >1.55 mmol/L)

    Normal------------------- 40-60 mg/dL (SI: 1.04-1.55 mmol/L)

    Low -------------------------- -<40 mg/dL (SI: <1.04 mmol/L)

Low-density lipoprotein (LDL) cholesterol

    Optimal -----------------------<100 mg/dL (SI: <2.59 mmol/L)

    Low --------------------100-129 mg/dL (SI: 2.59-3.34 mmol/L)

    Borderline-high --------130-159 mg/dL (SI: 3.37-4.12 mmol/L)

    High ------------------160-189 mg/dL (SI: 4.14-4.90 mmol/L)

    Very high ----------------------≥190 mg/dL (SI: ≥4.92 mmol/L)

Non-HDL cholesterol

    Optimal- -----------------------<130 mg/dL (SI: <3.37 mmol/L)

    Borderline-high --------130-159 mg/dL (SI: 3.37-4.12 mmol/L)

    High --------------------------≥240 mg/dL (SI: ≥6.22 mmol/L)

Total cholesterol

    Optimal -----------------------<200 mg/dL (SI: <5.18 mmol/L)

    Borderline-high --------200-239 mg/dL (SI: 5.18-6.19 mmol/L)

    High --------------------------≥240 mg/dL (SI: ≥6.22 mmol/L)

Triglycerides

    Optimal -----------------------<150 mg/dL (SI: <1.70 mmol/L)

    Borderline-high --------150-199 mg/dL (SI: 1.70-2.25 mmol/L)

    High ------------------200-499 mg/dL (SI: 2.26-5.64 mmol/L)

    Very high ----------------------≥500 mg/dL (SI: ≥5.65 mmol/L)

Lipoprotein (a) ----------------------≤30 mg/dL (SI: ≤1.07 μmol/L)

Apolipoprotein B ------------------ 50-110 mg/dL (SI: 0.5-1.1 g/L)

Hematologic Values

Erythrocyte sedimentation rate ------------------------0-20 mm/h

Haptoglobin ------------------ 30-200 mg/dL (SI: 300-2000 mg/L)

Hematocrit----------------------- 41%-51% (SI: 0.41-0.51) (male);

    35%-45% (SI: 0.35-0.45) (female)

Hemoglobin A_{1c}---------------------- 4.0%-5.6% (20-38 mmol/mol)

Hemoglobin --------------- 13.8-17.2 g/dL (SI: 138-172 g/L) (male);

    12.1-15.1 g/dL (SI: 121-151 g/L) (female)

International normalized ratio ------------------------------0.8-1.2

Mean corpuscular volume (MCV) ------80-100 μm³ (SI: 80-100 fL)

Platelet count------------- 150-450 x 10³/μL (SI: 150-450 x 10⁹/L)

Protein (total) -------------------------6.3-7.9 g/dL (SI: 63-79 g/L)

Reticulocyte count--- 0.5%-1.5% of red blood cells (SI: 0.005-0.015)

White blood cell count------ 4500-11,000/μL (SI: 4.5-11.0 x 10⁹/L)

Thyroid Values

Thyroglobulin ------ 3-42 ng/mL (SI: 3-42 μg/L) (after surgery and

    radioactive iodine treatment: <1.0 ng/mL [SI: <1.0 μg/L])

Thyroglobulin antibodies ---------------- ≤4.0 IU/mL (SI: ≤4.0 kIU/L)

Thyrotropin (TSH) ------------------------------------- 0.5-5.0 mIU/L

Thyrotropin-receptor antibodies (TRAb) ----------------≤1.75 IU/L

Thyroid-stimulating immunoglobulin----- ≤120% of basal activity

Thyroperoxidase (TPO) antibodies ----- <2.0 IU/mL (SI: <2.0 kIU/L)

Thyroxine (T_4) (free) -------0.8-1.8 ng/dL (SI: 10.30-23.17 pmol/L)

Thyroxine (T_4) (total)---- 5.5-12.5 μg/dL (SI: 94.02-213.68 nmol/L)

Free thyroxine (T_4) index ------------------------------------ 4-12

Triiodothyronine (T_3) (free)---- 2.3-4.2 pg/mL (SI: 3.53-6.45 pmol/L)

Triiodothyronine (T_3) (total)----70-200 ng/dL (SI: 1.08-3.08 nmol/L)

Triiodothyronine (T_3), reverse ---- 10-24 ng/dL (SI: 0.15-0.37 nmol/L)

Triiodothyronine uptake, resin -------------------------- 25%-38%

Radioactive iodine uptake---------------------3%-16% (6 hours);

    15%-30% (24 hours)

Endocrine Values
Serum

Aldosterone------------------ 4-21 ng/dL (SI: 111.0-582.5 pmol/L)

Alkaline phosphatase ---------- 50-120 U/L (SI: 0.84-2.00 μkat/L)

Alkaline phosphatase (bone-specific) ----------------------------

    ≤20 μg/L (adult male); ≤14 μg/L (premenopausal female);

    ≤22 μg/L (postmenopausal female)

Androstenedione --

    65-210 ng/dL (SI: 2.27-7.33 nmol/L) (adult male);

    30-200 ng/dL (SI:1.05-6.98 nmol/L) (adult female)

Antimullerian hormone --

    0.7-19.0 ng/mL (SI: 5.0-135.7 pmol/L) (male, >12 years);

    0.9-9.5 ng/mL (SI: 6.4-67.9 pmol/L) (female, 13-45 years);

    <1.0 ng/mL (SI: <7.1 pmol/L) (female, >45 years)

Calcitonin -------------<16 pg/mL (SI: <4.67 pmol/L) (basal, male);

    <8 pg/mL (SI: <2.34 pmol/L) (basal, female);

    ≤130 pg/mL (SI: ≤37.96 pmol/L) (peak calcium infusion, male);

    ≤90 pg/mL (SI: ≤26.28 pmol/L) (peak calcium infusion, female)

Carcinoembryonic antigen ------------- <2.5 ng/mL (SI: <2.5 μg/L)

Chromogranin A ------------------------- <93 ng/mL (SI: <93 μg/L)

Corticosterone --- 53-1560 ng/dL (SI: 1.53-45.08 nmol/L) (>18 years)

Corticotropin (ACTH) ---------- 10-60 pg/mL (SI: 2.2-13.2 pmol/L)

Cortisol (8 AM) -------------- 5-25 μg/dL (SI: 137.9-689.7 nmol/L)

Cortisol (4 PM) ----------------- 2-14 µg/dL (SI: 55.2-386.2 nmol/L)

C-peptide -------------------- 0.5-2.0 ng/mL (SI: 0.17-0.66 nmol/L)

C-reactive protein ----------- 0.8-3.1 mg/L (SI: 7.62-29.52 nmol/L)

Cross-linked N-telopeptide of type 1 collagen --------------------

    5.4-24.2 nmol BCE/mmol creat (male);

    6.2-19.0 nmol BCE/mmol creat (female)

Dehydroepiandrosterone sulfate (DHEA-S)

Patient Age	Female	Male
18-29 years	44-332 µg/dL (SI: 1.19-9.00 µmol/L)	89-457 µg/dL (SI: 2.41-12.38 µmol/L)
30-39 years	31-228 µg/dL (SI: 0.84-6.78 µmol/L)	65-334 µg/dL (SI: 1.76-9.05 µmol/L)
40-49 years	18-244 µg/dL (SI: 0.49-6.61 µmol/L)	48-244 µg/dL (SI: 1.30-6.61 µmol/L)
50-59 years	15-200 µg/dL (SI: 0.41-5.42 µmol/L)	35-179 µg/dL (SI: 0.95-4.85 µmol/L)
≥60 years	15-157 µg/dL (SI: 0.41-4.25 µmol/L)	25-131 µg/dL (SI: 0.68-3.55 µmol/L)

Deoxycorticosterone ---- <10 ng/dL (SI: <0.30 nmol/L) (>18 years)

1,25-Dihydroxyvitamin D_3 ---- 16-65 pg/mL (SI: 41.6-169.0 pmol/L)

Estradiol ------------- 10-40 pg/mL (SI: 36.7-146.8 pmol/L) (male);

    10-180 pg/mL (SI: 36.7-660.8 pmol/L) (follicular, female);

    100-300 pg/mL (SI: 367.1-1101.3 pmol/L) (midcycle, female);

    40-200 pg/mL (SI: 146.8-734.2 pmol/L) (luteal, female);

    <20 pg/mL (SI: <73.4 pmol/L) (postmenopausal, female)

Estrone ------------- 10-60 pg/mL (SI: 37.0-221.9 pmol/L) (male);

    17-200 pg/mL (SI: 62.9-739.6 pmol/L) (premenopausal female);

    7-40 pg/mL (SI: 25.9-147.9 pmol/L) (postmenopausal female)

α-Fetoprotein ----------------------------- <6 ng/mL (SI: <6 µg/L)

Follicle-stimulating hormone (FSH) -------------------------------

    1.0-13.0 mIU/mL (SI: 1.0-13.0 IU/L) (male);

    <3.0 mIU/mL (SI: <3.0 IU/L) (prepuberty, female);

    2.0-12.0 mIU/mL (SI: 2.0-12.0 IU/L) (follicular, female);

    4.0-36.0 mIU/mL (SI: 4.0-36.0 IU/L) (midcycle, female);

    1.0-9.0 mIU/mL (SI: 1.0-9.0 IU/L) (luteal, female);

    >30.0 mIU/mL (SI: >30.0 IU/L) (postmenopausal, female)

Free fatty acids -------------- 10.6-18.0 mg/dL (SI: 0.4-0.7 nmol/L)

Gastrin -------------------------------- <100 pg/mL (SI: <100 ng/L)

Growth hormone (GH)--- 0.01-0.97 ng/mL (SI: 0.01-0.97 µg/L) (male);

    0.01-3.61 ng/mL (SI: 0.01-3.61 µg/L) (female)

Homocysteine ----------------------- ≤1.76 mg/L (SI: ≤13 µmol/L)

β-Human chorionic gonadotropin (β-hCG) -----------------------

    <3.0 mIU/mL (SI: <3.0 IU/L) (nonpregnant female);

    >25 mIU/mL SI: >25 IU/L) indicates a positive pregnancy test

β-Hydroxybutyrate ---------------- <3.0 mg/dL (SI: <288.2 µmol/L)

17-Hydroxypregnenolone --- 29-189 ng/dL (SI: 0.87-5.69 nmol/L)

17α-Hydroxyprogesterone ---

    <220 ng/dL (SI: <6.67 nmol/L) (adult male);

    <80 ng/dL (SI: <2.42 nmol/L) (follicular, female);

    <285 ng/dL (SI: <8.64 nmol/L) (luteal, female);

    <51 ng/dL (SI: <1.55 nmol/L) (postmenopausal, female)

25-Hydroxyvitamin D --

    <20 ng/mL (SI: <49.9 nmol/L) (deficiency);

    21-29 ng/mL (SI: 52.4-72.4 nmol/L) (insufficiency);

    30-80 ng/mL (SI: 74.9-199.7 nmol/L) (optimal levels);

    >80 ng/mL (SI: >199.7 nmol/L) (toxicity possible)

Inhibin B ------------------------- 15-300 pg/mL (SI: 15-300 ng/L)

Insulinlike growth factor 1 (IGF-1)

Patient Age	Female	Male
18 years	162-541 ng/mL (SI: 21.2-70.9 nmol/L)	170-640 ng/mL (SI: 22.3-83.8 nmol/L)
19 years	138-442 ng/mL (SI: 18.1-57.9 nmol/L)	147-527 ng/mL (SI: 19.3-69.0 nmol/L)
20 years	122-384 ng/mL (SI: 16.0-50.3 nmol/L)	132-457 ng/mL (SI: 17.3-59.9 nmol/L)
21-25 years	116-341 ng/mL (SI: 15.2-44.7 nmol/L)	116-341 ng/mL (SI: 15.2-44.7 nmol/L)
26-30 years	117-321 ng/mL (SI: 15.3-42.1 nmol/L)	117-321 ng/mL (SI: 15.3-42.1 nmol/L)
31-35 years	113-297 ng/mL (SI: 14.8-38.9 nmol/L)	113-297 ng/mL (SI: 14.8-38.9 nmol/L)
36-40 years	106-277 ng/mL (SI: 13.9-36.3 nmol/L)	106-277 ng/mL (SI: 13.9-36.3 nmol/L)
41-45 years	98-261 ng/mL (SI: 12.8-34.2 nmol/L)	98-261 ng/mL (SI: 12.8-34.2 nmol/L)
46-50 years	91-246 ng/mL (SI: 11.9-32.2 nmol/L)	91-246 ng/mL (SI: 11.9-32.2 nmol/L)
51-55 years	84-233 ng/mL (SI: 11.0-30.5 nmol/L)	84-233 ng/mL (SI: 11.0-30.5 nmol/L)
56-60 years	78-220 ng/mL (SI: 10.2-28.8 nmol/L)	78-220 ng/mL (SI: 10.2-28.8 nmol/L)
61-65 years	72-207 ng/mL (SI: 9.4-27.1 nmol/L)	72-207 ng/mL (SI: 9.4-27.1 nmol/L)
66-70 years	67-195 ng/mL (SI: 8.8-25.5 nmol/L)	67-195 ng/mL (SI: 8.8-25.5 nmol/L)
71-75 years	62-184 ng/mL (SI: 8.1-24.1 nmol/L)	62-184 ng/mL (SI: 8.1-24.1 nmol/L)
76-80 years	57-172 ng/mL (SI: 7.5-22.5 nmol/L)	57-172 ng/mL (SI: 7.5-22.5 nmol/L)
>80 years	53-162 ng/mL (SI: 6.9-21.2 nmol/L)	53-162 ng/mL (SI: 6.9-21.2 nmol/L)

Insulinlike growth factor binding protein 3 ----------- 2.5-4.8 mg/L

Insulin ----------------------- 1.4-14.0 µIU/mL (SI: 9.7-97.2 pmol/L)

Islet-cell antibody assay--

    0 Juvenile Diabetes Foundation units

Luteinizing hormone (LH)--

    1.0-9.0 mIU/mL (SI: 1.0-9.0 IU/L) (male);

    <1.0 mIU/mL (SI: <1.0 IU/L) (prepuberty, female);

    1.0-18.0 mIU/mL (SI: 1.0-18.0 IU/L) (follicular, female);

    20.0-80.0 mIU/mL (SI: 20.0-80.0 IU/L) (midcycle, female);

    0.5-18.0 mIU/mL (SI: 0.5-18.0 IU/L) (luteal, female);

    >30.0 mIU/mL (SI: >30.0 IU/L) (postmenopausal, female)

Metanephrines (plasma fractionated)

    Metanephrine--------------------<99 pg/mL (SI: <0.50 nmol/L)

    Normetanephrine-------------- <165 pg/mL (SI: <0.90 nmol/L)

75-g oral glucose tolerance test blood glucose values -----------

    60-100 mg/dL (SI: 3.3-5.6 mmol/L) (fasting);

    <200 mg/dL (SI: <11.1 mmol/L) (1 hour);

    <140 mg/dL (SI: <7.8 mmol/L) (2 hour);

    between 140-200 mg/dL (SI: 7.8-11.1 mmol/L) is considered

    impaired glucose tolerance or prediabetes. Greater than

    200 mg/dL (SI: >11.1 mmol/L) is a sign of diabetes mellitus

50-g oral glucose tolerance test for gestational diabetes --------

    <140 mg/dL (SI: <7.8 mmol/L) (1 hour)

100-g oral glucose tolerance test for gestational diabetes -------

    <95 mg/dL (SI: <5.3 mmol/L) (fasting);

    <180 mg/dL (SI: <10.0 mmol/L) (1 hour);

    <155 mg/dL (SI: <8.6 mmol/L) (2 hour);

    <140 mg/dL (SI: <7.8 mmol/L) (3 hour)

Osteocalcin ---------------------9.0-42.0 ng/mL (SI: 9.0-42.0 µg/L)

Parathyroid hormone, intact (PTH) - 10-65 pg/mL (SI: 10-65 ng/L)

Parathyroid hormone–related protein (PTHrP) --------<2.0 pmol/L

Progesterone ------------------≤1.2 ng/mL (SI: ≤3.8 nmol/L) (male);

    ≤1.0 ng/mL (SI: ≤3.2 nmol/L) (follicular, female);

    2.0-20.0 ng/mL (SI: 6.4-63.6 nmol/L) (luteal, female);

    ≤1.1 ng/mL (SI: ≤3.5 nmol/L) (postmenopausal, female);

    >10.0 ng/mL (SI: >31.8 nmol/L) (evidence of ovulatory adequacy)

Proinsulin ------------------ 26.5-176.4 pg/mL (SI: 3.0-20.0 pmol/L)

Prolactin -----------------4-23 ng/mL (SI: 0.17-1.00 nmol/L) (male);

    4-30 ng/mL (SI: 0.17-1.30 nmol/L) (nonlactating female);

    10-200 ng/mL (SI: 0.43-8.70 nmol/L) (lactating female)

Prostate-specific antigen (PSA) ------------------------------------

    <2.0 ng/mL (SI: <2.0 µg/L) (≤40 years);

    <2.8 ng/mL (SI: <2.8 µg/L) (≤50 years);

    <3.8 ng/mL (SI: <3.8 µg/L) (≤60 years);

    <5.3 ng/mL (SI: <5.3 µg/L) (≤70 years);

    <7.0 ng/mL (SI: <7.0 µg/L) (≤79 years);

    <7.2 ng/mL (SI: <7.2 µg/L) (≥80 years)

Renin activity, plasma, sodium replete, ambulatory --------------

    0.6-4.3 ng/mL per h

Renin, direct concentration ------- 4-44 pg/mL (SI: 0.1-1.0 pmol/L)

Sex hormone–binding globulin (SHBG) ---------------------------

    1.1-6.7 µg/mL (SI: 10-60 nmol/L) (male);

    2.2-14.6 µg/mL (SI: 20-130 nmol/L) (female)

α-Subunit of pituitary glycoprotein hormones --------------------

    <1.2 ng/mL (SI: <1.2 µg/L)

Testosterone (bioavailable)--

    0.8-4.0 ng/dL (SI: 0.03-0.14 nmol/L)

    (20-50 years, female on oral estrogen);

    0.8-10.0 ng/dL (SI: 0.03-0.35 nmol/L)

    (20-50 years, female not on oral estrogen);

    83.0-257.0 ng/dL (SI: 2.88-8.92 nmol/L) (male 20-29 years);

    72.0-235.0 ng/dL (SI: 2.50-8.15 nmol/L) (male 30-39 years);

    61.0-213.0 ng/dL (SI: 2.12-7.39 nmol/L) (male 40-49 years);

    50.0-190.0 ng/dL (SI: 1.74-6.59 nmol/L) (male 50-59 years);

    40.0-168.0 ng/dL (SI: 1.39-5.83 nmol/L) (male 60-69 years)

Testosterone (free)-- 9.0-30.0 ng/dL (SI: 0.31-1.04 nmol/L) (male);

    0.3-1.9 ng/dL (SI: 0.01-0.07 nmol/L) (female)

Testosterone (total)- 300-900 ng/dL (SI: 10.4-31.2 nmol/L) (male);

    8-60 ng/dL (SI: 0.3-2.1 nmol/L) (female)

Vitamin B_{12} ----------------- 180-914 pg/mL (SI: 133-674 pmol/L)

Chemistry Values

Alanine aminotransferase ------- 10-40 U/L (SI: 0.17-0.67 µkat/L)

Albumin-------------------------------3.5-5.0 g/dL (SI: 35-50 g/L)

Amylase ------------------------ 26-102 U/L (SI: 0.43-1.70 µkat/L)

Aspartate aminotransferase ---- 20-48 U/L (SI: 0.33-0.80 µkat/L)

Bicarbonate ---------------------- 21-28 mEq/L (SI: 21-28 mmol/L)

Bilirubin (total) ---------------- 0.3-1.2 mg/dL (SI: 5.1-20.5 µmol/L)

Blood gases

    Po_2, arterial blood ---------80-100 mm Hg (SI: 10.6-13.3 kPa)

    Pco_2, arterial blood ------------35-45 mm Hg (SI: 4.7-6.0 kPa)

Blood pH--- 7.35-7.45

Calcium -----------------------8.2-10.2 mg/dL (SI: 2.1-2.6 mmol/L)

Calcium (ionized) ----------- 4.60-5.08 mg/dL (SI: 1.2-1.3 mmol/L)

Carbon dioxide ------------------- 22-28 mEq/L (SI: 22-28 mmol/L)

CD_4 cell count--------------------500-1400/µL (SI: 0.5-1.4 x 10^9/L)

Chloride----------------------- 96-106 mEq/L (SI: 96-106 mmol/L)

Creatine kinase ----------------- 50-200 U/L (SI: 0.84-3.34 µkat/L)

Creatinine-----------0.7-1.3 mg/dL (SI: 61.9-114.9 µmol/L) (male);

    0.6-1.1 mg/dL (SI: 53.0-97.2 µmol/L) (female)

Ferritin --------------------- 15-200 ng/mL (SI: 33.7-449.4 pmol/L)

Folate --------------------------------- ≥4.0 ng/mL (SI: ≥4.0 µg/L)

Glucose ------------------------ 70-99 mg/dL (SI: 3.9-5.5 mmol/L)

γ-Glutamyltransferase ------------ 2-30 U/L (SI: 0.03-0.50 µkat/L)

Iron --
50-150 µg/dL (SI: 9.0-26.8 µmol/L) (male);
35-145 µg/dL (SI: 6.3-26.0 µmol/L) (female)
Lactate dehydrogenase --------- 100-200 U/L (SI: 1.7-3.3 µkat/L)
Lactic acid --------------------5.4-20.7 mg/dL (SI: 0.6-2.3 mmol/L)
Lipase ------------------------- 10-73 U/L (SI: 0.17-1.22 µkat/L)
Magnesium -------------------- 1.5-2.3 mg/dL (SI: 0.6-0.9 mmol/L)
Osmolality ------------275-295 mOsm/kg (SI: 275-295 mmol/kg)
Phosphate --------------------- 2.3-4.7 mg/dL (SI: 0.7-1.5 mmol/L)
Potassium --------------------- 3.5-5.0 mEq/L (SI: 3.5-5.0 mmol/L)
Prothrombin time -------------------------------------8.3-10.8 s
Serum urea nitrogen--------------8-23 mg/dL (SI: 2.9-8.2 mmol/L)
Sodium -------------------- 136-142 mEq/L (SI: 136-142 mmol/L)
Transferrin saturation ----------------------------------- 14%-50%
Troponin I ------------------------------- <0.6 ng/mL (SI: <0.6 µg/L)
Tryptase --------------------------- <11.5 ng/mL (SI: <11.5 µg/L)
Uric acid ------------------- 3.5-7.0 mg/dL (SI: 208.2-416.4 µmol/L)

Urine

Albumin-----------30-300 µg/mg creat (SI: 3.4-33.9 µg/mol creat)
Albumin-to-creatinine ratio ----------------------- <30 mg/g creat
Aldosterone-------------------- 3-20 µg/24 h (SI: 8.3-55.4 nmol/d)
(should be <12 µg/24 h [SI: <33.2 nmol/d] with oral sodium
loading—confirmed with 24-hour urinary sodium >200 mEq)
Calcium -------------------- 100-300 mg/24 h (SI: 2.5-7.5 mmol/d)
Catecholamine fractionation
Normotensive normal ranges:
Dopamine ------------------- <400 µg/24 h (SI: <2610 nmol/d)
Epinephrine --------------------- <21 µg/24 h (SI: <115 nmol/d)
Norepinephrine ----------------- <80 µg/24 h (SI: <473 nmol/d)

Citrate ----------------- 320-1240 mg/24 h (SI: 16.7-64.5 mmol/d)
Cortisol ------------------------- 4-50 µg/24 h (SI: 11-138 nmol/d)
Cortisol following dexamethasone-suppression test
(low-dose: 2 day, 2 mg daily)---- <10 µg/24 h (SI: <27.6 nmol/d)
Creatinine-------------------- 1.0-2.0 g/24 h (SI: 8.8-17.7 mmol/d)
Glomerular filtration rate (estimated) ----->60 mL/min per 1.73 m^2
5-Hydroxyindole acetic acid---2-9 mg/24 h (SI: 10.5-47.1 µmol/d)
Iodine (random)--->100 µg/L
17-Ketosteroids----6.0-21.0 mg/24 h (SI: 20.8-72.9 µmol/d) (male);
4.0-17.0 mg/24 h (SI: 13.9-59.0 µmol/d) (female)
Metanephrine fractionation
Normotensive normal ranges:
Metanephrine -------- <261 µg/24 h (SI: <1323 nmol/d) (male);
<180 µg/24 h (SI: <913 nmol/d) (female)
Normetanephrine --------------------- age and sex dependent
Total metanephrine ------------------ age and sex dependent
Osmolality ---------- 150-1150 mOsm/kg (SI: 150-1150 mmol/kg)
Oxalate -------------------------- <40 mg/24 h (SI: <456 mmol/d)
Phosphate ------------------ 0.9-1.3 g/24 h (SI: 29.1-42.0 mmol/d)
Potassium --------------------17-77 mEq/24 h (SI: 17-77 mmol/d)
Sodium --------------------40-217 mEq/24 h (SI: 40-217 mmol/d)
Uric acid -------------------------<800 mg/24 h (SI: <4.7 mmol/d)

Saliva

Cortisol (salivary), midnight --------- <0.13 µg/dL (SI: <3.6 nmol/L)

Semen

Semen analysis-------------->20 million sperm/mL; >50% motility

COMMON ABBREVIATIONS USED IN ENDOCRINE BOARD REVIEW

ACTH = corticotropin

ACE inhibitor = angiotensin-converting enzyme inhibitor

ALT = alanine aminotransferase

AST = aspartate aminotransferase

BMI = body mass index

CNS = central nervous system

CT = computed tomography

DHEA = dehydroepiandrosterone

DHEA-S = dehydroepiandrosterone sulfate

DNA = deoxyribonucleic acid

DPP-4 inhibitor = dipeptidyl-peptidase 4 inhibitor

DXA = dual-energy x-ray absorptiometry

FDA = Food and Drug Administration

FGF-23 = fibroblast growth factor 23

FNA = fine-needle aspiration

FSH = follicle-stimulating hormone

GH = growth hormone

GHRH = growth hormone–releasing hormone

GLP-1 receptor agonist = glucagonlike peptide 1 receptor agonist

GnRH = gonadotropin-releasing hormone

hCG = human chorionic gonadotropin

HDL = high-density lipoprotein

HIV = human immunodeficiency virus

HMG-CoA reductase inhibitor = 3-hydroxy-3-methylglutaryl coenzyme A reductase inhibitor

IGF-1 = insulinlike growth factor 1

LDL = low-density lipoprotein

LH = luteinizing hormone

MCV = mean corpuscular volume

MIBG = *meta*-iodobenzylguanidine

MRI = magnetic resonance imaging

NPH insulin = neutral protamine Hagedorn insulin

PCSK9 inhibitor = proprotein convertase subtilisin/kexin 9 inhibitor

PET = positron emission tomography

PSA = prostate-specific antigen

PTH = parathyroid hormone

PTHrP = parathyroid hormone–related protein

SGLT-2 inhibitor = sodium-glucose cotransporter 2 inhibitor

SHBG = sex hormone–binding globulin

T_3 = triiodothyronine

T_4 = thyroxine

TPO antibodies = thyroperoxidase antibodies

TRH = thyrotropin-releasing hormone

TRAb = thyrotropin-receptor antibodies

TSH = thyrotropin

VLDL = very low-density lipoprotein

ENDOCRINE
BOARD
REVIEW 2021

Adrenal Board Review

Tobias Else, MD

1 A 46-year-old woman who has been cared for in your practice for several years for primary adrenal insufficiency and Hashimoto thyroiditis presents for follow-up. She takes hydrocortisone, 15 mg, upon awakening, and 5 mg in the early afternoon. She takes fludrocortisone, 0.1 mg every other day, and levothyroxine, 100 mcg daily. She reports some forgetfulness, minor lower-extremity weakness, and slipping of her footwear when walking. She has not had any diarrhea.

On physical examination, her blood pressure is 123/78 mm Hg and pulse rate is 72 beats/min. She appears tanned, slightly more than on previous exams, but no skin lesions are appreciated. Her ankle reflexes are diminished, and vibration sense is absent in the toes.

Laboratory evaluation:
Hemoglobin = 12.4 g/dL (12.1-15.1 g/dL)
  (SI: 124 g/L [121-151 g/L])
Mean corpuscular volume = 94 μm^3 (80-100 μm^3)
  (SI: 94 fL [80-100 fL])
White blood cell count = 4200/μL
  (4500-11,000/μL) (SI: 4.2 × 10^9/L
  [4.5-11.0 × 10^9/L]) (normal differential)
TSH = 5.2 mIU/L (0.5-5.0 mIU/L)
ACTH = 210 pg/mL (10-60 pg/mL)
  (SI: 46.2 pmol/L [2.2-13.2 pmol/L])
Renin (mass) = 20 pg/mL (4-44 pg/mL)
Vitamin B$_{12}$ = 220 pg/mL (180-914 pg/mL)
  (SI: 162.4 pmol/L [133-674 pmol/L])
Folate = 4.5 ng/mL (≥4.0 ng/mL)
  (SI: 4.5 μg/L [≥4.0 μg/L])
Tissue transglutaminase-IgA, IgG antibodies,
  negative

Which of the following is the best next test in the diagnostic workup?
A. Genetic testing for adrenoleukodystrophy
B. Free T$_4$ measurement
C. Esophagogastroduodenoscopy with deep duodenal biopsy
D. Homocysteine and methylmalonic acid measurement
E. IgA measurement

2 A 47-year-old woman has a recent diagnosis of breast cancer treated with a curative attempt by surgery. Multigene panel testing for cancer-associated predisposition reveals the *RET* p.V804M pathogenic variant, but no other changes. She is referred for further management.

Her mother was diagnosed with advanced breast cancer at age 59 years, and her 85-year-old father has prostate cancer. Her sister has a history of papillary thyroid cancer, and her 4 younger brothers are healthy. She has no family history of medullary thyroid cancer, pheochromocytoma, or hyperparathyroidism.

On physical examination, her blood pressure is 119/72 mm Hg and pulse rate is 69 beats/min with a regular rate and rhythm. Findings on abdominal examination are normal. Thyroid examination does not show a goiter, thyroid nodules, or enlarged lymph nodes.

Laboratory test results:
TSH = 2.8 mIU/L (0.55.0 mIU/L)
Sodium = 136 mEq/L (136-142 mEq/L)
  (SI: 134 mmol/L [136-142 mmol/L])
Potassium = 4.2 mEq/L (3.5-5.0 mEq/L)
  (SI: 4.2 mmol/L [3.5-5.0 mmol/L])
Calcium = 9.8 mg/dL (8.2-10.2 mg/dL)
  (SI: 2.5 mmol/L [2.1-2.6 mmol/L])

Albumin = 4.2 g/dL (3.5-5.0 g/dL)
(SI: 42 g/L [35-50 g/L])

25-Hydroxyvitamin D = 32 ng/mL (30-80 ng/mL
[optimal]) (SI: 79.9 nmol/L [74.9-199.7 nmol/L])

Phosphate = 2.9 mg/dL (2.3-4.7 mg/dL)
(SI: 0.9 mmol/L [0.7-1.5 mmol/L])

Plasma epinephrine and norepinephrine,
within normal range

Which of the following is the best next step in this patient's care?

A. Refer for total thyroidectomy
B. Perform whole-body MRI and measure plasma free metanephrines and calcitonin
C. Measure PTH, calcitonin, and 25-hydroxyvitamin D
D. Measure plasma free metanephrines, calcitonin, and carcinoembryonic antigen
E. Perform thyroid ultrasonography and abdominal MRI and measure calcitonin and carcinoembryonic antigen

3 A 36-year-old man is referred for evaluation by a head and neck surgeon. The patient was recently diagnosed with a right carotid body tumor measuring 1.8 cm. He has hypertension diagnosed 4 years ago and periodic lower back pain. He takes amlodipine, 10 mg daily, and occasionally cyclobenzaprine and ibuprofen (he last took these medications 2 weeks ago). He has had no episodes of palpitations, sweating, pallor or vision changes. He has occasional headaches. His maternal aunt has kidney cancer, and a maternal cousin has a neck tumor. The patient's 2 sisters, parents, and grandparents are healthy. On physical examination, his blood pressure is 152/92 mm Hg and pulse rate is 89 beats/min with a regular rate and rhythm. Findings on abdominal and neurologic examinations are normal.

The head and neck surgeon is concerned that the carotid body tumor is possibly producing hormones. The following plasma free metanephrine levels are obtained:

Plasma metanephrine = 39.4 pg/mL (<99 pg/mL)
(SI: 0.20 nmol/L [<0.50 nmol/L])

Plasma normetanephrine = 4542 pg/mL
(<165 pg/mL) (SI: 24.80 nmol/L [<0.90 nmol/L])

Which of the following is the best next step in this patient's management?

A. Hold cyclobenzaprine for at least 4 weeks and repeat plasma free metanephrine measurement
B. Measure urinary fractionated metanephrines
C. Perform MIBG scan
D. Perform CT of the chest, abdomen, and pelvis
E. Plan for carotid body surgery with initiation of α-blockade

4 A 39-year-old woman is diagnosed with a pheochromocytoma. She has a personal history of anxiety with significant symptoms, such as palpitations, headache, clamminess, and sweating, which in retrospect are most likely due to the catecholamine-secreting tumor. At age 24 years, a right-sided carotid body tumor was diagnosed, and she has postoperative Horner syndrome. Her brother has a history of pheochromocytoma. Her parents are healthy. Her father has 4 sisters and 3 brothers, all of whom are healthy. Two of the patient's paternal first cousins have glomus jugulare tumors. All of her paternal aunts' children are healthy (*see pedigree*).

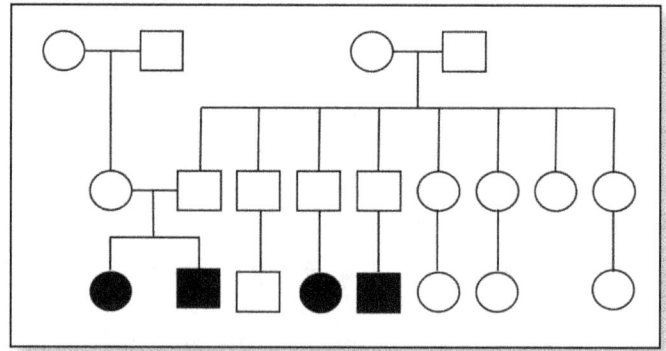

She requests genetic testing, and multigene panel testing is ordered to assess for pathogenic variants predisposing to pheochromocytoma and paraganglioma.

Which of the following genes most likely has a pathogenic variant?

A. *SDHC*
B. *SDHB*
C. *SDHD*
D. *VHL*
E. *RET*

5 A 42-year-old man with recent onset of reduced libido, muscle weakness, and fatigue was evaluated by another endocrinologist and found to have a cortisol concentration of 22 μg/dL (607 nmol/L) and an ACTH concentration of 23 pg/mL (5.1 pmol/L) after 1 mg of dexamethasone. He is referred for petrosal sinus sampling.

He describes onset of symptoms over the last 6 months. He is an avid cycler and runner and used to run marathons, but now he cannot complete a 5k due to weakness, fatigue, and exhaustion. He also comments on night sweats. He has unintentionally lost 15.4 lb (7 kg), and his current weight is 128 lb (58 kg) (BMI = 23 kg/m²). Twenty-five years ago, he had aortic valve replacement for a congenital bicuspid aortic valve. He has seasonal allergies for which he takes nasal fluticasone.

He was found to have low testosterone levels and was prescribed a trial of testosterone replacement for 3 months. However, his symptoms did not improve. Pituitary MRI showed a questionable 2-mm small cystic area posterior to the anterior pituitary. CT of the chest, abdomen, pelvis shows normal-appearing adrenal glands that are large, but still normal sized, and no pathologic findings.

On physical examination, his blood pressure is 118/78 mm Hg, pulse rate is 89 beats/min, and temperature is 100°F (37.8°C). He appears slightly older than his stated age.

Laboratory test results (without testosterone replacement):
> White blood cell count = 11,400/μL
> (4500-11,000/μL) (SI: 11.4 × 10⁹/L
> [4.5-11.0 × 10⁹/L])
> Neutrophil count, increased
> Lymphocyte count, normal
> Total testosterone = 42 ng/dL (300-900 ng/dL)
> (SI: 1.5 nmol/L [10.4-31.2 nmol/L])
> Prolactin = 20 ng/mL (4-23 ng/mL)
> (SI: 0.87 nmol/L [0.17-1.00 nmol/L])
> FSH = 3.7 mIU/mL (1.0-13.0 mIU/mL)
> (SI: 3.7 IU/L [1.0-13.0 IU/L])
> LH = 2.0 mIU/mL (1.0-9.0 mIU/mL)
> (SI: 2.0 IU/L [1.0-9.0 IU/L])

> IGF-1 = 67 ng/mL (98-261 ng/mL)
> (SI: 8.8 nmol/L [12.8-34.2 nmol/L])
> Serum cortisol (random) = 68 μg/dL
> (SI: 1876 nmol/L)
> Urinary cortisol = 158 μg/24 h (4-50 μg/24 h)
> (SI: 436 nmol/d [11-138 nmol/d])
> ACTH (random) = 27 pg/mL (10-60 pg/mL)
> (SI: 5.9 pmol/L [2.2-13.2 pmol/L])
> TSH = 7.7 mIU/L (0.5-5.0 mIU/L)
> Free T₄ = 0.7 ng/dL (0.8-1.8 ng/dL)
> (SI: 9.01 pmol/L [10.30-23.17 pmol/L])

Which of the following is the best next step in this patient's management?

A. Start mifepristone, 300 mg daily
B. Measure salivary cortisol (3 measurements)
C. Perform transesophageal echocardiography and blood cultures
D. Stop fluticasone, start thyroid hormone replacement and testosterone replacement
E. Refer to neuroradiology for petrosal sinus sampling

6 A 32-year-old man is referred for management of Cushing syndrome. A corticotroph adenoma was initially diagnosed when the patient was 24 years old, and he underwent transsphenoidal surgery with subsequent improvement for several years. However, he required repeated surgery 5 years ago. He now has symptoms and signs of hypercortisolism with central fat distribution, bruising, and active striae. The cortisol concentration following a 1-mg dexamethasone-suppression test is 12 μg/dL (331 nmol/L), and urinary free cortisol excretion is 240 μg/24 h (662 nmol/d). Salivary cortisol is measured 3 times and ranges from 0.98 to 1.20 μg/dL (27-33 nmol/L).

The neurosurgeon states that surgery is not possible, and osilodrostat is prescribed at a dosage of 2 mg twice daily. After 4 weeks, the patient's urinary free cortisol value is 98 μg/24 h (271 nmol/d), and the osilodrostat dosage is increased to 4 mg twice daily. The patient returns after 2 weeks with anorexia, headaches, and fatigue. Laboratory evaluation shows a potassium concentration of 3.2 mEq/L (3.2 mmol/L). Overall, the patient has lost 4.4 lb (2 kg).

On physical examination, he still has features of Cushing syndrome. His blood pressure is 150/90 mm Hg, and pulse rate is 84 beats/min.

Which of the following is the best next step in this patient's care?
- A. Administer hydrocortisone, 100 mg; hold osilodrostat; and send patient to the emergency department
- B. Increase the dosage of osilodrostat to 6 mg twice daily
- C. Obtain measurements of 24-hour urinary cortisol and plasma ACTH and start spironolactone
- D. Continue therapy and reevaluate in 2 weeks
- E. Hold osilodrostat and start mifepristone, 300 mg daily

7 A 27-year-old woman was diagnosed with classic 21-hydroxylase deficiency at birth and has been adherent to treatment with hydrocortisone and fludrocortisone acetate her entire life. She had vaginal reconstruction at age 19 years and has been using dilators periodically since then. For the last 18 months, she has been sexually active and wants to have children, but she has not conceived despite optimally timed intercourse. She currently takes hydrocortisone, 10 mg upon waking and 5 mg with both lunch and her evening meal, plus fludrocortisone acetate, 0.1 mg with breakfast. She has regular monthly menses and shaves her upper lip and chin once a month. Home urine testing documents monthly ovulation.

On physical examination, she has no moon facies, no striae or facial plethora, no acne, and a trace of shaved stubble.

Which of the following is the key laboratory parameter to monitor when adjusting her glucocorticoid therapy?
- A. Follicular-phase androstenedione
- B. Follicular-phase progesterone
- C. 17-Hydroxyprogesterone after her morning dose
- D. Periovulatory testosterone
- E. Luteal-phase 17-hydroxyprogesterone

8 A 45-year-old woman presents with resistant hypertension. She developed hypokalemia while taking amlodipine and hydrochlorothiazide. Lisinopril and potassium chloride supplements, 80 mEq daily, were added with eventual resolution of the hypokalemia but her blood pressure did not normalize. She has also gained 22 lb (10 kg) over the last 2 years and now has diet-controlled diabetes mellitus.

On physical examination, she has mild dermal atrophy and central fat distribution. Proximal muscle strength is normal. She has no plethora, dorsocervical fat pad, or striae. Her BMI is 34 kg/m², and blood pressure is 148/95 mm Hg.

Laboratory test results:
Serum sodium = 138 mEq/L (136-142 mEq/L) (SI: 138 mmol/L [136-142 mmol/L])
Serum potassium = 3.6 mEq/L (3.5-5.0 mEq/L) (SI: 3.6 mmol/L [3.5-5.0 mmol/L])
Serum glucose = 157 mg/dL (70-99 mg/dL) (SI: 8.7 mmol/L [3.9-5.5 mmol/L])
Serum aldosterone = 13 ng/dL (4-21 ng/dL) (SI: 361 pmol/L [111-583 pmol/L])
Plasma renin activity = <0.6 ng/mL per h (0.6-4.3 ng/mL per h)
Serum creatinine = 0.8 mg/dL (0.6-1.1 mg/dL) (SI: 70.7 μmol/L [53.0-97.2 μmol/L])
Plasma metanephrines, normal

Abdominal CT with contrast demonstrates a 3.8-cm left adrenal mass and an atrophic right adrenal gland (*see image, arrows*).

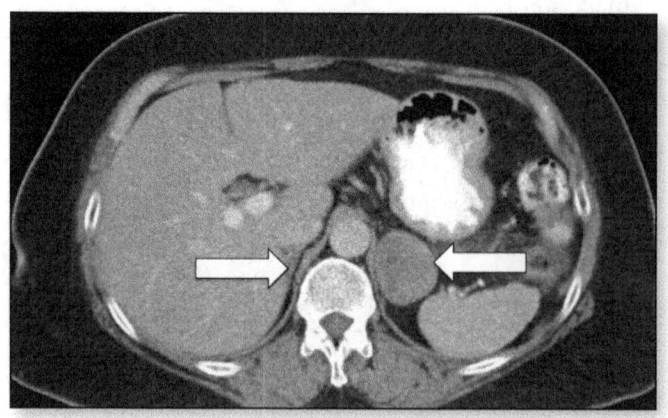

The patient is referred for further evaluation and recommendations.

Which of the following is the best next step?
- A. Prescribe spironolactone, 50 mg daily
- B. Recommend left adrenalectomy
- C. Biopsy the left adrenal gland
- D. Schedule adrenal venous sampling to measure aldosterone and cortisol
- E. Measure serum cortisol after 1 mg of dexamethasone

9 A 32-year-old woman has a history of Cushing disease status post surgery 3 years ago with subsequent improvement in her diabetes mellitus and hypertension. She has noted weight gain, poor sleep, irregular menses, and worsening glycemia for the past 6 months. Her medications include amlodipine, 10 mg daily, and metformin, 1500 mg daily.

On physical examination, her blood pressure is 145/85 mm Hg. She has facial plethora and moderate supraclavicular fat pads.

Laboratory test results:
Fasting glucose = 205 mg/dL (70-99 mg/dL) (SI: 11.4 mmol/L [3.9-5.5 mmol/L])
Potassium = 2.7 mEq/L (3.5-5.0 mEq/L) (SI: 2.7 mmol/L [3.5-5.0 mmol/L])
Serum cortisol (8 AM) = 18 µg/dL (5-25 µg/dL) (SI: 497 nmol/L [138-690 nmol/L])
Hemoglobin A$_{1c}$ = 8.5% (4.0%-5.6%) (69 mmol/mol [20-38 mmol/mol])
Plasma ACTH = 65 pg/mL (10-60 pg/mL) (SI: 14.3 pmol/L [2.2-13.2 pmol/L])
Late-night salivary cortisol = 0.32 µg/dL (<0.13 µg/dL) (SI: 8.8 nmol/L [<3.6 nmol/L])

Urinary free cortisol = 360 µg/24 h (4-50 µg/24 h) (SI: 994 nmol/d [11-138 nmol/d])
Serum hCG (qualitative), negative

Pituitary MRI shows only postoperative changes. After discussing treatment options, mifepristone, 300 mg daily, is prescribed.

Before starting mifepristone, she should be treated to achieve which of the following?
- A. Normal blood pressure
- B. Normal fasting glucose
- C. Normal serum potassium
- D. Normal plasma triglycerides
- E. No additional treatment is required

10 A 52-year-old man with hypertension and hypokalemia is undergoing evaluation for primary aldosteronism.

Screening laboratory test results:
Sodium = 147 mEq/L (136-142 mEq/L) (SI: 147 mmol/L [136-142 mmol/L])
Potassium = 3.2 mEq/L (3.5-5.0 mEq/L) (SI: 3.2 mmol/L [3.5-5.0 mmol/L])
Serum aldosterone = 24 ng/dL (4-21 ng/dL) (SI: 666 pmol/L [111-583 pmol/L]) (repeated measurement = 26 ng/dL [SI: 721 pmol/L])
Plasma renin activity = <0.6 ng/mL per h (0.6-4.3 ng/mL per h) (repeated measurement = <0.6 ng/mL per h)

CT with fine cuts of the adrenals demonstrate normal-appearing glands with slight thickening of the central part of the right adrenal gland.

He undergoes adrenal venous sampling with continuous infusion of cosyntropin at 50 mcg per hour. The results are shown (*see table*).

Measurement	Right adrenal vein	Left adrenal vein	Inferior vena cava
Aldosterone	3000 ng/dL (SI: 83,220 pmol/L)	456 ng/dL (SI: 12,649 pmol/L)	40 ng/dL (SI: 1109 pmol/L)
Cortisol	750 µg/dL (SI: 20,691 nmol/L)	120 µg/dL (SI: 3311 nmol/L)	20 µg/dL (SI: 552 nmol/L)
Aldosterone-to-cortisol ratio	4.0	3.8	2.0

How do you interpret the results of the adrenal venous sampling study?

A. Unsuccessful study: unable to localize

B. Successful study: left adrenal gland is the source (left adenoma)

C. Successful study: both adrenal glands are sources (bilateral hyperaldosteronism)

D. Unsuccessful study: however, there is enough information to localize the source to the right adrenal (right adenoma)

E. Insufficient information to interpret whether the study was successful

11 A 44-year-old woman presents with a 5-month history of rapidly progressive balding, voice deepening, and hirsutism. She has also had amenorrhea for 2 months and has a new diagnosis of hypertension.

Her primary care physician obtained the following laboratory test results:

Sodium = 144 mEq/L (136-142 mEq/L)
(SI: 144 mmol/L [136-142 mmol/L])

Potassium = 3.2 mEq/L (3.5-5.0 mEq/L)
(SI: 3.2 mmol/L [3.5-5.0 mmol/L])

Serum aldosterone = <4 ng/dL (4-21 ng/dL)
(SI: <111.0 pmol/L [111.0-582.5 pmol/L])

Plasma renin activity = <0.6 ng/mL per h
(0.6-4.3 ng/mL per h)

Plasma ACTH = 15 pg/mL (10-60 pg/mL)
(SI: 3.3 pmol/L [2.2-13.2 pmol/L])

Serum cortisol = 14 µg/dL (5-25 µg/dL)
(SI: 386.2 nmol/L [137.9-389.7 nmol/L])

Serum DHEA-S = 1630 µg/dL (18-244 µg/dL)
(SI: 44.17 µmol/L [0.49-6.61 µmol/L])

Serum total testosterone = 279 ng/dL (8-60 ng/dL)
(SI: 9.7 nmol/L [0.3-2.1 nmol/L])

SHBG = 1.3 µg/mL (2.2-14.6 µg/mL)
(SI: 12 nmol/L [20-130 nmol/L])

11-Deoxycortisol = 310 ng/dL (10-79 ng/dL)
(SI: 8.9 nmol/L [0.29-2.28 nmol/L])

Which of the following is the most likely diagnosis?

A. Macronodular adrenocortical hyperplasia

B. Nonclassic 11β-hydroxylase deficiency

C. Adrenocortical carcinoma

D. Hyperthecosis

E. Ovarian Sertoli-Leydig–cell tumor

12 A 6-cm left adrenal pheochromocytoma is diagnosed in a 55-year-old man. His urinary metanephrine and normetanephrine levels are 8 to 12 times the upper normal limit. His blood pressure is 165/105 mm Hg, and pulse rate is 85 beats/min. Phenoxybenzamine, 10 mg at bedtime, is initiated and is advanced to 10 mg twice daily the next day. The patient calls the clinic 4 days later with concerns of palpitations. Fluid intake has been 3.5 L per day. His blood pressure is now 140/90 mm Hg, and pulse rate is 85 beats/min sitting. When standing, his blood pressure is 110/70 mm Hg, and pulse rate is 115 beats/min.

Which of the following is the most important next step in his management?

A. Add metoprolol, 100 mg twice daily

B. Increase the phenoxybenzamine dosage to 20 mg twice daily

C. Substitute nicardipine for phenoxybenzamine

D. Maintain the same phenoxybenzamine dosage and refer for surgery

E. Increase sodium intake

13 A 24-year-old man is referred by a urologist for evaluation before surgery for testicular masses. The patient gives a history of taking hydrocortisone and fludrocortisone throughout childhood, but he stopped all medications at age 21 years.

On physical examination, he is a normal-appearing young man with a blood pressure of 106/72 mm Hg and pulse rate of 84 beats/min. Both testes have firm, irregular masses that are 4 to 6 cm in maximal dimension. His 8-AM cortisol concentration is 4 µg/dL (110.4 nmol/L) by immunoassay and 1 µg/dL (27.6 nmol/L) by tandem mass spectrometry. Semen analysis documents azoospermia.

Which of the following is the most likely pattern of laboratory test results in this patient?

Answer	Testosterone	Androstenedione	LH
A.	↑	↑	↑
B.	↓	↓	↓
C.	Normal	↑	↓
D.	↓	↓	↑
E.	Normal	Normal	Normal

14 A 52-year-old man is referred for evaluation of resistant hypertension. Chlorthalidone was discontinued 1 month ago due to hypokalemia. He is currently treated with nifedipine, candesartan, nebivolol, and clonidine. On this regimen, he was screened for primary aldosteronism 1 week ago.

Laboratory test results:
Sodium = 144 mEq/L (136-142 mEq/L)
(SI: 144 mmol/L [136-142 mmol/L])
Potassium = 2.9 mEq/L (3.5-5.0 mEq/L)
(SI: 2.9 mmol/L [3.5-5.0 mmol/L])
Serum aldosterone = 8 ng/dL (4-21 ng/dL)
(SI: 222 pmol/L [111.0-582.5 pmol/L])
Plasma renin activity = <0.6 ng/mL per h
(0.6-4.3 ng/mL per h)

Which of the following is the best conclusion about what needs to be done now on the basis of these screening tests?

A. No further testing; primary aldosteronism has been excluded
B. Rescreen after correcting hypokalemia
C. Rescreen after stopping candesartan
D. Rescreen after substituting doxazosin for nifedipine
E. No further testing; primary aldosteronism has been established

15 A 72-year-old man is referred for evaluation of primary aldosteronism. He has had resistant hypertension with difficult-to-control potassium for at least 15 years. The evaluation reveals a 0.9-cm left aldosterone-producing adenoma with concordant lateralization on adrenal venous sampling.

The patient is referred for laparoscopic adrenalectomy. His preoperative blood pressure is 150/90 mm Hg.

Preoperative laboratory test results:
Serum potassium = 3.9 mEq/L (3.5-5.0 mEq/L)
(SI: 3.9 mmol/L [3.5-5.0 mmol/L])
Baseline serum creatinine = 1.7 mg/dL
(0.7-1.3 mg/dL) (SI: 150.3 µmol/L
[61.9-114.9 µmol/L])
Urine albumin = 220 mg/24 h (<30 mg/24 h)

For which of the following complications is this patient at risk postoperatively?

A. Renal failure
B. Refractory hypotension
C. Prolonged hyperkalemia
D. Persistent hyperaldosteronism
E. Adrenal insufficiency

16 A 78-year-old woman is hospitalized for acute liver injury after unintentionally overdosing on acetaminophen-oxycodone for chronic pain. One year ago, an unclassified connective tissue disease was diagnosed that manifests as myositis and arthritis, and she has since been treated with prednisone, 20 mg daily. She increased the amount of pain medication she was taking over the last week due to worsening joint and muscle pain. On hospital admission, she was hypotensive with abdominal pain and nausea, and you are consulted about her corticosteroid regimen.

On physical examination, she is jaundiced and lethargic with dermal atrophy, bruising, muscle weakness, and prominent supraclavicular fat pads. Her blood pressure is 94/68 mm Hg, and pulse rate is 100 beats/min.

Laboratory test results:

Sodium = 128 mEq/L (136-142 mEq/L)
(SI: 128 mmol/L [136-142 mmol/L])

Potassium = 3.8 mEq/L (3.5-5.0 mEq/L)
(SI: 3.8 mmol/L [3.5-5.0 mmol/L])

Serum DHEA-S = <15 µg/dL (15-157 µg/dL)
(SI: <0.41 µmol/L [0.41-4.25 µmol/L])

Plasma ACTH = <2 pg/mL (10-60 pg/mL)
(SI: <0.4 pmol/L [2.2-13.2 pmol/L])

Serum aldosterone = 16 ng/dL (4-21 ng/dL)
(SI: 443.8 pmol/L [111.0-582.5 pmol/L])

Plasma renin activity = 8 ng/mL per h
(0.6-4.3 ng/mL per h)

Serum cortisol (8 AM) = <0.5 µg/dL (5-25 µg/dL)
(SI: <13.8 nmol/L [137.9-389.7 nmol/L])

Serum ALT = 2680 U/L (50-120 U/L)
(SI: 44.76 µkat/L [0.84-2.00 µkat/L])

In addition to fluid resuscitation, which of the following should be recommended?

A. Perform a cosyntropin-stimulation test
B. Add fludrocortisone, 0.1 mg twice daily
C. Increase the prednisone dosage to 20 mg twice daily
D. Substitute prednisolone, 20 mg daily, for prednisone
E. Perform adrenal CT

17 A 42-year-old woman with a history of Cushing disease is concerned about recurrence. Six years ago, she underwent transsphenoidal pituitary microsurgery for removal of a 5-mm corticotroph adenoma (confirmed with immunohistochemistry). Postoperatively, she had well-documented secondary adrenal insufficiency requiring glucocorticoid support for 11 months until her pituitary-adrenal axis recovered. Her signs and symptoms of hypercortisolism resolved. During the past 6 months, she has gained 25 lb (11.4 kg), but her menses remain regular. She feels more depressed and is having difficulty dealing with the stress of her job.

On physical examination, she has some facial rounding and subtle plethora. Her blood pressure is 148/96 mm Hg, and she has several small bruises on her legs. She has good muscle strength, no striae, and no edema. Her primary care physician measured a urinary cortisol excretion of 28 µg/24 h (77.3 nmol/d).

Which of the following tests is the most sensitive for detecting recurrence of her Cushing disease?

A. Another 24-hour urinary free cortisol measurement
B. Late-night salivary cortisol measurement
C. 1-mg overnight dexamethasone-suppression test
D. 8-mg overnight dexamethasone-suppression test
E. Inferior petrosal sinus sampling with ovine corticotropin-releasing hormone stimulation

18 A primary care physician refers a 45-year-old man from southern Illinois with bilateral adrenal enlargement. The physician is concerned about the possibility of bilateral pheochromocytoma, as plasma metanephrines measured in his office by venipuncture were slightly elevated. The patient's CT is shown, demonstrating adrenal enlargement *(see image, arrows)*.

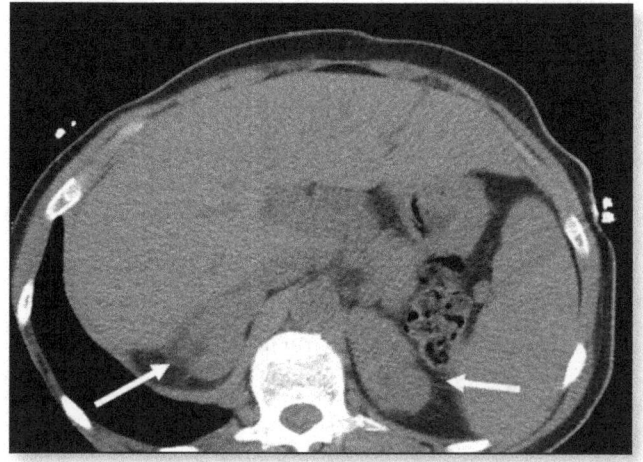

The patient's appetite has been poor, and he has lost 11 lb (5 kg) in the past 3 months. He has no family history of endocrinopathy. He is not taking any medications.

On physical examination, his blood pressure is 100/68 mm Hg with a pulse rate of 96 beats/min seated, and blood pressure is 88/50 mm Hg with a pulse rate of 120 beats/min standing. The rest of the examination findings are unremarkable.

Initial laboratory test results:

Plasma normetanephrine = 225 pg/mL
(<165 pg/mL) (SI: <1.23 nmol/L [<0.90 nmol/L])

Plasma metanephrine = <40 pg/mL (<99 pg/mL)
(SI: <0.21 nmol/L [<0.50 nmol/L])

After examining the patient, you obtain the following additional laboratory tests (sample drawn at 8 AM):

Sodium = 131 mEq/L (136-142 mEq/L)
(SI: 131 mmol/L [136-142 mmol/L])

Potassium = 4.4 mEq/L (3.5-5.0 mEq/L)
(SI: 4.4 mmol/L [3.5-5.0 mmol/L])

Creatinine = 0.6 mg/dL (0.7-1.3 mg/dL)
(SI: 53.0 µmol/L [61.9-114.9 µmol/L])

Aldosterone = 4 ng/dL ((4-21 ng/dL)
(SI: 111 pmol/L [111.0-582.5 pmol/L])

Plasma renin activity = 17 ng/mL per h
(0.6-4.3 ng/mL per h)

Plasma ACTH = 212 pg/mL (10-60 pg/mL)
(SI: 46.6 pmol/L [2.2-13.2 pmol/L])

Cortisol = 3.2 µg/dL (5-25 µg/dL) (SI: 88.3 nmol/L
[137.9-389.7 nmol/L])

Which of the following diagnostic tests is most likely to be helpful in the further diagnosis and management of this patient?

A. Measurement of 24-hour urinary free cortisol
B. Measurement of 21-hydroxylase antibodies
C. Pituitary-directed MRI
D. Bilateral adrenal venous sampling for cortisol, aldosterone, and catecholamines
E. CT-guided percutaneous adrenal biopsy

19 A 25-year-old recently married woman has a well-documented diagnosis of nonclassic 21-hydroxylase deficiency (21-OHD). Her cosyntropin-stimulated 17-hydroxyprogesterone concentration is 3400 ng/dL (103.0 nmol/L), and her cortisol concentration is 21 µg/dL (579 nmol/L). She has not had DNA testing for genotyping. No members of her family or her husband's family have classic 21-OHD, there is no suspicious family history, and neither the patient nor her husband is of an ethnicity with an unusually high prevalence of classic or nonclassic 21-OHShe now wants to start a family, and she asks about the risk of having an affected child.

Which of the following statements best characterizes her risk of having a child with classic 21-OHD?

A. Her risk of having a child with *classic* 21-OHD is <0.01%
B. Her risk of having a child with *classic* 21-OHD is >0.5%
C. She cannot have a child with *classic* 21-OHD because she has the *nonclassic* form
D. She can have a child with *classic* 21-OHD only if her partner also has a clinical diagnosis of *nonclassic* 21-OHD

20 At your hospital's weekly clinical endocrine conference, a colleague asks for your opinion regarding a 44-year-old man with metastatic pheochromocytoma. He had a left adrenalectomy 2 years earlier to treat a 6.8-cm pheochromocytoma. Postoperative studies showed a solitary metastasis to T12, and CT of the lungs showed two 1.5-cm lesions in the right upper lobe. He underwent external beam radiation therapy for the bone metastasis in T12. He was then lost to follow-up because of lack of health insurance. He is currently asymptomatic. He has continued to take doxazosin, 2 mg daily, and metformin, 500 mg daily (initiated because of hyperglycemia at the time of presentation 2 years ago). He is unaware of any family history of endocrine disorders.

On physical examination, his blood pressure is 128/84 mm Hg, pulse rate is 78 beats/min, and BMI is 24.4 kg/m². He has no mucosal neuromas, café-au-lait spots, or axillary freckling.

Laboratory test results:

Chemistry profile, normal
Complete blood cell count, normal
Hemoglobin A_{1c} = 4.8% (4.0%-5.6%) (29 mmol/mol [20-38 mmol/mol])
Thyroid function, normal
Morning fasting calcitonin, normal
Urinary catecholamines, normal

Measurement	At diagnosis 2 years ago	At today's visit
Urinary metanephrine	615 µg/24 h (SI: 3.12 nmol/d)	587 µg/24 h (SI: 2.98 nmol/d)
Urinary normetanephrine	2120 µg/24 h (SI: 11.58 nmol/d)	1146 µg/24 h (SI: 6.26 nmol/d)

Imaging with *meta*-iodobenzylguanidine shows some uptake in the previously described T12 lesion, as well as faint uptake in 2 small (1.5-cm) right upper lobe lung nodules (identical in size to those found 2 years earlier). Fluorodeoxyglucose single-photon emission CT and PET show uptake in the same locations, as well as intense segmental uptake in the large intestine.

Which of the following is the best course of action now?
- A. [131]*meta*-iodobenzylguanidine therapy
- B. External beam radiotherapy to the colon
- C. Cytotoxic chemotherapy with cyclophosphamide, vincristine, doxorubicin, or capecitabine and temozolomide
- D. Cabozantinib therapy
- E. Antiresorptive therapy with a bisphosphonate or denosumab

21 A colleague whose daughter recently received a diagnosis of Cushing syndrome asks you for a second opinion. The patient is a 25-year-old woman who has gained 20 lb (9.1 kg) in the past 5 months with associated facial fullness and plethora. She has new-onset hypertension and oligomenorrhea. She is not taking any medications.

On physical examination, she is a cushingoid-appearing young woman with a blood pressure of 142/94 mm Hg. Pulse rate is 76 beats/min, and BMI is 28.1 kg/m². She has substantial supraclavicular and dorsocervical fat accumulation. With the exception of some slight edema, the rest of the examination findings are normal.

Laboratory test results:
Pregnancy test, negative
Sodium = 141 mEq/L (136-142 mEq/L) (SI: 141 mmol/L [136-142 mmol/L])
Potassium = 3.7 mEq/L (3.5-5.0 mEq/L) (SI: 3.7 mmol/L [3.5-5.0 mmol/L])
Chloride = 99 mEq/L (96-106 mEq/L) (SI: 99 mmol/L [96-106 mmol/L])
Bicarbonate = 28 mEq/L (21-28 mEq/L) (SI: 28 mmol/L [21-28 mmol/L])
Fasting glucose = 99 mg/dL (70-99 mg/dL) (SI: 5.5 mmol/L [3.9-5.5 mmol/L])
Serum urea nitrogen = 15 mg/dL (8-23 mg/dL) (SI: 5.4 mmol/L [2.9-8.2 mmol/L])
Creatinine = 0.9 mg/dL (0.6-1.1 mg/dL) (SI: 8.0 µmol/L [53.0-97.2 µmol/L])
Calcium = 9.5 mg/dL (8.2-10.2 mg/dL) (SI: 2.4 mmol/L [2.1-2.6 mmol/L])
Late-night salivary cortisol = 0.41 µg/dL (<0.13 µg/dL) (SI: 11.3 nmol/L [<3.6 nmol/L])
Urinary free cortisol = 129 µg/24 h (4-50 µg/24 h) (SI: 356 nmol/d [11-138 nmol/d])
Serum cortisol (8 AM) = 17.6 µg/dL (5-25 µg/dL) (SI: 485.5 nmol/L [137.9-389.7 nmol/L])
Serum cortisol (8 AM) after overnight 1-mg dexamethasone-suppression test = 17.4 µg/dL (SI: 480.0 nmol/L)
Serum cortisol (8 AM) after overnight 8-mg dexamethasone-suppression test = 17.1 µg/dL (SI: 471.8 nmol/L)
DHEA-S = 5.0 µg/dL (44-332 µg/dL) (SI: 0.14 µmol/L [1.19-9.00 µmol/L])
Basal plasma ACTH = 14.0 pg/mL (10-60 pg/mL) (SI: 3.1 pmol/L [2.2-13.2 pmol/L])

Pituitary MRI is interpreted to show a 2-mm hypodense lesion in the left side of the pituitary gland. She has been referred to a neurosurgeon who has scheduled transsphenoidal pituitary surgery.

Which of the following should you recommend?
- A. Octreotide acetate scintigraphy
- B. Bilateral inferior petrosal ACTH sampling with corticotropin-releasing hormone stimulation
- C. CT of the adrenal glands
- D. CT of the chest
- E. Pituitary surgery as scheduled

22 A 67-year-old woman has a right adrenal mass that was incidentally discovered on an annual surveillance CT performed for a medical history of colon cancer. She was treated with partial colectomy and adjuvant chemotherapy 6 years ago. The adrenal mass measures 2.2 cm in maximal diameter with a precontrast attenuation value of 25 Hounsfield units and 30% contrast washout at 10 minutes. The mass was not visible on CT 1 year ago.

On physical examination, her blood pressure is 123/84 mm Hg and pulse rate is 70 beats/min. She is clinically well and has no cushingoid features.

Laboratory test results:
Serum glucose = 90 mg/dL (70-99 mg/dL)
  (SI: 5.0 mmol/L [3.9-5.5 mmol/L])
Serum potassium = 4.0 mEq/L (3.5-5.0 mEq/L)
  (SI: 4.0 mmol/L [3.5-5.0 mmol/L])
Plasma metanephrine = <39 pg/mL (<99 pg/mL)
  (SI: <0.20 nmol/L [<0.50 nmol/L])
Plasma normetanephrine = <147 pg/mL
  (<165 pg/mL) (SI: 0.80 nmol/L [<0.90 nmol/L])
Serum cortisol after 1-mg dexamethasone =
  0.8 µg/dL (SI: 22.1 nmol/L)

Which of the following is the best next step?
A. Perform ^{18}F-fluorodeoxyglucose PET
B. Perform MRI of the adrenal mass with in-phase and out-of-phase images
C. Refer for laparoscopic right adrenalectomy
D. Perform another CT in 1 year
E. Measure serum aldosterone and plasma renin activity

Calcium and Bone Board Review

Natalie E. Cusano, MD, MS

1 A 53-year-old man with osteoporosis and a history of multiple medical problems presents to establish care. His bone density was initially measured because of a low testosterone level; however, testosterone has subsequently been within range without therapy. He has had fatigue; weakness; chronic dental issues; headaches; dizziness; and diffuse arthralgias, myalgias, and bone pain since childhood. He has had no issues with morning erections or maintenance of erections. He has no personal history of fracture and no parental history of hip fracture. He received teriparatide, 20 mcg daily, for 2 years followed by denosumab, 60 mg subcutaneously, every 6 months for 4 years (last dose 2 years ago).

On physical examination, his height is 62 in (157 cm) and weight is 140 lb (63.6 kg).

Recent bone density assessment was notable for T-scores of –3.2 at the lumbar spine, –1.4 at the femoral neck, and –1.1 at the total hip.

Laboratory test results:
- Serum calcium = 9.3 mg/dL (8.2-10.2 mg/dL) (SI: 2.3 mmol/L [2.1-2.6 mmol/L])
- PTH = 50 pg/mL (10-65 pg/mL) (SI: 50 ng/L [10-65 ng/L])
- 25-Hydroxyvitamin D = 26 ng/mL (30-80 ng/mL [optimal]) (SI: 64.9 nmol/L [74.9-199.7 nmol/L])
- Magnesium = 2.3 mg/dL (1.5-2.3 mg/dL) (SI: 0.95 mmol/L [0.6-0.9 mmol/L])
- Phosphate = 3.0 mg/dL (2.3-4.7 mg/dL) (SI: 1.0 mmol/L [0.7-1.5 mmol/L])
- Serum alkaline phosphatase = 27 U/L (50-120 U/L) (SI: 0.45 μkat/L [0.84-2.00 μkat/L])

Which of the following is the best next step in this patient's care?
- A. Measure a morning fasting testosterone level
- B. Restart denosumab, 60 mg subcutaneously every 6 months
- C. Order genetic testing for *PHEX* pathogenic variants
- D. Measure vitamin B$_6$ and order genetic testing for *ALPL* pathogenic variants
- E. Provide reassurance no treatment is needed since his low bone density is due to small bone size

2 A 65-year-old man presents for a second opinion regarding management of normocalcemic primary hyperparathyroidism. He has had elevated PTH concentrations for the past 2 years with consistently normal serum total and ionized calcium. Secondary causes of hyperparathyroidism have been excluded, including vitamin D deficiency, kidney failure, medication effect, hypercalciuria, and malabsorption. Normocalcemic primary hyperparathyroidism was diagnosed in the setting of a kidney stone, and he was noted to have osteoporosis on recent bone density testing, significant for T-scores of –2.7 at the lumbar spine, –2.1 at the femoral neck, and –2.0 at the distal radius. Ultrasonography and sestamibi imaging have not localized an adenoma.

Laboratory test results:
- Serum calcium = 9.3 mg/dL (8.2-10.2 mg/dL) (SI: 2.3 mmol/L [2.1-2.6 mmol/L])
- PTH = 100 pg/mL (10-65 pg/mL) (SI: 100 ng/L [10-65 ng/L])
- 25-Hydroxyvitamin D = 40 ng/mL (30-80 ng/mL [optimal]) (SI: 99.8 nmol/L [74.9-199.7 nmol/L])
- Magnesium = 2.3 mg/dL (1.5-2.3 mg/dL) (SI: 0.95 mmol/L [0.6-0.9 mmol/L])

Phosphate = 3.0 mg/dL (2.3-4.7 mg/dL)
(SI: 1.0 mmol/L [0.7-1.5 mmol/L])
Creatinine = 0.8 mg/dL (0.7-1.3 mg/dL)
(SI: 70.2 μmol/L [53.0-97.2 μmol/L])
Urinary calcium = 275 mg/24 h (100-300 mg/24 h)
(SI: 6.9 mmol/d [2.5-7.5 mmol/d])

Which of the following is the best next step in this patient's management?
A. Refer to a parathyroid surgeon for bilateral neck exploration
B. Repeat ultrasonography and sestamibi imaging in 1 year
C. Refer for selective venous sampling
D. Start hydrochlorothiazide, 25 mg daily
E. Start alendronate, 70 mg weekly

3 A 54-year-old woman is brought to the emergency department with seizures. She has had previous emergency department visits for alcohol intoxication. Her medical history and medications are otherwise unknown.

Physical examination demonstrates tongue biting and positive Chvostek sign. She has no neck scars, mucocutaneous candidiasis, or vitiligo.

Laboratory test results:
Serum calcium = 5.4 mg/dL (8.2-10.2 mg/dL)
(SI: 1.4 mmol/L [2.1-2.6 mmol/L])
PTH = <3 pg/mL (10-65 pg/mL)
(SI: <3 ng/L [10-65 ng/L])
25-Hydroxyvitamin D = 6 ng/mL (30-80 ng/mL
[optimal]) (SI: 15.0 nmol/L [74.9-199.7 nmol/L])
Magnesium = 0.6 mEq/L (1.5-2.3 mEq/L)
(SI: 0.25 mmol/L [0.6-0.9 mmol/L])
Phosphate = 1.8 mg/dL (2.3-4.7 mg/dL)
(SI: 0.6 mmol/L [0.7-1.5 mmol/L])
Albumin = 2.8 g/dL (3.5-5.0 g/dL)
(SI: 28 g/dL [35-50 g/L])
Amylase = 105 U/L (26-102 U/L)
(SI: 1.75 μkat/L [0.43-1.70 μkat/L])
Lipase = 75 U/L (10-73 U/L)
(SI: 1.25 μkat/L [0.17-1.22 μkat/L])

Which of the following is the primary cause of this patient's hypocalcemia?
A. Alcohol withdrawal
B. Chronic hypoparathyroidism
C. Hypomagnesemia
D. Vitamin D deficiency
E. Pancreatitis

4 A 63-year-old woman with bipolar disorder is referred for hypercalcemia. She has been treated with lithium since the time bipolar disorder was diagnosed at age 23 years. She was noted to have hypercalcemia 2 years ago on routine laboratory testing. She has no history of nephrolithiasis. Recent bone density assessment demonstrated osteoporosis at the femoral neck and distal radius. She has limited dairy intake and is taking calcium supplements, 500 mg twice daily, and vitamin D, 1000 IU daily.

Laboratory test results:
Serum calcium = 11.3 mg/dL (8.2-10.2 mg/dL)
(SI: 2.8 mmol/L [2.1-2.6 mmol/L])
PTH = 101 pg/mL (10-65 pg/mL)
(SI: 101 ng/L [10-65 ng/L])
25-Hydroxyvitamin D = 32 ng/mL (30-80 ng/mL
[optimal]) (SI: 79.9 nmol/L [74.9-199.7 nmol/L])
Magnesium = 1.8 mg/dL (1.5-2.3 mg/dL)
(SI: 0.74 mmol/L [0.6-0.9 mmol/L])
Phosphate = 2.4 mg/dL (2.3-4.7 mg/dL)
(SI: 0.8 mmol/L [0.7-1.5 mmol/L])
24-Hour urinary calcium clearance-to-creatinine
clearance ratio = 0.01

Which of the following is the best next step in this patient's management?
A. Recommend no therapy since she has familial hypocalciuric hypercalcemia
B. Recommend no therapy since most patients on long-term lithium treatment develop hypercalcemia
C. Discontinue lithium
D. Discontinue all calcium intake
E. Refer for parathyroid surgery for primary hyperparathyroidism

5 A 70-year-old woman with type 2 diabetes mellitus presents for follow-up after screening bone density testing. She has been taking metformin, 1000 mg twice daily, and pioglitazone, 45 mg daily, for many years. She has 2 servings of dairy per day and takes supplements with 600 mg of calcium and 800 IU vitamin D daily. She has no personal history of fracture, no parental history of hip fracture, and no other known risk factors for osteoporosis.

On physical examination, her height is 62 in (157.5 cm) and weight is 140 lb (63.6 kg) (BMI = 25.6 kg/m²).

Laboratory test results:
Complete blood count, normal
Comprehensive metabolic panel, normal
Hemoglobin A_{1c} = 7.9% (4.0%-5.6%)
(63 mmol/mol [20-38 mmol/mol])
25-Hydroxyvitamin D = 29 ng/mL (30-80 ng/mL [optimal]) (SI: 72.4 nmol/L [74.9-199.7 nmol/L])

Recent bone density testing is notable for T-scores of −1.8 at the lumbar spine, −2.0 at the femoral neck, and −2.1 at the total hip. Her 10-year risk of fracture calculated by FRAX is 12% for major osteoporotic fracture and 2.5% for hip fracture. Trabecular bone score is 1.150 (degraded).

Which of the following is the best next step for management of her bone health?
A. Change pioglitazone to canagliflozin
B. Adjust FRAX score for trabecular bone score
C. Increase vitamin D supplementation
D. Add dulaglutide to her regimen
E. Repeat bone density testing in 2 years

6 An 18-year-old man is referred to endocrinology. He recently immigrated, established medical care, and was noted to have abnormalities on routine blood tests. He has no known relevant medical history and is not taking any medications. Review of systems is positive for perioral and extremity numbness/tingling.

On physical examination, his height is 64 in (162.5 cm) and weight is 180 lb (81.8 kg) (BMI = 30.9 kg/m²). He has round facies and mild cognitive impairment. His hand is shown in the photograph (*see image*). He states his mother has a similar height and physical phenotype.

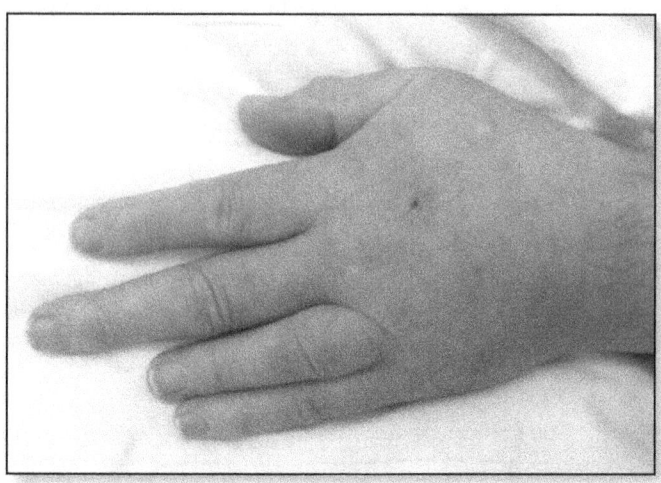

Which of the following patterns would be expected from the results of his laboratory testing?

Answer	Calcium	PTH	Phosphate
A.	Low	Low	Low
B.	Low	Low	High
C.	Low	High	Low
D.	Low	High	High
E.	Normal	Normal	Normal

7 A 41-year-old pregnant woman with a history of postoperative hypoparathyroidism presents at 39 weeks' gestation with headache, nausea, and vomiting. She developed hypoparathyroidism after parathyroid surgery for primary hyperparathyroidism at age 35 years. Genetic evaluation at that time was negative for pathogenic variants in the *MEN1* and *RET* genes. Her treatment regimen for hypoparathyroidism before pregnancy consisted of calcium, 600 mg 4 times daily; calcitriol, 0.75 mcg twice daily; and vitamin D, 1000 IU daily. On this regimen, her serum calcium concentration was 8.4 mg/dL (2.1 mmol/L) before pregnancy. She is currently taking calcium, 600 mg 3 times daily; calcitriol, 0.5 mcg twice daily; and vitamin D, 1000 IU daily.

Because of gastroesophageal reflux, she has been substituting several chewable calcium carbonate tablets per day instead of her usual calcium supplement.

Laboratory test results:
- Serum calcium = 10.8 mg/dL (8.2-10.2 mg/dL) (SI: 2.7 mmol/L [2.1-2.6 mmol/L])
- 25-Hydroxyvitamin D = 34 ng/mL (30-80 ng/mL [optimal]) (SI: 84.9 nmol/L [74.9-199.7 nmol/L])
- 1,25-Dihydroxyvitamin D = 82 pg/mL (16-65 pg/mL) (SI: 213.2 pmol/L [41.6-169.0 pmol/L])
- PTHrP = 4.0 pmol/L (<2.0 pmol/L)
- Bicarbonate = 24 mEq/L (21-28 mEq/L) (SI: 24 mmol/L [21-28 mmol/L])
- Albumin = 3.3 g/dL (3.5-5.0 g/dL) (SI: 33 g/L [35-50 g/L])
- Phosphate = 5.0 mg/dL (2.3-4.7 mg/dL) (SI: 1.6 mmol/L [0.7-1.5 mmol/L])
- Creatinine = 0.6 mg/dL (0.6-1.1 mg/dL) (SI: 53.0 μmol/L [53.0-97.2 μmol/L])

Which of the following is the most likely cause of this patient's hypercalcemia?
- A. Recurrence of primary hyperparathyroidism
- B. Milk-alkali syndrome
- C. Granulomatous disease
- D. Humoral hypercalcemia of malignancy
- E. Reduced calcium and calcitriol requirements during pregnancy

8 An 80-year-old White woman presents for a second opinion regarding management of osteoporosis. Osteoporosis was diagnosed after bone density assessment documented a T-score of −3.3 at the femoral neck. She has no personal or family history of fracture and has never been treated with glucocorticoids. Her primary care provider recommended bisphosphonate therapy, but the patient declined due to concern for adverse effects, stating, "Don't those medications just make the bone stiffer and actually cause hip fractures?"

How do you counsel this patient regarding the estimated benefits of antiresorptive therapy vs risks of atypical femoral fracture and osteonecrosis of the jaw?

Answer	Fracture risk reduction	Atypical femoral fracture risk	Osteonecrosis of the jaw risk
A.	75%	1/100,000	5/10,000
B.	50%	1/100,000	5/10,000
C.	50%	5/10,000	1/100,000
D.	25%	1/100,000	5/10,000
E.	25%	5/10,000	1/100,000

9 A 55-year-old man is referred to the emergency department by his primary care provider for hypercalcemia. He was recently seen for evaluation of fatigue that he had been experiencing for the past 3 months. He has hypertension treated with amlodipine but otherwise has no notable medical history. He is not taking any additional medications or supplements. He has had no anorexia, nausea, vomiting, abdominal pain, polyuria, polydipsia, or other new symptoms.

Physical examination demonstrates pallor of the mucus membranes. He is alert and oriented to person, place, and time.

Laboratory test results:
- Serum calcium = 18.4 mg/dL (8.2-10.2 mg/dL) (SI: 4.6 mmol/L [2.1-2.6 mmol/L])
- Ionized calcium = 4.90 (4.60-5.08 mg/dL) (SI: 1.23 mmol/L [1.2-1.3 mmol/L])
- PTH = 23 pg/mL (10-65 pg/mL) (SI: 23 ng/L [10-65 ng/L])
- 25-Hydroxyvitamin D = 22 ng/mL (30-80 ng/mL [optimal]) (SI: 54.9 nmol/L [74.9-199.7 nmol/L])
- Albumin = 3.9 g/dL (3.5-5.0 g/dL) (SI: 39 g/L [35-50 g/L])
- Hemoglobin = 9.9 g/dL (13.8-17.2 g/dL) (SI: 99 g/L [138-172 g/L])
- Creatinine = 1.5 mg/dL (0.6-1.1 mg/dL) (SI: 132.6 μmol/L [53.0-97.2 μmol/L])
- Serum protein electrophoresis, positive for monoclonal protein

Which of the following is the best next step for treatment of this patient's elevated calcium?
- A. Normal saline intravenously
- B. Cinacalcet, 30 mg orally 3 times daily
- C. Pamidronate, 60 mg intravenously
- D. Emergency plasmapheresis
- E. No treatment necessary

10 A 56-year-old woman with end-stage kidney disease due to hypertension has been on hemodialysis for 8 years. She is referred due to a pelvic fracture and a femoral neck T-score of −2.2. Medications for the past 6 years include calcitriol, 0.5 mcg twice daily, and cinacalcet, 90 mg twice daily.

Laboratory test results:
Serum calcium = 8.1 mg/dL (8.2-10.2 mg/dL)
(SI: 2.0 mmol/L [2.1-2.6 mmol/L])
Phosphate = 5.2 mg/dL (2.3-4.7 mg/dL)
(SI: 1.7 mmol/L [0.7-1.5 mmol/L])
25-Hydroxyvitamin D = 24 ng/mL (25-80 ng/mL [optimal]) (SI: 59.9 nmol/L [62.4-199.7 nmol/L])
PTH = 78 pg/mL (10-65 pg/mL) (SI: 78 ng/L [10-65 ng/L])
Total alkaline phosphatase = 48 U/L (50-120 U/L) (SI: 0.80 μkat/L [0.84-2.00 μkat/L])

An iliac crest biopsy is performed after double-tetracycline labeling.

Which of the following is most likely to be found on the bone biopsy?
- A. Osteitis fibrosa cystica
- B. Osteomalacia
- C. Adynamic bone disease
- D. Mixed renal osteodystrophy
- E. Osteoporosis

11 A 37-year-old woman is admitted to the hospital with hypercalcemia. She moved 6 months ago from Los Angeles where she worked in the entertainment industry. She has a 2-month history of progressive anorexia, 15-lb (6.8-kg) weight loss, nausea, fatigue, polyuria, and polydipsia. She has had no fevers or night sweats.

She has no notable medical history and has never had kidney stones, bone pain, or fractures. She takes no medications and states that she has not recently used alcohol, tobacco, or illicit drugs.

On physical examination, she is afebrile, oriented but lethargic, and dehydrated. Findings on breast examination are normal. There is no palpable lymphadenopathy. Nodularity in both buttocks is noted.

Laboratory test results:
Calcium = 14.5 mg/dL (8.2-10.2 mg/dL)
(SI: 3.63 mmol/L [2.1-2.6 mmol/L])
Albumin = 4.1 g/dL (3.5-5.0 g/dL)
(SI: 41 g/L [35-50 g/L])
Creatinine = 2.0 mg/dL (0.6-1.1 mg/dL)
(SI: 176.8 μmol/L [53.0-97.2 μmol/L])
Phosphate = 4.9 mg/dL (2.3-4.7 mg/dL)
(SI: 1.6 mmol/L [0.7-1.5 mmol/L])
PTH = <10 pg/mL (10-65 pg/mL)
(SI: <10 ng/L [10-65 ng/L])
25-Hydroxyvitamin D = 15 ng/mL (25-80 ng/mL [optimal]) (SI: 37.4 nmol/L [62.4-199.7 nmol/L])
1,25-Dihydroxyvitamin D = 82 pg/mL (16-65 pg/mL) (SI: 213.2 pmol/L [41.6-169.0 pmol/L])

CT of the buttocks is shown (*see image*).

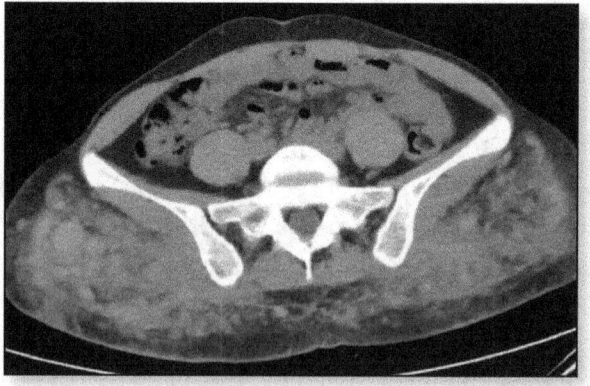

Which of the following is the most likely diagnosis?
- A. Foreign-body granulomas
- B. T-cell lymphoma
- C. Sarcoidosis
- D. Calciphylaxis
- E. Fibrodysplasia ossificans progressiva

12 A 25-year-old man presents for follow-up of hypoparathyroidism. He initially presented at age 3 years with a seizure and severe hypocalcemia. Since then, he has taken calcium and calcitriol. He has also been treated for intermittent oral candidiasis and fungal infections of his fingernails and toenails since childhood. He otherwise feels well.

On physical examination, he has some tinea of the nails and negative Chvostek and Trousseau signs.

In addition to measuring calcium, phosphate, and kidney function, which of the following should be measured now?

A. Antiphospholipid antibodies
B. Glutamic acid decarboxylase (GAD-65) antibodies
C. 21-Hydroxylase antibodies
D. Tissue transglutaminase antibodies
E. TPO antibodies

13 A 59-year-old woman with osteoporosis has been on daily calcium plus vitamin D and alendronate, 70 mg orally weekly, for the past 2 years. She entered menopause 5 years ago and did not take hormone therapy. Despite excellent adherence to the regimen, her repeated DXA shows significant declines in bone mineral density at both the spine (4% decline) and hip (6% decline). On review of systems, she notes an 8-lb (3.6-kg) weight loss and mild fatigue.

Laboratory test results:
Calcium = 8.9 mg/dL (8.2-10.2 mg/dL)
(SI: 2.2 mmol/L [2.1-2.6 mmol/L])
Albumin = 3.8 g/dL (3.5-5.0 g/dL)
(SI: 38 g/L [35-50 g/L])
Creatinine = 0.8 mg/dL (0.6-1.1 mg/dL)
(SI: 70.2 μmol/L [53.0-97.2 μmol/L])
Intact PTH = 90 pg/mL (10-65 pg/mL)
(SI: 90 ng/L [10-65 ng/L])
25-Hydroxyvitamin D = 20 ng/mL (30-80 ng/mL [optimal]) (SI: 49.9 nmol/L [74.9-199.7 nmol/L])
Hemoglobin = 11.5 g/dL (12.1-15.1 g/dL)
(SI: 115 g/L [121-151 g/L])

Which of the following laboratory studies would be most useful for diagnosing the cause of this patient's poor response to therapy?

A. Serum protein electrophoresis
B. Measurement of urinary calcium excretion (24-hour urine collection)
C. Cosyntropin-stimulation test
D. Tissue transglutaminase antibody assessment
E. Fasting serum C-telopeptide measurement

14 A 74-year-old man is admitted to the hospital with altered mental status, nausea, vomiting, and dehydration. His medical history is notable for chronic obstructive pulmonary disease, coronary artery disease, and an 80 pack-year smoking history.

On physical examination, he is barely arousable. His blood pressure is 96/65 mm Hg, and pulse rate is 120 beats/min. He has dry mucus membranes, and there is no lymphadenopathy.

Chest x-ray in the emergency department reveals a 3-cm spiculated mass in the right upper lung lobe with destruction of an adjacent rib.

Laboratory tests results:
Calcium = 16.8 mg/dL (8.2-10.2 mg/dL)
(SI: 4.2 mmol/L [2.1-2.6 mmol/L])
Ionized calcium = 7.25 mg/dL (4.60-5.08 mg/dL)
(SI: 1.8 mmol/L [1.2-1.3 mmol/L])
Serum urea nitrogen = 50 mg/dL (8-23 mg/dL)
(SI: 17.9 mmol/L [2.9-8.2 mmol/L])
Creatinine = 3.5 mg/dL (0.7-1.3 mg/dL)
(SI: 309.4 μmol/L [61.9-114.9 μmol/L])
Serum protein electrophoresis, normal
Urine protein electrophoresis, normal
Intact PTH = <10 pg/mL (10-65 pg/mL)
(SI: <10 ng/L [10-65 ng/L])

The patient receives vigorous intravenous saline hydration (2 L in the first 4 hours followed by 150 cc/h); calcitonin, 4 units/kg every 6 hours; and zoledronic acid, 4 mg intravenously × 1 dose. Forty-eight hours after admission, he is more alert and responsive, blood pressure is 140/85 mm Hg, and pulse rate is 90 beats/min. His serum calcium concentration is now 13.8 mg/dL (3.5 mmol/L) and his creatinine concentration is 1.8 mg/dL (159.1 µmol/L).

Which of the following is the best next step?
- A. Increase the rate of intravenous saline to 200 cc/h and add furosemide
- B. Stop calcitonin and continue current hydration and monitoring
- C. Administer another dose of zoledronic acid, 4 mg intravenously
- D. Administer denosumab, 60 mg subcutaneously
- E. Begin hydrocortisone, 50 mg intravenously every 6 hours

15 A 72-year-old woman has been taking alendronate, 70 mg weekly, for the past 2 years to treat osteoporosis of the lumbar spine. She says that she has taken it correctly except for missing a few doses and that she has had no adverse effects. A another DXA was performed at the same center as her initial study. The report indicates a significant loss of bone mineral density (decline of 7%) at the total hip, a significant increase of bone mineral density at the lumbar spine (+4%), and no change at the femoral neck. The most recent DXA results for the hip are shown (*see image*).

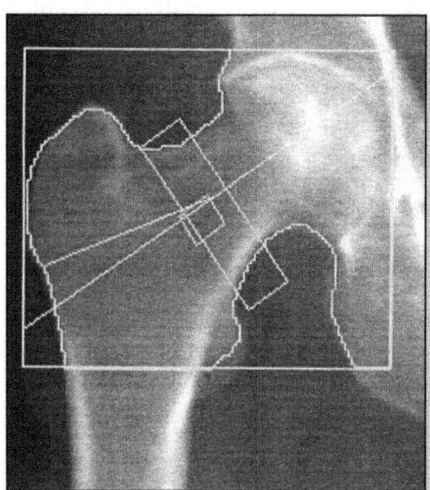

DXA Results Summary:

Region	Area (cm²)	BMC (g)	BMD (g/cm²)	T-Score	PR (%)	Z-Score	AM (%)
Neck	5.78	3.89	0.672	-1.9	72	-0.5	92
Troch	13.42	9.58	0.714	-0.5	92	0.2	103
Inter	17.24	15.09	0.875	-1.8	73	-0.9	85
Total	**36.45**	**28.55**	**0.783**	**-1.7**	**76**	**-0.7**	**88**
Ward's	1.08	0.45	0.422	-2.6	54	-0.4	89

Total BMD CV 1.0%, ACF = 1.019, BCF = 1.001, TH = 5.863

BMC = bone mineral content; BMD = bone mineral density.

Which of the following is the best next step in this patient's management?
- A. Continue current regimen
- B. Do an extensive workup for secondary causes of bone loss
- C. Prescribe an intensive weight-bearing exercise program
- D. Revise the region of interest for the total hip measurement
- E. Switch from alendronate to intravenous zoledronic acid

16 A 55-year-old woman is referred after results of a screening DXA. Her last menstrual period was 3 years ago, and she has occasional mild hot flashes that do not interfere with her quality of life. Her BMI is 20 kg/m². She is generally healthy, but she fractured 2 ribs last year after missing a step. She does not smoke cigarettes, she drinks 1 glass of wine nightly, and she takes no medications. Her daily intake provides 1200 mg of calcium and 800 IU of vitamin Her mother fractured a hip.

The patient's DXA documents the following:

Site	BMD, g/cm²	T-score
Total hip	0.698	−1.5
Femoral neck	0.658	−1.7
L1-L4	0.983	−0.3

Vertebral fracture assessment is negative for spinal compression fractures. Her FRAX 10-year risk is 12% for any major osteoporotic fracture and 0.7% for hip fracture.

Which of the following is the correct management plan?
   A. Start alendronate and repeat DXA in 1 year
   B. Continue calcium and vitamin D and repeat DXA in 2 years
   C. Start raloxifene and perform DXA in 1 year
   D. Start estrogen replacement therapy
   E. Start nasal calcitonin therapy

17 A 69-year-old woman has been treated with alendronate, 70 mg weekly, for 2 years. Her recent DXA scan shows a femoral neck T-score of –2.7 and no change in bone mineral density compared with findings from 2 years ago. She says she is 3 in (7.6 cm) shorter than her young adult height, but she does not know whether her height has changed over the past few years. Vertebral fracture assessment shows a compression fracture of L1 (*see image*). No baseline testing is available. For the past several years, she has had back pain almost every day, some days more than others, but she does not recall an incident that might explain this finding.

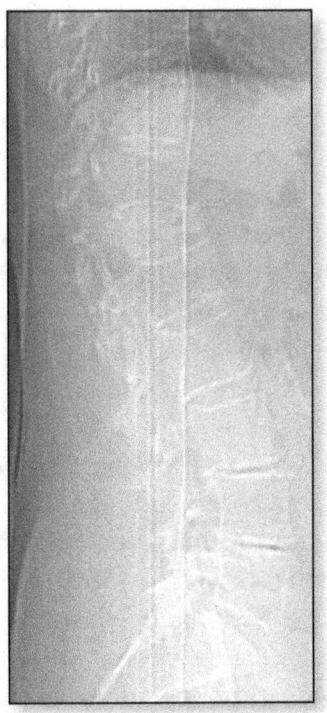

Which of the following tests is most likely to give useful information regarding the age of this fracture if it occurred more than 6 months ago?
   A. Nuclear medicine bone scan
   B. Lumbar spine radiograph
   C. MRI
   D. CT
   E. Bone-specific alkaline phosphatase measurement

18 A 28-year-old man presents with fatigue, and primary hyperparathyroidism is subsequently diagnosed.

Laboratory test results:
   Serum calcium = 11.9 mg/dL (8.2-10.2 mg/dL)
      (SI: 3.0 mmol/L [2.1-2.6 mmol/L])
   Serum PTH = 120 pg/mL (10-65 pg/mL)
      (SI: 120 ng/L [10-65 ng/L])
   Urinary calcium = 400 mg/24 h (100-300 mg/24 h)
      (SI: 10 mmol/d [2.5-7.5 mmol/d])

His family history is positive for recurrent hyperparathyroidism and chronic diarrhea in his father, as well as kidney stones and peptic ulcers in 1 of his 3 siblings.

Which of the following is the most likely underlying diagnosis in this case?
   A. Familial "idiopathic" hyperparathyroidism
   B. Hereditary "renal leak" hypercalciuria
   C. Hereditary activation of the calcium-sensing receptor
   D. Multiple endocrine neoplasia type 1
   E. Hyperparathyroidism–jaw tumor syndrome

19 An 18-year-old male refugee presents with a history of bone pain, joint deformities, and severe dental problems since childhood. On physical examination, he has short stature, severe genu varum (bow-leggedness), and very poor dentition, but no abnormal skin pigmentation. Family history is unavailable because he was separated from his family and grew up in an orphanage.

Laboratory blood test results:

Calcium = 8.8 mg/dL (8.2-10.2 mg/dL)
(SI: 2.2 mmol/L [2.1-2.6 mmol/L])

Albumin = 4.0 g/dL (3.5-5.0 g/dL)
(SI: 40 g/L [35-50 g/L])

Phosphate = 1.3 mg/dL (2.3-4.7 mg/dL)
(SI: 0.4 mmol/L [0.7-1.5 mmol/L])

25-Hydroxyvitamin D = 24 ng/mL (30-80 ng/mL
[optimal]) (SI: 59.9 nmol/L [74.9-199.7 nmol/L])

1,25-Dihydroxyvitamin D = 30 pg/mL
(16-65 pg/mL) (SI: 78 pmol/L
[41.6-169.0 pmol/L])

Intact PTH = 110 pg/mL (10-65 pg/mL)
(SI: 110 ng/L [10-65 ng/L])

Which of the following is the most likely diagnosis?

A. X-linked hypophosphatemic rickets

B. Oncogenic osteomalacia (tumor-induced osteomalacia)

C. McCune-Albright syndrome

D. Vitamin D–resistant rickets

E. Vitamin D–deficient rickets

20 A 75-year-old man with primary hyperparathyroidism is referred for management. He is asymptomatic and generally feels well. He has not experienced kidney stones, fractures, or loss of height. His BMI is 22 kg/m². DXA shows T-scores of –1.8 at the lumbar spine, –1.6 at the femoral neck, and –2.2 at the one-third distal radius.

Laboratory test results:

Serum calcium = 10.8 mg/dL (8.2-10.2 mg/dL)
(SI: 2.7 mmol/L [2.1-2.6 mmol/L])

Albumin = 4.0 g/dL (3.5-5.0 g/dL)
(SI: 40 g/L [35-50 g/L])

Intact PTH = 88 pg/mL (10-65 pg/mL)
(SI: 88 ng/L [10-65 ng/L])

25-Hydroxyvitamin D = 18 ng/mL (30-80 ng/mL
[optimal]) (SI: 44.9 nmol/L [74.9-199.7 nmol/L])

1,25-Dihydroxyvitamin D = 50 pg/mL
(16-65 pg/mL) (SI: 130 pmol/L
[41.6-169.0 pmol/L])

Urinary calcium = 180 mg/24 h (100-300 mg/24 h)
(SI: 4.5 mmol/d [2.5-7.5 mmol/d])

Which of the following is the best recommendation with respect to oral vitamin D₃ (cholecalciferol) therapy in this patient?

A. 400 IU daily

B. 1000 IU daily

C. 4000 IU daily

D. 50,000 IU weekly

E. No supplementation

21 A 75-year-old woman had a hip fracture after a fall from standing height. She has no notable medical history other than borderline hypertension. Recent DXA was significant for T-scores of –2.1 at the lumbar spine, –1.9 at the femoral neck, and –1.7 at the total hip. She is a former cigarette smoker. She has no parental history of hip fracture. She takes a daily supplement with 1200 mg of calcium in divided doses and 800 IU of vitamin

Which of the following is the best recommendation for this patient regarding pharmacologic osteoporosis therapy?

A. Not needed because she has osteopenia, not osteoporosis

B. Treatment only if her FRAX-derived 10-year risk of major osteoporotic fracture is ≥20% or hip fracture risk is ≥3%

C. Strongly recommended based on her age

D. Strongly recommended because of her history of tobacco use

E. Strongly recommended because of her hip fracture

22 A 76-year-old woman in whom osteoporosis was diagnosed at age 67 years presents for follow-up. Since her diagnosis, she has been treated with an oral bisphosphonate. Menopause was at age 53 years, and she has not taken estrogen. Results from a laboratory evaluation (including a complete blood cell count; chemistry panel; and measurements of PTH, 25-hydroxyvitamin D, and 24-hour urinary calcium excretion) were normal 2 years ago and again last month. Ten years ago, breast cancer was diagnosed, and she was treated with surgery, chemotherapy, radiation, and tamoxifen for 5 years. Over the past 2 years, her bone mineral density has decreased. She has lost 2 in (5.1 cm) in height. Vertebral fracture assessment shows 2 thoracic compression fractures of uncertain age. The patient asks about treatment with teriparatide.

Which of the following is a contraindication to the use of teriparatide in this patient?
   A. Age older than 70 years
   B. History of radiation treatment
   C. Previous bisphosphonate therapy
   D. History of breast cancer
   E. She has no contraindications

23 A 70-year-old woman with recently diagnosed osteoporosis presents for follow-up. She is going to start therapy with alendronate, 70 mg weekly. Results from laboratory evaluation include a normal complete blood cell count, chemistry panel, and 24-hour urinary calcium excretion. Her serum 25-hydroxyvitamin D level is 18 ng/mL (44.9 nmol/L). A vitamin D supplement of 2000 IU daily is recommended.

The soonest her 25-hydroxyvitamin D level should be checked again to determine the full effect of this additional supplement is:
   A. 2 weeks
   B. 1 month
   C. 3 months
   D. 6 months
   E. 12 months

24 An 80-year-old woman with Paget disease is referred for evaluation. Ten years ago, a nuclear bone scan showed increased uptake limited to the right tibia, and radiographs showed pagetic changes of the tibia. Her alkaline phosphatase level at that time was 125 U/L (50-120 U/L) (SI: 2.09 μkat/L [0.84-2.00 μkat/L]). She has not received treatment. She now describes severe pain in her right tibia and a radiograph shows coarsened trabeculae and a periosteal reaction. Her alkaline phosphatase concentration is 250 U/L (4.18 μkat/L). Her γ-glutamyltranspeptidase level is normal.

Which of the following is the best next step?
   A. C-telopeptide measurement
   B. Percutaneous biopsy of the tibia
   C. Whole-body bone scan
   D. MRI of the right tibia
   E. Zoledronic acid, 5 mg intravenously

25 A 43-year-old man has had 2 episodes of calcium-containing kidney stones. His workup reveals normal serum calcium and PTH levels, with a 24-hour urinary calcium excretion of 335 mg/24 h (100-300 mg/24 h) (SI: 8.4 mmol/d [2.5-7.5 mmol/d]), but normal 24-hour urinary oxalate, uric acid, sodium, and citrate levels. His urine volume is 2650 mL/24 h. Kidney stone analysis reveals calcium oxalate.

Which of the following recommendations would provide the greatest reduction in his risk of future calcium oxalate stone disease?
   A. Sodium citrate, 500 mg 4 times daily
   B. Allopurinol, 300 mg daily
   C. Hydrochlorothiazide, 25 mg once daily
   D. Reduced dietary sodium
   E. Reduced dietary oxalate

26 A 48-year-old man is referred for evaluation and management of muscle pain, fatigue, and weakness. On physical examination, he has proximal muscle weakness. His lumbar spine T-score is −3.3.

Laboratory test results:
   Chemistry panel, normal
   25-Hydroxyvitamin D = 28 ng/mL (30-80 ng/mL [optimal]) (SI: 69.9 nmol/L [74.9-199.7 nmol/L])
   1,25-Dihydroxyvitamin D = 12 pg/mL (16-65 pg/mL) (SI: 31.2 pmol/L [41.6-169.0 pmol/L])
   PTH = 98 pg/mL (10-65 pg/mL) (SI: 98 ng/L [10-65 ng/L])
   Serum and urine protein electrophoresis, free kappa and lambda light chains, normal
   Serum phosphate = 1.1 to 1.3 mg/dL (2.3-4.7 mg/dL) [SI: 0.36 to 0.41 mmol/L [0.72-1.52 mmol/L])
   Serum FGF-23 = 350 RU/mL (<180 RU/mL)

Which of the following treatments should be recommended now?
- A. Potassium phosphate and calcitriol
- B. Cholecalciferol and calcitriol
- C. Potassium phosphate alone
- D. Alendronate
- E. Zoledronic acid

27 A 57-year-old woman with osteoporosis has been on risedronate, 35 mg orally weekly, for the past 2 years. Her diet provides more than 1000 mg of elemental calcium each day, and she takes 1000 IU of cholecalciferol daily. Her last menstrual period occurred 5 years ago, and she has never taken hormone therapy. A follow-up DXA on the same machine now shows significant declines in bone mineral density at both the spine (6% decline) and hip (5% decline) compared with values obtained 2 years ago. On review of systems, she feels well and has no new symptoms. BMI is 23 kg/m², and physical examination findings are unchanged.

Laboratory test results, including serum calcium, albumin, creatinine, intact PTH, 25-hydroxyvitamin D, electrolytes, ferritin, and 24-hour urinary calcium excretion, are normal.

Which of the following is the most likely reason for her poor response to therapy?
- A. Nonadherence to treatment
- B. Malabsorption
- C. Undiagnosed eating disorder
- D. Positioning error by the DXA technician
- E. Lack of potency of risedronate to stop rapid postmenopausal bone loss

28 A 48-year-old woman undergoes total thyroidectomy for papillary carcinoma of the thyroid and is left with permanent surgical hypoparathyroidism. She is an avid daily exerciser and experiences "muscle cramps" unless she takes 1 to 2 extra calcium chews (400 mg elemental calcium per chew) before and after vigorous exercise. This is in addition to 1800 mg of elemental calcium daily in divided doses; calcitriol, 1.0 mcg twice daily; and levothyroxine, 150 mcg daily.

On physical examination, she has a well-healed thyroidectomy scar and negative Chvostek and Trousseau signs.

Laboratory test results 6 months after surgery:
Serum calcium = 8.2 mg/dL (8.2-10.2 mg/dL)
  (SI: 2.1 mmol/L [2.1-2.6 mmol/L])
Albumin = 4.0 g/dL (3.5-5.0 g/dL)
  (SI: 40 g/L [35-50 g/L])
Phosphate = 4.9 mg/dL (2.3-4.7 mg/dL)
  (SI: 1.6 mmol/L [0.7-1.5 mmol/L])
25-Hydroxyvitamin D = 40 ng/mL (25-80 ng/mL
  [optimal]) (SI: 99.8 nmol/L [62.4-199.7 nmol/L])
Urinary calcium = 380 mg/24 h (100-300 mg/24 h)
  (SI: 9.5 mmol/d [2.5-7.5 mmol/d])

Which of the following should be recommended now?
- A. Continue current regimen
- B. Increase calcium by 50%
- C. Increase calcitriol by 50%
- D. Begin sevelamer
- E. Begin hydrochlorothiazide

Diabetes Mellitus, Section 1 Board Review

Serge A. Jabbour, MD

1 A 32-year-old woman with a 10-year history of type 1 diabetes is self-referred because of high glycemic variability. She has been on insulin pump therapy for 6 years, with a recent hemoglobin A_{1c} level of 8.0% (64 mmol/mol). Pregnancy test is negative. Recently, she started using continuous glucose monitoring (CGM). CGM downloads over the past 2 weeks show the following:

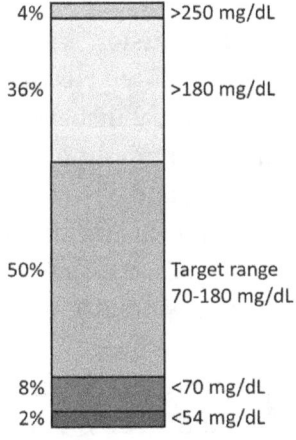

Which of the following should be her CGM-based targets?

A.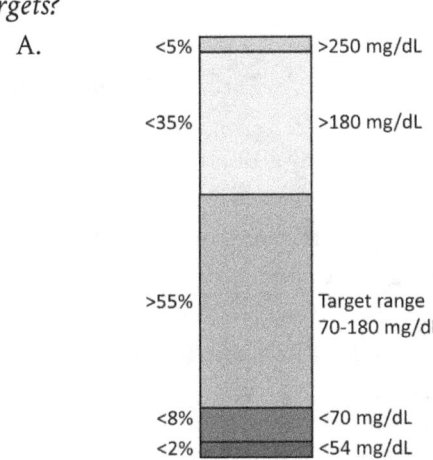

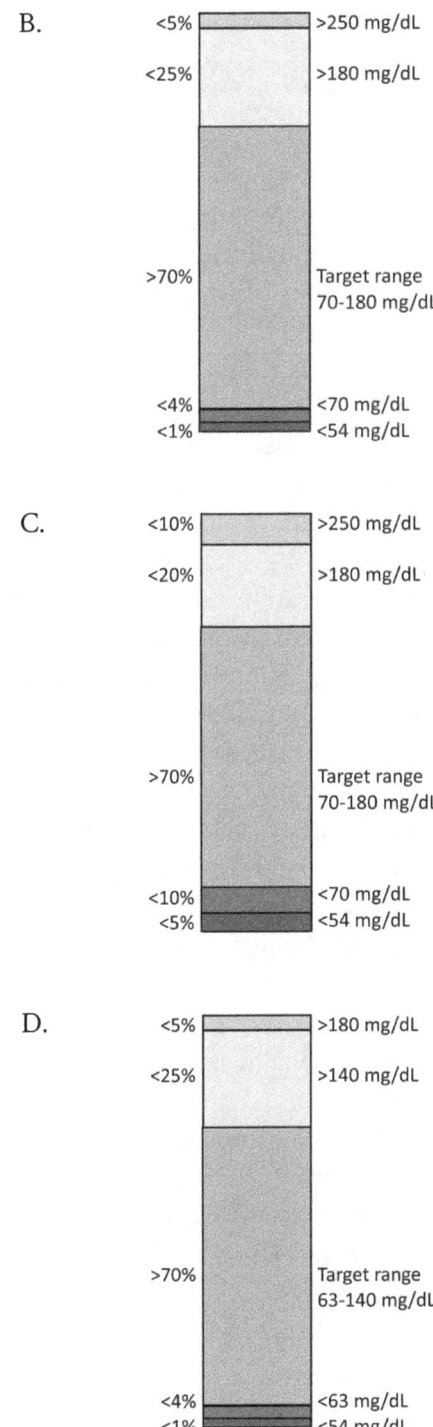

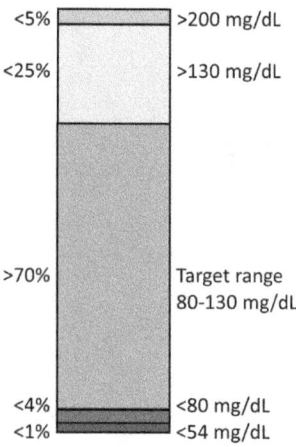

E.

<5%	>200 mg/dL
<25%	>130 mg/dL
>70%	Target range 80-130 mg/dL
<4%	<80 mg/dL
<1%	<54 mg/dL

2 A 65-year-old man presents for evaluation 3 months after hospitalization for diabetic ketoacidosis. He has a 5-year history of type 2 diabetes mellitus. He also has dyslipidemia, hypertension, polymyalgia rheumatica, and recently diagnosed metastatic melanoma.

His diabetes has been well controlled on metformin, 2000 mg daily, and empagliflozin, 25 mg daily, with hemoglobin A_{1c} values ranging between 6.5% and 7.2% (48-55 mmol/mol). His estimated glomerular filtration rate is 68 mL/min per 1.73 m². His other medications include atorvastatin, 40 mg daily, and ramipril, 10 mg daily. Prednisone, 10 mg daily, was added 3 months ago to treat polymyalgia rheumatica. His BMI fluctuates between 26 and 28 kg/m².

His oncologist decides to start nivolumab and ipilimumab. He is able to tolerate these drugs without adverse effects, but 2 months later, he is admitted to the hospital with diabetic ketoacidosis.

Laboratory test results on admission:
Blood glucose = 850 mg/dL (70-99 mg/dL) (SI: 47.2 mmol/L [3.9-5.5 mmol/L])
Serum β-hydroxybutyrate = 85 mg/dL (<3.0 mg/dL) (SI: 8165 μmol/L [<288.2 μmol/L])
Hemoglobin A_{1c} = 7.6% (4.0%-5.6%) (60 mmol/mol [20-38 mmol/mol])
Serum glutamic acid decarboxylase 65 antibodies, negative

After hydration and intravenous insulin, he recovers and is discharged on a basal and mealtime insulin regimen, in addition to atorvastatin and ramipril. You see him a week later in the outpatient setting.

Which of the following is the best next step?
A. Restart metformin and empagliflozin and wean him off insulin over the next weeks to months
B. Restart metformin, add once-weekly semaglutide, and wean him off insulin over the next weeks to months
C. Restart metformin, add dulaglutide, add repaglinide, and stop mealtime insulin
D. Continue insulin indefinitely
E. Add metformin, add glimepiride, and stop mealtime insulin

3 A 66-year-old man presents for diabetes management 1 week after hospital discharge. This was his second admission within a month for heart failure with reduced ejection fraction (HFrEF). He has had type 2 diabetes for 2 years. He also has hypertension, dyslipidemia, stage 3 chronic kidney disease, and obstructive sleep apnea.

His current medications are ramipril, metoprolol, furosemide, sacubitril-valsartan, and rosuvastatin.

Review of systems is notable for shortness of breath on exertion and fatigue.

On physical examination, his blood pressure is 120/70 mm Hg and BMI is 29 kg/m². He has a few crackles at the lung bases and 1+ edema in his lower extremities.

Laboratory test results:
Hemoglobin A_{1c} = 6.8% (4.0%-5.6%) (51 mmol/mol [20-38 mmol/mol])
Estimated glomerular filtration rate = 38 mL/min per 1.73 m² (>60 mL/min per 1.73 m²)
Urinary albumin-to-creatinine ratio = 140 mg/g creat (<30 mg/g creat)

Which of the following is the best next step?
A. Add saxagliptin
B. Add liraglutide
C. Add dulaglutide
D. Add dapagliflozin
E. No change

4 A 56-year-old Black man with end-stage kidney disease due to hypertensive nephropathy will be undergoing kidney transplant in few weeks. In addition to hypertension, he has a history of obesity, prediabetes (recent hemoglobin A_{1c} = 6.3% [45 mmol/mol]), dyslipidemia, sleep apnea, fatty liver, and hepatitis C virus infection. Because this patient is at high risk for posttransplant diabetes, his nephrologist asks for your guidance.

In addition to lifestyle intervention and, if possible, a quick taper of prednisone to a maintenance dosage, which of the following agents would be best avoided?

A. Azathioprine
B. Cyclosporine
C. Tacrolimus
D. Mycophenolate mofetil
E. Belatacept

5 A 54-year-old woman is seen for follow-up regarding type 1 diabetes mellitus. She has had diabetes since age 10 years, complicated by nephropathy, nonproliferative retinopathy, neuropathy, and gastroparesis. She is on a basal-mealtime insulin regimen but is not adherent and misses insulin injections on a regular basis. She has declined insulin pumps and glucose sensors. Her hemoglobin A_{1c} level has ranged between 8.5% and 12.0% (69-108 mmol/mol) in recent years.

Her new concerns are blurred vision, decreased visual acuity, and floaters for the past few months. She has not seen an ophthalmologist in 3 years.

A fundoscopic examination is performed (*see image*).

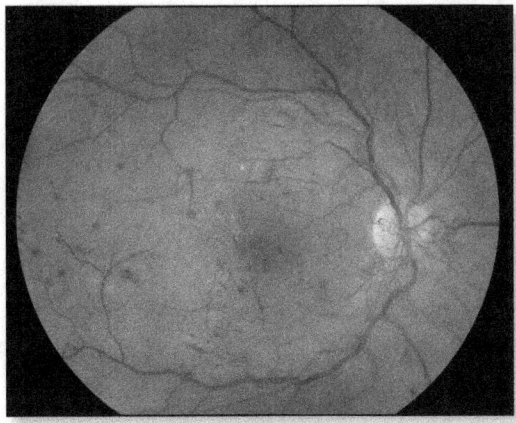

You immediately refer her to ophthalmology.

Based on her nonadherence history and the fundoscopic findings, which of the following is the best next step?

A. Focal laser photocoagulation
B. Anti-VEGF (vascular endothelial growth factor) agents
C. Vitrectomy
D. Panretinal laser photocoagulation
E. Intravitreal glucocorticoids

6 A 23-year-old woman with a 10-year history of type 1 diabetes mellitus has just learned that she is 4 weeks pregnant (G1,P0). Her diabetes is well controlled on insulin detemir, 12 units in the morning and 8 units in the evening, and insulin lispro based on an insulin-to-carbohydrate ratio of 1:15 and a sensitivity factor of 1:40. She has no known diabetes-related complications.

On physical examination, her blood pressure is 110/70 mm Hg and BMI is 22 kg/m^2. Examination findings are unremarkable.

Laboratory test results:
Hemoglobin A_{1c} = 6.8% (4.0%-5.6%)
   (51 mmol/mol [20-38 mmol/mol])
Serum creatinine, normal
Electrolytes, normal
TSH, normal
Urinary albumin-to-creatinine ratio, normal

Average self-monitoring blood glucose values over the past 2 weeks:
Fasting = 110 mg/dL (SI: 6.1 mmol/L)
1-Hour postprandial = 155 mg/dL
   (SI: 8.6 mmol/L) after breakfast, 150 mg/dL
   (SI: 8.3 mmol/L) after lunch, 160 mg/dL
   (SI: 8.9 mmol/L) after dinner
2-Hour postprandial = 140 mg/dL
   (SI: 7.8 mmol/L) after breakfast, 130 mg/dL
   (SI: 7.2 mmol/L) after lunch, 145 mg/dL
   (SI: 8.0 mmol/L) after dinner

Which of the following insulin regimens would be best?

Answer	Morning detemir	Evening detemir	Insulin-to-carbohydrate ratio	Insulin sensitivity factor
A.	16 units	8 units	1:20	1:50
B.	12 units	8 units	1:15	1:40
C.	12 units	10 units	1:12	1:40
D.	14 units	10 units	1:6	1:20
E.	12 units	10 units	1:15	1:40

7 A 32-year-old woman with a 10-year history of type 1 diabetes mellitus attends a follow-up visit. She does not have any other medical problems. Findings on her last eye examination 6 months ago were normal. Her menses are regular. She is not planning pregnancy soon. She uses an insulin pump with a continuous glucose monitor. Her only medication is insulin aspart.

On physical examination, her BMI is 22 kg/m² and blood pressure is 110/60 mm Hg. Examination findings are unremarkable.

Laboratory test results:

Measurement	3 Months ago	Current
Hemoglobin A$_{1c}$	6.4% (46 mmol/mol)	6.9% (52 mmol/mol)
Serum creatinine	0.6 mg/dL (SI: 53.0 µmol/L)	0.6 mg/dL (SI: 53.0 µmol/L)
Electrolytes, TSH, liver enzymes, complete blood cell count	Normal	Normal
Urine albumin-to-creatinine ratio	22 mg/g creat	345 mg/g creat
Pregnancy test	...	Negative

Which of the following is the best next step?
- A. Lower hemoglobin A$_{1c}$ to less than 6.5% (<48 mmol/mol)
- B. Add ramipril
- C. Add losartan
- D. Add canagliflozin
- E. Repeat measurement of the urinary albumin-to-creatinine ratio

8 A 36-year-old man with a 10-year history of type 1 diabetes mellitus was admitted to the hospital 7 days ago with diabetic ketoacidosis due to pump failure. On admission, he had acute pancreatitis caused by severe hypertriglyceridemia. After receiving intravenous fluids and insulin infusion, his serum ketones and anion gap normalized. His serum triglyceride concentration is now 350 mg/dL (3.96 mmol/L). However, his amylase and lipase levels are still elevated, and he is unable to tolerate enteral nutrition.

Total parenteral nutrition (TPN) is started. Two days later, his insulin infusion rate is 2 units/h with blood glucose values ranging between 140 and 180 mg/dL (7.8-10.0 mmol/L). The medical team decides to stop the intravenous insulin infusion because of difficult venous access.

Which of the following is the best next step?
- A. Add 40 units of regular insulin to TPN bag
- B. Add 20 units of regular insulin to TPN bag and 20 units of subcutaneous insulin glargine daily
- C. Add 30 units of insulin lispro to TPN bag and 10 units of subcutaneous insulin glargine daily
- D. Start subcutaneous regular insulin sliding scale
- E. Start subcutaneous insulin lispro, 10 units every 6 hours

9 A 62-year-old woman seeks an opinion on how she can prevent diabetes in the future. She has a strong family history of type 2 diabetes mellitus. She also has hypertension and dyslipidemia.

Her only medications are rosuvastatin and amlodipine.

On physical examination, her BMI is 34 kg/m² and blood pressure is 120/60 mm Hg. She has 2+ edema in both lower extremities. Findings are otherwise unremarkable.

Recent laboratory test results:
Hemoglobin A$_{1c}$ = 6.1% (4.0%-5.6%) (43 mmol/mol [20-38 mmol/mol])
Estimated glomerular filtration rate = 76 mL/min per 1.73 m² (>60 mL/min per 1.73 m²)

On the basis of available studies, which of the following is the best option?

A. Dulaglutide
B. Empagliflozin
C. Metformin
D. Lifestyle intervention
E. Pioglitazone

10 A 52-year-old man with a 10-year history of type 2 diabetes mellitus is referred for a second opinion. He has been treated with once-daily insulin glargine and insulin glulisine with meals. His self-monitoring blood glucose values range between 80 and 120 mg/dL (4.4-6.7 mmol/L) before meals and between 120 and 140 mg/dL (6.7-7.8 mmol/L) 2 hours after meals. He reports rare hypoglycemic episodes.

His review of systems is notable for recent fatigue. His medications include aspirin, lisinopril, and atorvastatin. For years, his hemoglobin A_{1c} level has been in the range of 6.5% to 6.9% (48-52 mmol/mol), but 4 months ago it was 7.8% (62 mmol/mol) and a recent value was 8.2% (66 mmol/mol).

Laboratory test results:
Hemoglobin = 8.9 g/dL (13.8-17.2 g/dL)
(SI: 89 g/L [13.8-17.2 g/L])
Serum creatinine = 0.8 mg/dL (0.7-1.3 mg/dL)
(SI: 70.7 µmol/L [61.9-114.9 µmol/L])
Liver function, normal
TSH, normal
Urinary albumin-to-creatinine ratio = 205 mg/g creat (<30 mg/g creat)

Which of the following is the most likely cause of this patient's high hemoglobin A_{1c}?

A. Iron deficiency
B. Laboratory error
C. Hemolysis
D. Albuminuria
E. High nighttime blood glucose levels

11 A 65-year-old man with a 20-year history of type 2 diabetes mellitus and hypertension complicated by nephropathy is referred for help achieving better glycemic control. His regimen consists of premixed NPH/regular insulin, 40 units at breakfast and 30 units at dinner. He performs self-monitoring of blood glucose twice daily, with values ranging between 200 and 300 mg/dL (11.1-16.7 mmol/L). His hemoglobin A_{1c} level has been between 8.5% and 10.0% (69-86 mmol/mol). His medications include ramipril, amlodipine, metoprolol, rosuvastatin, and biotin.

Laboratory test results:
Hemoglobin A_{1c} = 9.0% (4.0%-5.6%)
(75 mmol/mol [20-38 mmol/mol])
Serum creatinine = 2.2 mg/dL (0.7-1.3 mg/dL)
(SI: 194.5 µmol/L [61.9-114.9 µmol/L])
Urinary albumin-to-creatinine ratio = 3886 mg/g creat (<30 mg/g creat)
Liver function, normal
TSH = 7.5 mIU/L (0.5-5.0 mIU/L)
Serum fructosamine = 210 µmol/L
(200-285 µmol/L)

The discrepancy between this patient's hemoglobin A_{1c} and fructosamine levels is most likely caused by which of the following?

A. Laboratory error
B. Biotin
C. Hemolysis
D. Hypothyroidism
E. Proteinuria

12 An 18-year-old girl is referred for recent diagnosis of diabetes mellitus. Her father has confirmed type 1 diabetes and wanted her to be screened for diabetes. A hemoglobin A_{1c} measurement was 6.9% (52 mmol/mol) and a fasting glucose value was 91 mg/dL (5.1 mmol/L). Tests for islet-cell antibodies, insulin autoantibodies, and glutamic acid decarboxylase autoantibodies were negative. The patient began a low-carbohydrate diet and has been exercising regularly for 3 months, but her repeated hemoglobin A_{1c} level is now 7.4%

(57 mmol/mol) and many of her postprandial glucose measurements are in the range of 200 to 250 mg/dL (11.1-13.9 mmol/L). She has no symptoms of hyperglycemia.

On physical examination, she has no skin tags or acanthosis nigricans. Her BMI is 23 kg/m².

Which of the following should be ordered next?
   A. Fructosamine measurement
   B. Zinc transporter 8 (ZnT8) antibody testing
   C. Genetic testing for pathogenic variants in the *GCK* gene (glucokinase)
   D. Genetic testing for pathogenic variants in the *HNF1A* gene (hepatocyte nuclear factor-1 alpha)
   E. 1,5-anhydroglucitol measurement

13 A 33-year-old woman with a 20-year history of type 1 diabetes mellitus presents for a follow-up visit. She starts to cry because of major stress due to recent divorce. She reports having intermittent nausea for the last few days. She tells you that she feels unwell and attributes it to stress. She uses insulin pump therapy with insulin aspart at a basal rate of 1.2 units/h, an insulin-to-carbohydrate ratio of 1:15, and a sensitivity factor of 1:40. She has not been doing glucose fingerstick readings at home on a regular basis, but when she does, the values range between 70 and 250 mg/dL (3.9-13.9 mmol/L) without a real pattern. She had declined the use of a continuous glucose sensor in the past. A glucose fingerstick measurement in the office today is 385 mg/dL (21.4 mmol/L).

Laboratory tests from 2 weeks ago show a hemoglobin A_{1c} value of 9.3% (78 mmol/mol) with a normal basic metabolic panel. A pregnancy test is negative.

Which of the following is the best immediate next step?
   A. Basal rate testing
   B. Diabetes education
   C. Assessment for ketones
   D. Initiation of a continuous glucose sensor
   E. Therapy for stress management

14 An 18-year-old boy is referred for management of type 1 diabetes mellitus, which was recently diagnosed during a hospital admission for diabetic ketoacidosis. He is on basal and mealtime insulins. He is currently doing well, with most blood glucose measurements within range. He uses a continuous glucose sensor. He has no symptoms or concerns.

If testing for other autoimmune conditions, which of the following antibodies will this patient most likely have?
   A. Tissue transglutaminase antibodies
   B. Autoantibodies to intrinsic factor
   C. 21-Hydroxylase antibodies
   D. Gliadin antibodies
   E. TPO antibodies

15 A 31-year-old woman has a 16-year history of type 1 diabetes mellitus. She is referred for management of suboptimal glycemic control. She is on basal and mealtime insulins. Her glycemic control was initially acceptable with hemoglobin A_{1c} values around 7.0% (53 mmol/mol), but over the past few years, she has missed appointments and her hemoglobin A_{1c} levels have reached 9.0% to 10.0% (75-86 mmol/mol). She has had 2 episodes of diabetic ketoacidosis in the past 8 months. Recurrent hypoglycemic events have been occurring without a specific pattern. She states she has intentionally lost 8 lb (3.6 kg) over the past year. Her menses are regular on hormonal contraception. She has a strong family history of Graves disease.

Current medications include insulin glargine, insulin lispro, an oral contraceptive, and biotin.

On physical examination, her blood pressure is 110/60 mm Hg and BMI is 19 kg/m². Examination findings are unremarkable.

Laboratory test results:
   Hemoglobin A_{1c} = 9.1% (4.0%-5.6%)
      (76 mmol/mol [20-38 mmol/mol])
   Estimated glomerular filtration rate = 75 mL/min per 1.73 m² (>60 mL/min per 1.73 m²)
   Serum sodium = 141 mEq/L (136-142 mEq/L)
      (SI: 141 mmol/L [3.9-5.5 mmol/L])

Serum potassium = 3.6 mEq/L (3.5-5.0 mEq/L)
   (SI: 3.6 mmol/L [3.5-5.0 mmol/L])
Serum cortisol, not done due to laboratory error
ACTH = 38 pg/mL (10-60 pg/mL)
   (SI: 8.4 pmol/L [2.2-13.2 pmol/L])
TSH = 2.0 mIU/L (0.5-5.0 mIU/L)
Tissue transglutaminase antibodies, negative

Which of the following is the best next step?
   A. Initiate insulin pump therapy
   B. Perform a cosyntropin-stimulation test
   C. Measure TSH again after stopping biotin
      for 5 days
   D. Refer for psychological evaluation

16 A 66-year-old woman is referred for management of type 2 diabetes mellitus. She has been treated with metformin for 4 years. She has dyslipidemia, hypertension, and chronic kidney disease. Her medications are metformin, rosuvastatin, amlodipine, carvedilol, and lisinopril.

On physical examination, her BMI is 29 kg/m^2 and blood pressure is 138/84 mm Hg.

Laboratory test results:
   Hemoglobin A$_{1c}$ = 7.4% (4.0%-5.6%)
      (57 mmol/mol [20-38 mmol/mol])
   Estimated glomerular filtration rate = 53 mL/min
      per 1.73 m^2 (>60 mL/min per 1.73 m^2)

You decide to add linagliptin. You explain that this drug, by increasing GLP-1 levels, will target which of the following pathogenic defects:
   A. Insulin resistance and β-cell dysfunction
   B. Hepatic glucose output and satiety
   C. Renal glucose reabsorption and satiety
   D. Glucagon secretion and insulin resistance
   E. Hepatic glucose output and β-cell dysfunction

17 A 72-year-old woman has a 22-year history of type 2 diabetes mellitus. She also has hypertension and chronic kidney disease. She is referred for suboptimal glycemic control with hemoglobin A$_{1c}$ values ranging between 8.5% and 10.0% (69-86 mmol/mol). She is taking 58 units of insulin glargine U100 twice daily and 42 units of insulin lispro U100 3 times

daily with meals. She misses 1 to 2 of her insulin doses every week. Her other medications are oral semaglutide, 14 mg daily; pravastatin; enalapril; metoprolol; hydrochlorothiazide; pantoprazole; and escitalopram.

On physical examination, her blood pressure is 142/90 mm Hg. Her BMI is 38 kg/m^2. She has a 2/6 systolic ejection murmur and 2+ edema in her lower extremities.

Laboratory test results:
   Hemoglobin A$_{1c}$ = 9.0% (4.0%-5.6%) (75 mmol/mol
      [20-38 mmol/mol])
   Estimated glomerular filtration rate = 48 mL/min
      per 1.73 m^2 (>60 mL/min per 1.73 m^2)
   Urine albumin-to-creatinine ratio = 154 mg/g creat
      (<30 mg/g creat)

Which of the following is the best next step in this patient's glycemic management?
   A. Switch insulin glargine to insulin degludec
   B. Increase each of her insulin doses by 20%
   C. Add ertugliflozin
   D. Switch insulin glargine and lispro to U500
      regular insulin
   E. Add dulaglutide

18 An 82-year-old woman with a 6-year history of type 2 diabetes mellitus is referred for recurrent hypoglycemic events. She has not been able to tolerate metformin, SGLT-2 inhibitors, or GLP-1 receptor agonists. Her current diabetes treatment regimen consists of insulin degludec, 50 units at bedtime; alogliptin, 25 mg daily; and nateglinide, 120 mg before meals. She measures her blood glucose 3 times daily. Over the past few weeks, she has documented several blood glucose values less than 50 mg/dL (<2.8 mmol/L) before and after meals, but she has not felt any symptoms of hypoglycemia. Her hemoglobin A$_{1c}$ level is 6.2% (44 mmol/mol).

Blood chemistries, urinalysis, and liver function tests are within normal limits.

Which of the following is the best next step in this patient's care?

Answer	Insulin degludec	Nateglinide	Alogliptin
A.	Decrease to 40 units at bedtime	Continue	Discontinue
B.	Decrease to 40 units at bedtime	Discontinue	Continue
C.	Replace with 50 units of insulin detemir	Discontinue	Discontinue
D.	Replace with 25 units of twice-daily NPH insulin	Discontinue	Continue

19 A 68-year-old man with a 22-year history of type 2 diabetes mellitus is admitted to the hospital with severe hyperglycemia and change in mental status. The patient lives alone and was found by his neighbor in a confused state.

On physical examination, the patient is lethargic and unable to answer any questions. His temperature is 100.5°F (38.1°C), blood pressure is 100/60 mm Hg, and pulse rate is 130 beats/min. His weight is 220 lb (100 kg), and BMI is 32 kg/m². Skin and mucous membranes are dry. There is no focal neurologic deficit.

Laboratory test results:
Hemoglobin A_{1c} = 10.5% (4.0%-5.6%)
(91 mmol/mol [20-38 mmol/mol])
Plasma glucose = 1300 mg/dL (70-99 mg/dL)
(SI: 72.2 mmol/L [3.9-5.5 mmol/L])
Serum sodium = 126 mEq/L (136-142 mEq/L)
(SI: 126 mmol/L [136-142 mmol/L])
Serum potassium = 4.5 mEq/L (3.5-5.0 mEq/L)
(SI: 4.5 mmol/L [3.5-5.0 mmol/L])
Serum bicarbonate = 21 mEq/L (21-28 mEq/L)
(SI: 21 mmol/L [21-28 mmol/L])
Serum chloride = 106 mEq/L (96-106 mEq/L)
(SI: 106 mmol/L [96-106 mmol/L])
Serum creatinine = 1.9 mg/dL (0.7-1.3 mg/dL)
(SI: 168.0 μmol/L [61.9-114.9 μmol/L])
Arterial pH = 7.35 (7.35-7.45)
Serum β-hydroxybutyrate = 2.6 mg/dL
(<3.0 mg/dL) (SI: 249.8 μmol/L [<288.2 μmol/L])

Effective serum osmolality = 324 mOsm/kg
(275-295 mOsm/kg) (SI: 324 mmol/kg
[275-295 mmol/kg])

Which of the following is the best next step?

Answer	Fluids over the first hour	Intravenous insulin
A.	1.5 L of 0.9% NaCl	Bolus of 10 units, then 10 units per h
B.	1.5 L of 0.9% NaCl	Bolus of 4 units, then 2 units per h
C.	1.5 L of 0.45% NaCl	Bolus of 10 units, then 10 units per h
D.	1.5 L of 0.45% NaCl	10 units per h
E.	1.5 L of 3.0% NaCl	Bolus of 10 units, then 10 units per h

20 A 64-year-old cardiologist is self-referred for diabetes management. He has had type 2 diabetes mellitus for 3 years and takes metformin, 2000 mg daily. His medical history includes hypertension, dyslipidemia, myocardial infarction, and ischemic stroke. In addition to metformin, current medications are benazepril, rosuvastatin, metoprolol, amlodipine, and aspirin.

On physical examination, his blood pressure is 132/84 mm Hg and BMI is 33 kg/m². He has a soft systolic ejection murmur and weak pedal pulses. There are no focal neurologic deficits.

Laboratory test results:
Hemoglobin A_{1c} = 8.2% (4.0%-5.6%) (66 mmol/mol [20-38 mmol/mol])
Estimated glomerular filtration rate = 66 mL/min per 1.73 m² (>60 mL/min per 1.73 m²)
Liver function, normal
TSH, normal
Urine albumin-to-creatinine ratio = 35 mg/g creat (<30 mg/g creat)

Which of the following agents should be added next?
  A. Sitagliptin
  B. Glimepiride
  C. Insulin glargine
  D. Liraglutide
  E. Repaglinide

21 A 48-year-old man with longstanding type 1 diabetes mellitus and peripheral neuropathy presents for a follow-up visit. He has had a right plantar ulcer in the past. His hemoglobin A_{1c} level is 7.6% (60 mmol/mol). On foot examination, he has absent sensation to 10-g monofilament, absent ankle reflexes, callus formation on the plantar aspect of the second and third metatarsal heads, and absent pedal pulses.

Which of the following is the strongest predictor of the development of future foot ulcers in this patient?
  A. History of previous ulceration
  B. Absent pedal pulses
  C. Absent ankle reflexes
  D. Abnormal monofilament testing
  E. Callus formation

22 A 45-year-old woman has a skin lesion on her left lower extremity (*see image*). A similar but smaller lesion is also present on her right lower extremity.

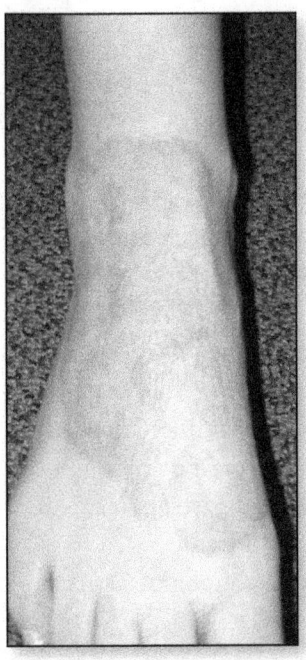

Biopsy shows an inflammatory granulomatous dermatitis with collagen degeneration and fat deposition.

Which of the following diagnoses does this patient most likely have?
  A. Diabetes mellitus
  B. Graves disease
  C. Glucagonoma
  D. Pseudohypoparathyroidism
  E. Familial hypercholesterolemia

23 A 32-year-old Asian American man presents to his primary care physician for an annual visit. He feels well and has no concerns. He has no known medical conditions. He does not take any medications. He has no known family history of diabetes mellitus and does not smoke cigarettes or drink alcohol.

On physical examination, his blood pressure is 120/70 mm Hg and BMI is 24 kg/m². The rest of his examination findings are unremarkable.

In addition to lifestyle management counseling regarding diet and physical activity, when should screening be performed with respect to his prediabetes/diabetes risk?
  A. Now
  B. At age 45 years
  C. When symptomatic
  D. At age 45 years if BMI is greater than 25 kg/m²
  E. Only if BMI is greater than 25 kg/m²

24 A 52-year-old man presents for evaluation of hypoglycemia. He has been having frequent hyperadrenergic symptoms over the last 6 months with a recent episode of confusion. Two weeks ago, he was taken to the emergency department following a syncopal event during which his blood glucose concentration was documented to be 39 mg/dL (2.2 mmol/L). The neuroglycopenic episodes can occur when fasting or during the day, and his symptoms always improve with carbohydrate intake. He has gained 18 lb (8.2 kg) over the past 6 months.

He does not use illicit drugs or drink alcohol. He is on pravastatin, pantoprazole, amlodipine, metoprolol, aspirin, biotin, cinnamon, chromium, and vitamin He is married but is in the process of divorcing and has been significantly stressed.

On physical examination, his BMI is 31 kg/m². He has no other notable features.

Laboratory results during the emergency department visit 2 weeks ago:
Plasma glucose = 40 mg/dL (70-99 mg/dL) (SI: 2.2 mmol/L [3.9-5.5 mmol/L])
Plasma insulin = 28 µIU/mL (1.4-14.0 µIU/mL) (SI: 194.5 pmol/L [9.7-97.2 pmol/L])
Plasma C-peptide = 3.0 ng/mL (0.5-2.0 ng/mL) (SI: 0.99 nmol/L [0.17-0.66 nmol/L])
TSH = 1.2 mIU/L (0.5-5.0 mIU/L)
Plasma proinsulin = 88.1 pg/mL (26.5-176.4 pg/mL) (SI: 10.0 pmol/L [3.0-20.0 pmol/L])
Plasma β-hydroxybutyrate = 1.2 mmol/L
Insulin antibodies, negative
Estimated glomerular filtration rate = 85 mL/min per 1.73 m² (>60 mL/min per 1.73 m²)

On the basis of this patient's history and test results, which of the following is the best next management step?
A. Abdominal CT
B. Sulfonylurea screen
C. Cosyntropin-stimulation test
D. Standard supervised 72-hour fast
E. IGF-2 measurement

25 An 18-year-old man presents for continued management of diabetes mellitus. Diabetes was diagnosed at age 16 years when glycosuria and a hemoglobin A$_{1c}$ level of 6.9% (52 mmol/mol) were documented on a yearly checkup. Insulin therapy was started immediately. His current insulin dose is approximately 0.3 units/kg per day, administered as basal and mealtime insulins, and his current hemoglobin A$_{1c}$ level is 6.2% (44 mmol/mol) with occasional hypoglycemia. His family history is positive for diabetes in his mother, maternal grandfather, and an older sibling, all diagnosed at age 22 years or younger. His BMI is 23 kg/m².

Tests for glutamic acid decarboxylase antibodies, islet-cell antibodies, insulinoma-associated protein 2 antibodies, and zinc transporter 8 antibodies are negative. He did not have antibody testing at the time of diagnosis. His serum C-peptide concentration is 1.1 ng/mL (0.36 nmol/L).

Which of the following is the optimal management of this patient's diabetes?
A. Insulin administration via insulin pump therapy
B. Discontinuation of insulin and initiation of dapagliflozin
C. Discontinuation of insulin and initiation of glimepiride
D. Discontinuation of insulin and initiation of metformin
E. Continuation of current insulin regimen

26 A 25-year-old woman with a 15-year history of type 1 diabetes mellitus is considering an isolated pancreas transplant. Her blood glucose values have been very erratic and labile. Her hemoglobin A$_{1c}$ level has ranged from 8.0% to 10.0% (64 to 86 mmol/mol), and she has hypoglycemic unawareness despite being on a sensor-augmented insulin pump. She has nephropathy, proliferative retinopathy, gastroparesis, and peripheral neuropathy.

Laboratory test results:
Hemoglobin A$_{1c}$ = 8.8% (4.0%-5.6%) (73 mmol/mol [20-38 mmol/mol])
Creatinine = 1.3 mg/dL (0.6-1.1 mg/dL) (SI: 114.9 µmol/L [53.0-97.2 µmol/L])
Urinary albumin-to-creatinine ratio = 345 mg/g creat (<30 mg/g creat)

Which of the following outcomes can this patient expect within 5 years after a successful pancreas transplant?
A. Regression of retinopathy
B. Recovery of peripheral sensation
C. Regression of gastroparesis
D. Reduced albuminuria
E. Reduced likelihood of future pregnancies

27 A 58-year-old man with type 2 diabetes mellitus presents for a routine follow-up visit and is accompanied by his wife. His medical history is notable for hypertension, dyslipidemia, and fatty liver. His main concern is fatigue, which he has been experiencing for the past few months. One of his friends told him he should have testing for "adrenal fatigue." He has erectile dysfunction despite normal libido. His medications include metformin, sitagliptin, rosuvastatin, ramipril, and baby aspirin. He does not smoke cigarettes or drink alcohol.

On physical examination, his BMI is 42 kg/m² and blood pressure is 120/60 mm Hg.

Laboratory test results:
Hemoglobin A_{1c} = 7.2% (4.0%-5.6%)
  (55 mmol/mol [20-38 mmol/mol])
Hemoglobin = 17.1 g/dL (13.8-17.2 g/dL)
  (SI: 171 g/L [138-172 g/L])
Serum sodium = 141 mEq/L (136-142 mEq/L)
  (SI: 141 mmol/L [3.9-5.5 mmol/L])
Serum potassium = 4.0 mEq/L (3.5-5.0 mEq/L)
  (SI: 4.0 mmol/L [3.5-5.0 mmol/L])
Serum creatinine = 0.6 mg/dL (0.7-1.3 mg/dL)
  (SI: 53.0 μmol/L [61.9-114.9 μmol/L])
TSH = 3.8 mIU/L (0.5-5.0 mIU/L)
Serum cortisol (8 AM) = 12 μg/dL (5-25 μg/dL)
  (SI: 331.1 nmol/L [137.9-689.7 nmol/L])
Total testosterone = 250 ng/dL (300-900 ng/dL)
  (SI: 8.7 nmol/L [10.4-31.2 nmol/L])
LH = 4.0 mIU/mL (1.0-9.0 mIU/mL) (SI: 4.0 IU/L
  [1.0-9.0 IU/L])
FSH = 9.0 mIU/mL (1.0-13.0 mIU/mL) (SI: 9.0
  IU/L [1.0-13.0 IU/L])

Which of the following assessments should be ordered next?
  A. Polysomnography
  B. Pituitary MRI
  C. Serum prolactin measurement
  D. Cosyntropin-stimulation test
  E. Free T_4 measurement

28 A 61-year-old woman with an 8-year history of type 2 diabetes mellitus returns for a follow-up visit. She also has hypertension, dyslipidemia, and migraines. Her blood glucose is well controlled on basal and mealtime insulins, and she checks her blood glucose 6 to 8 times daily. Her blood glucose values are at goal, and her most recent hemoglobin A_{1c} value is 7.0% (53 mmol/mol). Her BMI is 29 kg/m².

Her current medications are insulin degludec, 30 units at bedtime; insulin lispro, 1 unit/8 g of carbohydrate; metformin, 2000 mg daily; atorvastatin, 40 mg daily; ramipril, 10 mg daily; cinnamon, 2000 mg daily; vitamin C, 1000 mg daily; chromium, 1 mg daily; and occasionally acetaminophen.

You prescribe the flash glucose monitoring system. The patient wears the new sensor on her arm. The next day, she sees an unusual reading of 350 mg/dL (19.4 mmol/L) on her sensor; a concomitant blood glucose fingerstick value is 110 mg/dL (6.1 mmol/L). The same discrepancy keeps happening for the next few days. The patient calls the clinic for guidance.

Which of the following is the best recommendation?
  A. Adjust the insulin based on the sensor data, as blood glucose fingerstick measurements are inaccurate
  B. Change the site of the sensor from the arm to the abdomen
  C. Stop cinnamon, as it can interfere with sensor glucose readings
  D. Stop acetaminophen, as it can interfere with sensor glucose readings
  E. Stop vitamin C, as it can interfere with sensor glucose readings

Diabetes Mellitus, Section 2 Board Review

Marie E. McDonnell, MD

29 A 77-year-old man with suboptimally controlled type 2 diabetes mellitus and a history of mild cognitive impairment is accompanied to his visit by his daughter. His home regimen includes insulin glargine, 100 units administered at bedtime; insulin lispro, 15 units administered before meals; and metformin, 1000 mg twice daily. Additional medications include lisinopril, amlodipine, and atorvastatin.

On physical examination, he is alert. Mucous membranes are somewhat dry. His weight is 180.4 lb (82 kg). His blood pressure is 168/88 mm Hg. Examination findings are unremarkable.

Laboratory test results:
Estimated glomerular filtration rate = 52 mL/min per 1.73 m^2 (>60 mL/min per 1.73 m^2)
Hemoglobin A$_{1c}$ = 9.8% (4.0%-5.6%) (84 mmol/mol [20-38 mmol/mol])

He brings his glucose meter, which has only 10 values in the last 3 months. The only time he checks his blood glucose is when his daughter helps him on the mornings when she is able to visit. All values from the glucose meter are between 80 and 130 mg/dL (4.4-7.2 mmol/L), and his daughter is not aware of hypoglycemia detected in the last 3 months. Professional continuous glucose monitoring is performed, and you review the ambulatory glucose profile (*see image*).

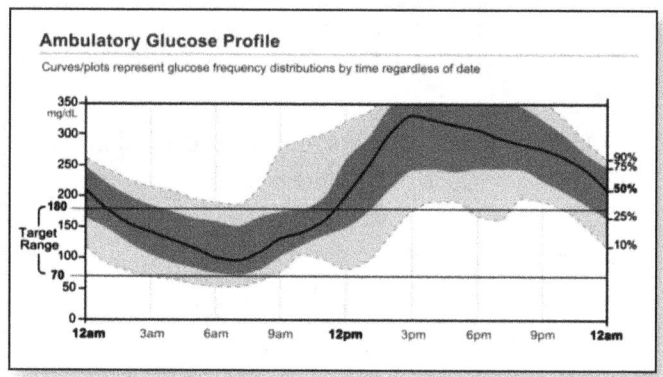

Which of the following is the correct interpretation of these data?

  A. The mean glucose value is 180 mg/dL (10.0 mmol/L) and the lowest measured glucose value is 50 mg/dL (2.8 mmol/L)

  B. Approximately 10% of glucose values at 6 AM are below 50 mg/dL (<2.8 mmol/L)

  C. The time-in-range is 25%

  D. Approximately 25% of the glucose values at 6 PM are above 250 mg/dL (>13.9 mmol/L)

  E. No hypoglycemic events (glucose <70 mg/dL [<3.9 mmol/L]) occur at 12 PM

30 A 69-year-old veterinarian presents for an urgent consult with a written report from an emergency department visit 2 weeks ago. She had a witnessed tonic-clonic seizure, and her plasma glucose measured by emergency medical services was 34 mg/dL (1.9 mmol/L). Following treatment with intravenous dextrose, her condition improved quickly. After transport to the emergency department, she declined hospitalization.

Other laboratory tests performed in the emergency department:

White blood cell count = 9000/μL
(4500-11,000/μL) (SI: 9.0 × 10⁹/L
[4.5-11.0 × 10⁹/L])
Hemoglobin = 10 g/dL (13.8-17.2 g/dL)
(SI: 100 g/dL [138-172 g/L])
Sodium = 132 mEq/L (136-142 mEq/L)
(SI: 132 mmol/L [136-142 mmol/L])
Potassium = 3.4 mEq/L (3.5-5.0 mEq/L)
(SI: 3.4 mmol/L [3.5-5.0 mmol/L])
Bicarbonate = 24 mEq/L (21-28 mEq/L)
(SI: 24 mmol/L [21-28 mmol/L])
Chloride = 101 mEq/L (96-106 mEq/L)
(SI: 101 mmol/L [96-106 mmol/L])

She reports unintentional weight loss of 8 lb (3.6 kg) in the past 2 months and a feeling of general malaise, prompting her to resign from her job 1 month ago. She has had 2 to 3 episodes of spontaneous diaphoresis resolved with sweet foods such as chocolate.

On physical examination, her blood pressure is 128/72 mm Hg without orthostasis, and her pulse rate is 102 beats/min. Examination findings are otherwise unremarkable.

Shes agrees to be admitted to the hospital for a supervised fast. At hour 19, she reports perioral numbness, and her point-of-care glucose measurement is 42 mg/dL (2.3 mmol/L). The fast is terminated. Intravenous glucagon, 1 mg, is administered and the measured plasma glucose 30 minutes later is 76 mg/dL (4.2 mmol/L).

The following laboratory values are obtained before glucagon administration and treating her with oral glucose:

Plasma glucose = 36 mg/dL (70-99 mg/dL)
(SI: 2.0 mmol/L [3.9-5.5 mmol/L])
Insulin = 1.2 μIU/mL (1.4-14.0 μIU/mL)
(SI: 8.3 pmol/L [9.7-97.2 pmol/L])
C-peptide = 0.1 ng/mL (0.5-2.0 ng/mL)
(SI: 0.03 nmol/L [0.17-0.66 nmol/L])
Proinsulin = 10.6 pg/mL (26.5-176.4 pg/mL)
(SI: 1.2 pmol/L [3.0-20.0 pmol/L])
β-Hydroxybutyrate = 2.2 mg/dL (<3.0 mg/dL)
(SI: 211.3 μmol/L [<288.2 μmol/L])

Sulfonylurea panel (plasma), negative
Insulin antibodies, negative
Insulin analogues, not measured

Which of the following is most likely to confirm the diagnosis?

A. Request ACTH and cortisol measurement from the drawn tube saved in the laboratory
B. Perform CT of the chest, abdomen, and pelvis
C. Measure IGF-1
D. Seek permission to search the patient's room and personal belongings for insulin
E. Perform abdominal ultrasonography

31 A 43-year-old previously healthy man presents with a history of multiple episodes of documented hypoglycemia responsive to orange juice. He reports that none of these episodes required assistance from another person to self-administer glucose, but he has now learned to carry candy or juice boxes when he is outside his home in order to avoid feeling unwell. He reports a 12-lb (5.5-kg) weight gain over the last 6 months and attributes that to waking overnight in response to hunger and eating snacks. As instructed, he returns to your office after an 8-hour fast performed at home. Upon arrival, his point-of-care glucose is 64 mg/dL (3.6 mmol/L). After an additional 45 minutes of supervised fasting, he reports feeling extreme fatigue and diaphoresis. A point-of-care glucose measurement is 34 mg/dL (1.9 mmol/L). A laboratory panel is immediately obtained before treating him with glucose tablets:

Plasma glucose = 46 mg/dL (70-99 mg/dL)
(SI: 2.6 mmol/L [3.9-5.5 mmol/L])
Insulin = 22.7 μIU/mL (1.4-14.0 μIU/mL)
(SI: 157.7 pmol/L [9.7-97.2 pmol/L])
C-peptide = 6.2 ng/mL (0.5-2.0 ng/mL)
(SI: 2.05 nmol/L [0.17-0.66 nmol/L])
Proinsulin = 599.6 pg/mL (26.5-176.4 pg/mL)
(SI: 68 pmol/L [3.0-20.0 pmol/L])
β-Hydroxybutyrate = 1.2 mg/dL (<3.0 mg/dL)
(SI: 115.3 μmol/L [<288.2 μmol/L])
Sulfonylurea panel (plasma), negative
Insulin antibodies, negative

Which of the following is this patient's most likely diagnosis?

    A. Hirata disease

    B. Insulinoma

    C. Adrenal insufficiency

    D. Factitious insulin administration

    E. Noninsulinoma pancreatogenous hypoglycemia syndrome

32 A 24-year-old woman who has had type 1 diabetes mellitus for 12 years seeks help with glycemic control in preparation for pregnancy. She has used a "pod" insulin pump for 8 years and has used a continuous glucose monitoring device for 4 years that is not integrated with her pump. She monitors her blood glucose by fingerstick on average twice daily. She reports significant stress at work, and her primary care physician recently prescribed medication for anxiety and depression.

Her current pump settings include a basal rate of 1.1 unit/h 24 hours a day, a correction factor of 1:15, and an insulin-to-carbohydrate ratio of 1:8. Per the downloaded pump report, she receives on average 26 units of basal insulin and 14 units of bolus insulin. She reports missing boluses on work days, as she has difficulty waking up on time and is often late.

Her current hemoglobin A_{1c} value is 7.4% (57 mmol/mol).

On physical examination, her weight is 163 lb (74 kg). She has an area of lipohypertrophy to the right of the umbilicus.

Her pump data are downloaded. She delays a pod change at least once per month, resulting in marked hyperglycemia for several hours. She has a glucose pattern (*see image*) that recurs in a similar fashion most weekends.

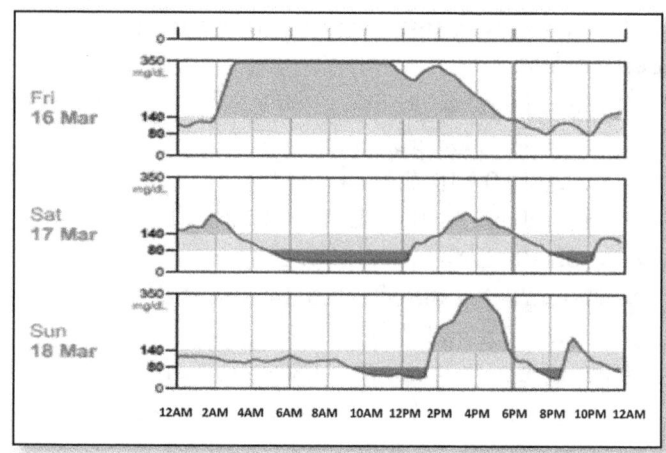

In addition to inquiring about her sleep and exercise habits on the weekends, asking about which of the following is most likely to explain her presentation?

    A. Inquire if she uses her pump's internal dosing tool to arrive at correction doses

    B. Determine if she changes her continuous glucose monitoring sensor routinely on Friday evenings

    C. Inquire about acetaminophen intake

    D. Inquire about alcohol intake at the end of the work week

    E. Determine if she is more likely to bolus before meals on the weekends than during the week

33 A 72-year-old woman seeks advice for hyperglycemia management to help her remain in a cancer clinical trial. Metastatic breast cancer was initially diagnosed at age 66 years. One month ago, she started a new chemotherapy medication and within 2 days she reported nausea, polyuria, and polydipsia with glucose values between 250 and 450 mg/dL (13.9-25.0 mmol/L). Her primary care physician prescribed intermittent insulin lispro per a "sliding scale." One day after self-administering 50 units of insulin lispro, her fasting glucose concentration was 280 mg/dL (15.5 mmol/L). The chemotherapeutic drug was discontinued, and 3 days later her fasting glucose concentration measured on her glucose meter was 122 mg/dL (6.8 mmol/L).

Type 2 diabetes mellitus was diagnosed 2 years ago based on a hemoglobin A_{1c} value of 6.8% (51 mmol/mol). However, after losing nearly 60 lb (27.3 kg) in the setting of cancer, her most recent hemoglobin A_{1c} level prior to recent chemotherapy was 5.7% (39 mmol/mol). She was not taking any antidiabetes medications before her cancer diagnosis. Other laboratory data include a recent estimated glomerular filtration rate of 64 mL/min per 1.73 m².

Which of the following chemotherapeutic drug classes most likely explains her presentation?
 A. PD-1 inhibitor
 B. mTOR inhibitor
 C. PI3 kinase inhibitor
 D. CTLA-4 inhibitor
 E. Platinum-based antineoplastic

34 A 28-year-old woman with a 10-year history of type 1 diabetes mellitus is referred by her nephrologist for better glycemic control in the setting of progressive decline in kidney function. Type 1 diabetes was initially diagnosed after glucose was identified in her urine during an evaluation for urinary tract infection. She does not recall if antibody testing was performed. She is not aware of other family members with diabetes and reports her mother was adopted. Her only sibling died shortly after birth due to renal agenesis.

After diagnosis, her diabetes was managed with basal insulin (without nutritional insulin) for 2 years. She recalls sometimes missing doses for more than a week when in college. Over the subsequent 6 years, her diabetes progressed and she eventually required meal-time insulin. She is currently on insulin pump therapy (total insulin dose = 0.2 units/kg per day). She has never had episodes of ketoacidosis or marked hyperglycemia.

On physical examination, her BMI is 24 kg/m². Her blood pressure is 129/78 mm Hg, and pulse rate is 88 beats/min. Her insulin pump site is intact. She has no symptoms or signs of neuropathy. Findings on recent retinal examination are normal without retinopathy.

Her hemoglobin A$_{1c}$ level is 7.3% (56 mmol/mol). Five years ago, her glomerular filtration rate was greater than 60 mL/min per 1.73 m², but it is now 26 mL/min per 1.73 m². On renal ultrasonography, both kidneys are severely hypoplastic. Her nephrologist has discussed the possibility of a future kidney/pancreas transplant.

Which of the following is the most likely etiology of her diabetes?
 A. Pathogenic variant in the *HNF1B* gene
 B. Pathogenic variant in the *GCK* gene
 C. Pancreatic divisum
 D. Type 1 diabetes
 E. Antibodies to the insulin receptor

35 A 20-year-old college student with a history of depression and attention deficit–hyperactivity disorder presents with his parents to discuss a recent diagnosis of prediabetes. At a visit with his primary care physician 2 weeks ago, he described fatigue, 7-lb (3.2-kg) weight loss in 3 months, lightheadedness, and difficulty getting out of bed for classes. He failed 2 classes in the last semester. His primary care physician prescribed escitalopram, 10 mg daily, and advised that the patient use his as-needed amphetamine more frequently to help him perform better in school.

Laboratory test results:
 TSH = 4.6 mIU/L (0.5-5.0 mIU/L)
 Hemoglobin A$_{1c}$ = 6.2% (4.0%-5.6%) (44 mmol/mol [20-38 mmol/mol])
 Sodium = 133 mEq/L (136-142 mEq/L) (SI: 133 mmol/L [136-142 mmol/L])
 Potassium = 5.6 mEq/L (3.5-5.0 mEq/L) (SI: 5.6 mmol/L [3.5-5.0 mmol/L])
 Bicarbonate = 20 mEq/L (21-28 mEq/L) (SI: 20 mmol/L [21-28 mmol/L])
 Random glucose = 166 mg/dL (SI: 9.2 mmol/L)
 Hematocrit = 42% (41%-51%) (SI: 0.42 [0.41-0.51])

On physical examination, he appears fatigued and prefers to lie down. His BMI is 25 kg/m². Mucous membranes are dry. While lying down, his blood pressure is 118/68 mm Hg, and pulse rate is 78 beats/min. After 1 minute of standing, his blood pressure is 90/58 mm Hg, and pulse rate is 92 beats/min.

Which of the following is the best immediate next step?
A. Measure tissue transglutaminase antibodies
B. Encourage fluid intake and repeat hemoglobin A_{1c} measurement in 3 months
C. Perform a cosyntropin-stimulation test
D. Measure TPO antibodies
E. Discontinue amphetamine

36 A 62-year-old man with a 25-year history of type 1 diabetes mellitus presents for urgent consultation. He reports waking up with pain and tingling occurring on the lateral aspect of his left thigh 3 days ago.

He has never felt this before and wonders if it is related to occasional insulin injections in that area of his leg. He otherwise feels well and has no difficulty walking or climbing stairs. He has a history of transient ischemic attack and myocardial infarction. Blood pressure and lipids are well controlled.

On physical examination, his blood pressure is 128/78 mm Hg, pulse rate is 82 beats/min, and BMI is 24 kg/m². He is alert and oriented. Findings on cranial nerve examination are normal. The painful area is nontender, and the skin is smooth and intact without eruption or rash. Neurologic examination findings are consistent with those of a recent visit indicating polyneuropathy, with poor vibration sensation in the fingertips and below the ankles. Vascular examination of the lower extremities reveals normal skin tone and peripheral pulses without notable edema or tenderness.

Which of the following is the best next step in this patient's management?
A. Provide reassurance
B. Start acyclovir
C. Perform a nerve conduction study
D. Perform Doppler ultrasonography
E. Perform MRI

37 A 28-year-old man presents for follow-up of newly diagnosed diabetes. One month ago, he presented to the hospital with 3 days of fever, mild headache, sore throat, dry cough, and polyuria and polydipsia. He was found to have a glucose concentration of 360 mg/dL (20.0 mmol/L) and diabetes was diagnosed. He was discharged on 0.15 units/kg of insulin glargine and metformin, 500 mg twice daily. He reports feeling overwhelmed and confused by the diagnosis of diabetes, as his primary physician told him that a recent screening test was normal. He missed a follow-up appointment and performed a few fingerstick blood glucose tests in the fasting state, which have ranged between 140 and 190 mg/dL (7.8-10.5 mmol/L).

Family history reveals that his mother had type 2 diabetes diagnosed in her 30s.

On physical examination, his blood pressure is 120/80 mm Hg, pulse rate is 80 beats/min, and BMI is 30 kg/m².

Laboratory test results:
Random plasma glucose = 230 mg/dL (SI: 12.8 mmol/L)
Creatinine = 0.8 mg/dL (0.7-1.3 mg/dL) (SI: 70.7 μmol/L [61.9-114.9 μmol/L])
Urinary albumin-to-creatinine ratio = 15 mg/g creat (<30 mg/g creat)
Urine ketones, negative
White blood cell count = 8200 μL (4500-11,000/μL) (SI: 8.2 × 10⁹/L [4.5-11.0 × 10⁹/L])
Hematocrit = 28% (41%-51%) (SI: 0.28 [0.41-0.51])
Hemoglobin = 9.2 g/dL (13.8-17.2 g/dL) (SI: 92 g/dL [138-172 g/L])
Hemoglobin A_{1c} = 4.2% (4.0%-5.6%) (22 mmol/mol [20-38 mmol/mol])
AST = 95 U/L (20-48 U/L) (SI: 1.59 μkat/L [0.33-0.80 μkat/L])
ALT = 45 U/L (10-40 U/L) (SI: 0.75 μkat/L [0.17-0.67 μkat/L])

Which of the following is the best next step in this patient's management?

A. Discontinue insulin, continue metformin, and follow-up in 3 months
B. Measure fructosamine
C. Discontinue both insulin and metformin
D. Measure C-peptide
E. Recommend genetic testing for monogenic diabetes

38 A patient with longstanding type 1 diabetes mellitus reports that he is considering enrolling in a study to receive cadaveric islet-cell transplant.

Which of the following is the most likely outcome 1 year after islet-cell transplant?

A. Elimination of insulin injections
B. Reduced occurrence of severe hypoglycemia events
C. Normalization of hemoglobin A_{1c}
D. Reduced quality of life

39 A 74-year-old Black woman inquires about her risk of developing diabetes. She has mostly been in good health. She lives independently, enjoys taking long walks, cooks for herself, and has no difficulty managing activities of daily living. Her medical history includes hypertension, which was diagnosed in her 50s and has been recently well controlled. She has a strong family history of type 2 diabetes and hypertension.

Medications include lisinopril, 20 mg once daily, and vitamin D, 2000 IU once daily.

On physical examination, her blood pressure is 142/82 mm Hg and BMI is 27.4 kg/m².

Laboratory test results:
Plasma glucose (fasting) = 112 mg/dL
(70-99 mg/dL) (SI: 6.2 mmol/L
[3.9-5.5 mmol/L])
LDL cholesterol = 142 mg/dL (<100 mg/dL)
(SI: 3.68 mmol/L [<2.59 mmol/L])
HDL cholesterol = 32 mg/dL (>60 mg/dL)
(SI: 0.83 mmol/L [>1.55 mmol/L])
Triglycerides = 196 mg/dL (<150 mg/dL)
(SI: 2.21 mmol/L [<1.70 mmol/L])

Which of the following is the best next test to determine whether this patient has diabetes?

A. Hemoglobin A_{1c} measurement
B. 2-Hour 75-g oral glucose tolerance test
C. Fructosamine measurement
D. 2-Hour postprandial fingerstick glucose measurement

40 A 39-year-old man is referred for evaluation after a fingerstick blood glucose measurement at a health screening fair was documented to be 178 mg/dL (9.9 mmol/L). He had recently eaten lunch. His medical history is notable for dyslipidemia that is well controlled on simvastatin, gout, and obesity.

On physical examination, his blood pressure is 132/78 mm Hg and BMI is 41.5 kg/m². Acanthosis nigricans is present, but there are no other notable findings on physical examination.

You reassess his glycemic status:
Fasting plasma glucose (laboratory) = 119 mg/dL
(70-99 mg/dL) (SI: 6.6 mmol/L
[3.9-5.5 mmol/L])
Hemoglobin A_{1c} = 6.6% (4.0%-5.6%) (49 mmol/mol
[20-38 mmol/mol])

Repeated sampling 1 week later:
Fasting plasma glucose = 107 mg/dL
(SI: 5.9 mmol/L)
Hemoglobin A_{1c} = 6.8% (51 mmol/mol)

Which of the following is this patient's most likely diagnosis?

A. Prediabetes
B. Impaired glucose tolerance
C. Impaired fasting glucose
D. Type 2 diabetes mellitus

41 An 82-year-old woman with a 22-year history of type 2 diabetes mellitus and hypertension is referred for glycemic management following an emergency department visit for severe hypoglycemia with loss of consciousness. Emergency medical technicians report that her initial blood glucose value was 34 mg/dL (1.9 mmol/L).

Her current home diabetes treatment regimen consists of 25 units of insulin detemir at bedtime, 9 units of rapid-acting insulin with meals, and correction doses for blood glucose values greater than 180 mg/dL (>10.0 mmol/L). She does not record the insulin doses taken. She would like to review how and when to take correction insulin doses.

Her home blood glucose measurements are as follows (*see table*).

On physical examination, her BMI is 19 kg/m² and blood pressure is 142/78 mm Hg. She has markedly reduced sensation in both feet. Her mood and affect are normal, and her memory appears to be sharp.

Laboratory test results:
Hemoglobin A_{1c} = 8.7% (4.0%-5.6%)
(72 mmol/mol [20-38 mmol/mol])
(estimated average glucose value 203 mg/dL [SI: 11.3 mmol/L])
Estimated glomerular filtration rate = 52 mL/min per 1.73 m² (<60 mL/min per 1.73 m²)
C-peptide = 3.6 ng/mL (0.9-4.3 ng/mL)
(SI: 1.2 nmol/L [0.30-1.42 nmol/L])

Which of the following would you recommend to reduce the risk for further episodes of severe hypoglycemia in this older woman?

A. Refer to a diabetes educator to help her better understand how to take her insulins
B. Reduce basal insulin to 20 units and keep meal boluses at 9 units
C. Reduce basal insulin to 20 units, stop the mealtime insulin, and start linagliptin
D. Stop the basal and meal insulins and start repaglinide with meals

42 A 29-year-old woman with a 6-year history of type 1 diabetes mellitus without microvascular complications is referred to establish care. She has no diabetes-related complications and is not planning pregnancy. Her treatment regimen consists of insulins degludec and aspart. She takes an oral contraceptive. She exercises regularly. There is no family history of heart disease.

On physical examination, her blood pressure is 120/70 mm Hg and BMI is 27 kg/m².

Laboratory test results (nonfasting):
Glucose = 192 mg/dL (SI: 10.7 mmol/L)
Hemoglobin A_{1c} = 6.9% (4.0%-5.6%)
(52 mmol/mol [20-38 mmol/mol])
Total cholesterol = 206 mg/dL (<200 mg/dL)
(SI: 5.34 mmol/L [<5.18 mmol/L])
LDL cholesterol = 126 mg/dL (<100 mg/dL)
(SI: 3.26 mmol/L [<2.59 mmol/L])
HDL cholesterol = 40 mg/dL (>60 mg/dL)
(SI: 1.04 mmol/L [>1.55 mmol/L])
Triglycerides = 210 mg/dL (<150 mg/dL)
(SI: 2.37 mmol/L [<1.70 mmol/L])
Serum creatinine = 0.86 mg/dL (0.6-1.1 mg/dL)
(SI: 76.0 μmol/L [53.0-97.2 μmol/L])
Urinary albumin-to-creatinine ratio = 32 mg/g creat (<30 mg/g creat)

Which of the following should be advised as the best course of action?

A. Start omega-3 fatty acids (460 mg eicosapentaenoic acid and 380 mg docosahexaenoic acid), 1 g daily
B. Start atorvastatin, 10 mg daily
C. Start ramipril, 10 mg daily
D. Start fenofibrate, 145 mg daily
E. Refer to a nutritionist

Blood glucose values and observations	Fasting	Prelunch	Predinner	Bedtime
Blood glucose values	150-199 mg/dL (SI: 8.3-11.0 mmol/L)	150-199 mg/dL (SI: 8.3-11.0 mmol/L)	100-199 mg/dL (SI: 5.6-11.0 mmol/L)	150-225 mg/dL (SI: 8.3-12.5 mmol/L)
Observations	Occasional values in the range of 68-75 mg/dL (SI: 3.8-4.2 mmol/L) or 211-274 mg/dL (SI: 11.7-15.2 mmol/L)	If lunch is late, values are 90-125 mg/dL (SI: 5.0-6.9 mmol/L)	N/A	Occasional value in the range of 110-130 mg/dL (SI: 6.1-7.2 mmol/L)

43 A 26-year-old woman with polycystic ovary syndrome would like to establish care, as her former endocrinologist left the area. She has had irregular menses since menarche, facial hirsutism, and acne. She has had a good clinical response to hormonal contraception and spironolactone. She has no concerns at this time and has no pregnancy plans.

On physical examination, her BMI is 32 kg/m² and blood pressure is 110/60 mm Hg. She has acanthosis nigricans on her neck.

Electrolytes, creatinine, and TSH are normal.

Which of the following is the most appropriate test to evaluate her risk for diabetes?
- A. 2-Hour oral glucose tolerance test
- B. Serum insulin measurement
- C. Hemoglobin A$_{1c}$ measurement
- D. Fasting glucose measurement
- E. HOMA-IR (Homeostatic Model Assessment of Insulin Resistance)

44 A 69-year-old man with longstanding type 1 diabetes mellitus presents for a follow-up visit. His blood glucose is managed using U100 insulin lispro delivered via a personal insulin pump and continuous glucose monitoring. He follows a low-carbohydrate and low-fat diet and exercises 5 to 6 days a week.

The basal insulin delivery rates are shown (*see table*).

Time segment	Basal insulin rate
12 AM-2 AM	0.75 units/h
2 AM-9 AM	0.65 units/h
9 AM-12 PM	1.75 units/h
12 PM-12 AM	0.7 units/h

He eats breakfast at 9 AM and eats his evening meal between 6 PM and 7 PM. He administers an insulin bolus at the beginning of meals using a 1:20 insulin-to-carbohydrate ratio and takes small correction boluses as needed for hyperglycemia using a 1:60 insulin correction factor.

He has no history of severe hypoglycemia. His hemoglobin A$_{1c}$ level is 6.9% (52 mmol/mol) today and was 6.5% (48 mmol/mol) 3 months ago. His continuous glucose monitoring daily overlay report for the week before the visit is shown (*see image*).

Which of the following would you recommend to help attenuate the marked postprandial glycemic excursions this patient is experiencing?
- A. Advise him to take his insulin bolus 10 to 15 minutes before meals
- B. Reduce the grams of carbohydrate eaten with each meal by 25%
- C. Perform a basal rate test from 9 AM to 9 PM
- D. Adjust his insulin-to-carbohydrate ratio to 1:6 for breakfast and the evening meal

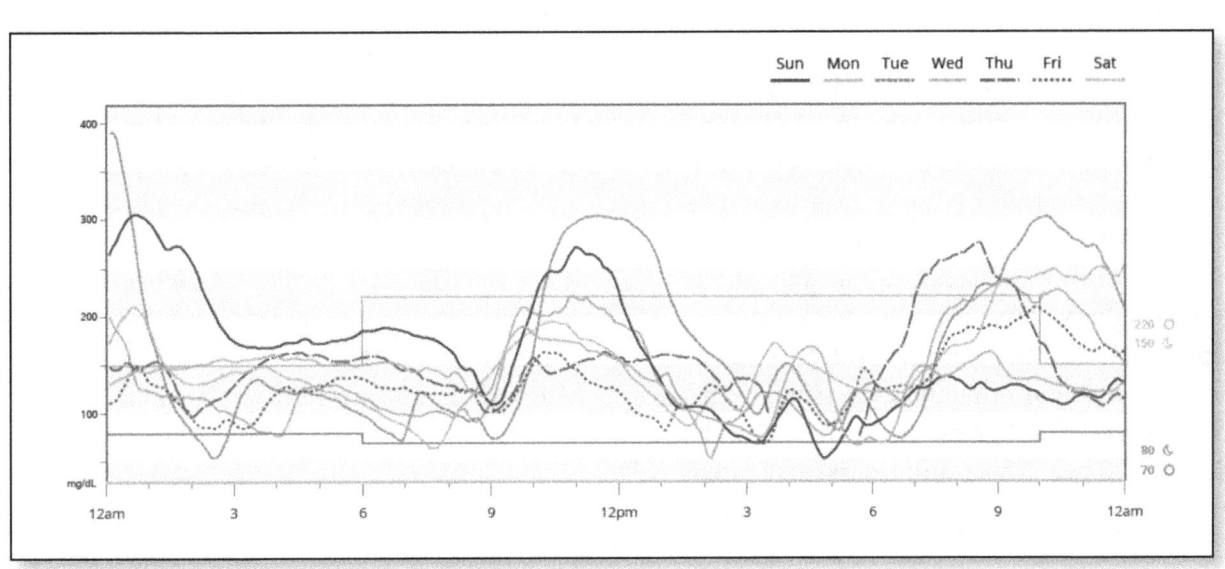

45 A 34-year-old man with type 1 diabetes mellitus is in the clinic waiting room when the receptionist notes he seems confused when his name is called, speaks with slurred words, and is unable to follow commands. He is found to have a fingerstick blood glucose value of 39 mg/dL (2.2 mmol/L). After recovery with oral glucose, he reports that despite careful monitoring, including use of his continuous glucose monitor, he has had 5 or 6 episodes of hypoglycemia with blood glucose levels between 40 and 50 mg/dL (2.2-2.8 mmol/L) in the past 2 weeks, without any warning symptoms that he can recall. Over his 16-year history of diabetes, he has always aimed for tight glycemic control because he fears developing long-term complications. His current hemoglobin A_{1c} level is 5.9% (41 mmol/mol), and his treatment regimen consists of multiple daily insulin injections.

Which of the following is the most important next step in this patient's care?

A. Temporarily relax his tight glucose targets

B. Instruct him to always carry a glucagon emergency kit

C. Begin using an insulin pump for insulin administration

D. Recommend attending a diabetes education class focused on hypoglycemia avoidance

E. Set his continuous glucose monitor hypoglycemia alarm threshold to 80 mg/dL (4.4 mmol/L)

46 A 26-year-old previously well man with type 1 diabetes mellitus is found unresponsive in his apartment by a friend. He moved out of his family's home 2 months ago to live on his own. He manages his diabetes with multiple daily insulin injections. Four months ago, his hemoglobin A_{1c} level was 6.9% (52 mmol/mol).

Upon arrival to the emergency department, he is obtunded and minimally responsive. He is afebrile, and his blood pressure is 110/72 mm Hg, pulse rate is 90 beats/min, and respiratory rate is 30 breaths/min.

Laboratory test results:

Plasma glucose = 220 mg/dL (70-99 mg/dL) (SI: 12.2 mmol/L [3.9-5.5 mmol/L])

Hemoglobin A_{1c} = 8.2% (4.0%-5.6%) (66 mmol/mol [20-38 mmol/mol])

Serum sodium = 152 mg/dL (136-142 mEq/L) (SI: 152 mmol/L [136-142 mmol/L])

Bicarbonate = 16 mEq/L (21-28 mEq/L) (SI: 16 mmol/L [21-28 mmol/L])

Serum pH = 7.19 (7.35-7.45)

Serum urea nitrogen = 34 mg/dL (8-23 mg/dL) (SI: 12.1 mmol/L [2.9-8.2 mmol/L])

Serum creatinine = 1.9 mg/dL (0.7-1.3 mg/dL) (SI: 168.0 μmol/L [61.9-114.9 μmol/L])

Serum potassium = 5.3 mEq/L (3.5-5.0 mEq/L) (SI: 5.3 mmol/L [3.5-5.0 mmol/L])

Urinalysis = 4+ glucose, large ketones, few white blood cells, no red blood cells, no blood

Which of the following most likely precipitated his condition?

A. Adrenal insufficiency

B. Canagliflozin

C. Rationing his insulin

D. Alcohol intoxication

47 A 39-year-old man is referred for evaluation of metabolic syndrome. The patient has gained 26 lb (11.8 kg) over the past year and has developed hypertension and dyslipidemia. His medical history is notable for schizoaffective disorder that has required medication. His current antipsychotic medications are olanzapine and trazodone, which he has taken for the past 15 months. He also takes hydrochlorothiazide and a calcium-channel blocker for hypertension.

On physical examination, he has a flat affect. His blood pressure is 128/68 mm Hg. His weight is 238 lb (108.2 kg) (BMI = 34.1 kg/m²), and waist circumference is 41.5 in (105 cm). He has central obesity, and there are pale striae on his abdomen. Muscle bulk and strength are normal.

Laboratory test results (fasting):

TSH = 1.1 mIU/L (0.5-5.0 mIU/L)

Glucose = 119 mg/dL (70-99 mg/dL)
(SI: 6.6 mmol/L [3.9-5.5 mmol/L])

Total cholesterol = 224 mg/dL (<200 mg/dL)
(SI: 5.80 mmol/L [<5.18 mmol/L])

Triglycerides = 427 mg/dL (<150 mg/dL)
(SI: 4.83 mmol/L [<1.70 mmol/L])

LDL cholesterol = 92 mg/dL (<100 mg/dL)
(SI: 2.38 mmol/L [<2.59 mmol/L])

HDL cholesterol = 38 mg/dL (>60 mg/dL)
(SI: 0.98 mmol/L [>1.55 mmol/L])

Which of the following should be recommended as the best next step in this patient's care?

- A. Consult with psychiatrist to change olanzapine to clozapine
- B. Consult with psychiatrist to change olanzapine to aripiprazole
- C. Start gemfibrozil
- D. Start metformin
- E. Start phentermine/topiramate

48 A 23-year-old man who has had type 1 diabetes mellitus since age 5 years is hospitalized for diabetic ketoacidosis. He also has bipolar disorder that is well controlled when he takes his medications. He is homeless. Most days, he eats 2 meals at a food kitchen. He has had 4 other hospital admissions for diabetic ketoacidosis this year. His current insulin regimen consists of insulin detemir, 15 units once daily, and insulin glulisine with meals. He keeps his insulins at a shelter where he spends most nights. He has health insurance.

Which of the following changes should be made to his insulin delivery regimen to help prevent further episodes of diabetic ketoacidosis?

- A. Hybrid closed-loop continuous subcutaneous insulin infusion pump with sensor system
- B. U200 basal insulin degludec once daily plus mealtime insulin
- C. A tubeless insulin pump
- D. U500 regular insulin twice daily

49 A 19-year-old man with type 1 diabetes mellitus reports a 6-month history of diarrhea, unintentional weight loss, poor glycemic control, and a rash. On physical examination, he has no abdominal tenderness, normal sensation to 1-g monofilament testing, and a rash that is characterized by erythematous, papular, small and large blisters that burn and itch intensely (*see image*).

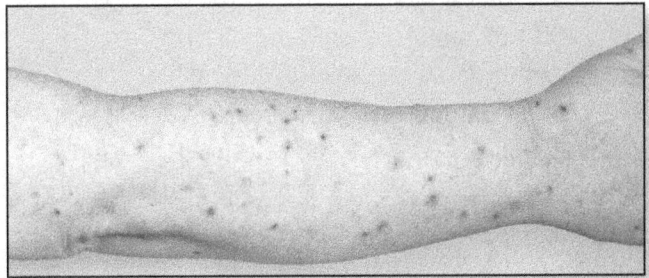

Which of the following is the best initial approach to evaluate his symptoms and rash?

- A. Colonoscopy
- B. Measurement of tissue transglutaminase antibodies
- C. Measurement of TPO antibodies
- D. Upper gastrointestinal series with small-bowel follow-through
- E. Skin biopsy

50 An 88-year-old man with type 2 diabetes mellitus, hypertension, dyslipidemia, chronic kidney disease, and coronary artery disease presents for follow-up. Although he has intentionally lost 6.6 lb (3 kg) in the past 6 months, his hemoglobin A$_{1c}$ level has increased from 6.7% to 8.3% (50 to 67 mmol/mol). He occasionally has blurred vision and polyuria after large meals. He has no shortness of breath but does report some ankle swelling at the end of the day.

Current medications include amlodipine, atenolol, aspirin, atorvastatin, isosorbide, furosemide, vitamins B$_{12}$ and D$_3$, and allopurinol.

On physical examination, his height is 65 in (165 cm) and weight is 189 lb (85.9 kg) (BMI = 31.4 kg/m^2). His blood pressure is 143/74 mm Hg, and pulse rate is 68 beats/min. Findings on cardiorespiratory examination are normal. His abdomen is rotund, pedal pulses are 1+, and there is no ankle edema.

Laboratory test results:
  Random glucose = 155 mg/dL (SI: 8.6 mmol/L)
  Creatinine = 2.2 mg/dL (0.7-1.3 mg/dL)
    (SI: 194.5 μmol/L [61.9-114.9 μmol/L])
  Estimated glomerular filtration rate = 30 mL/min
    per 1.73 m² (>60 mL/min per 1.73 m²)
  Urinary albumin-to-creatinine ratio = 1620 mg/g
    (<30 mg/g)
  LDL cholesterol = 53 mg/dL (<100 mg/dL)
    (SI: 1.37 mmol/L [<2.59 mmol/L])
  Aspartate aminotransferase, normal
  Alanine aminotransferase, normal
  Hematocrit = 37% (41%-51%) (SI: 0.37 [0.41-0.51])

*Which of the following medications is most likely to
reduce his risk for hospitalization due to heart failure?*
  A. Metformin
  B. Saxagliptin
  C. Empagliflozin
  D. Insulin
  E. Liraglutide

51 A 23-year-old woman was treated for
gestational diabetes during a previous
pregnancy and maintained her hemoglobin
A_{1c} level less than 6.5% (<48 mmol/mol). After
delivery, she did not have follow-up glycemic
testing. Now, 10 months later, she has a positive
pregnancy test 6 weeks after her last menstrual
period. She has no symptoms of diabetes at this
time. Her blood glucose value is 143 mg/dL
(7.9 mmol/L) about 90 minutes after breakfast.

Laboratory test results:
  Hemoglobin A_{1c} = 5.7% (4.0%-5.6%)
    (39 mmol/mol [20-38 mmol/mol])
  2-Hour plasma glucose (75-g oral glucose tolerance
    test) = 210 mg/dL (SI: 11.7 mmol/L)

*Which of the following is the best assessment of this
woman's current glycemic status?*
  A. Gestational diabetes mellitus
  B. Type 2 diabetes mellitus
  C. Prediabetes
  D. Indeterminate

52 A 67-year-old man with a 15-year history
of type 2 diabetes with retinopathy has
been admitted to the hospital after presenting with
an isolated concern of new-onset double vision and
feeling unsteady when walking since this morning.
He notes occasional blurry vision after large meals,
some tingling in his feet, and decreased libido. He
has no symptoms suggestive of thyroid disease or
adrenal insufficiency.

On neurologic examination, he is awake and
responsive and oriented to person, place, and time.
His right eye is deviated "down and out." Left eye
movements are normal. The rest of the cranial
nerves are intact. There is no ptosis or nystagmus,
and pupils are equal and reactive to light. He has
mild reduction of sensation bilaterally in the feet.

Laboratory test results (blood drawn at admission):
  Blood glucose = 203 mg/dL (70-99 mg/dL)
    (SI: 11.3 mmol/L [3.9-5.5 mmol/L])
  Hemoglobin A_{1c} = 8.5% (4.0%-5.6%)
    (69 mmol/mol [20-38 mmol/mol])

You are asked to see him after head CT reveals
no evidence of hemorrhage or infarct but shows
an enhancing suprasellar mass involving the
superior pituitary stalk. MRI with sellar and
suprasellar cuts confirms the presence of a pituitary
mass with suprasellar extension, but it does not
show evidence of optic or oculomotor nerve
impingement. Diplopia is still present on the third
hospital day.

*Which of the following is the most likely explanation
for his diplopia?*
  A. Unilateral endocrine ophthalmopathy
  B. Pituitary macroadenoma
  C. Mononeuritis affecting the third cranial nerve
  D. Reversible ischemic neurologic deficit
  E. Macular edema

53 A 42-year-old man with type 1 diabetes mellitus since age 21 years has been experiencing an increased frequency of early hypoglycemia and late hyperglycemia associated with certain meals. Otherwise, his home glucose values (fingerstick) are within range. He has been on insulin pump therapy for years with insulin aspart. His current hemoglobin A_{1c} level is 6.9% (52 mmol/mol). His hypoglycemic episodes occur mostly within an hour after eating his favorite large meal (pizza with extra cheese and ice cream). The early hypoglycemia is followed by high blood glucose values (200-300 mg/dL [11.1-16.7 mmol/L]) hours after the meal. He has gained weight in recent years, and his BMI is 28 kg/m².

His basal rate is 1.0 unit/h from midnight to 6 AM and 1.2 units/h from 6 AM to midnight. His mealtime boluses are 1 unit per 10 g of carbohydrate.

Which of the following is the best recommendation?
   A. Change his insulin-to-carbohydrate ratio to 1 unit per 12 g for high-fat meals
   B. Change the insulin bolus to extended for high-fat meals
   C. Eat more carbohydrates with high-fat meals
   D. Change insulin aspart to insulin aspart-niacinamide
   E. Take metoclopramide with high-fat meals

54 A 20-year-old woman with cystic fibrosis affecting her lungs and liver is seeing you for the first time after a hemoglobin A_{1c} level of 6.2% (44 mmol/mol) was documented and oral glucose tolerance testing resulted in a 2-hour plasma glucose concentration of 245 mg/dL (13.6 mmol/L). Three months later, her hemoglobin A_{1c} level is 6.1% (43 mmol/mol) and 2-hour plasma glucose concentration is 260 mg/dL (14.4 mmol/L). She has no family history of diabetes. Her BMI is 23 kg/m².

Which of the following therapeutic options should be started as the best next step?
   A. Metformin
   B. Repaglinide
   C. Dulaglutide
   D. Rapid-acting insulin
   E. Referral to nutritionist

55 A 43-year-old woman presents for evaluation of an episode of hypoglycemia. She underwent Roux-en-Y gastric bypass surgery several months ago for treatment of morbid obesity complicated by hypertension and type 2 diabetes. Two years ago, her BMI was 42 kg/m² and she was treated for gestational diabetes during her last pregnancy. Since having surgery and establishing her postoperative meal regimen, she notes that approximately 1 hour after certain meals, she feels nauseated and has diaphoresis followed rapidly by a loose stool. Her symptoms are relieved by sipping apple juice. She used her glucose meter to monitor her blood glucose during one of these episodes and a recent measurement was 58 mg/dL (3.2 mmol/L).

Which of the following is the most likely etiology of her hypoglycemia?
   A. Insulinoma
   B. Noninsulinoma pancreatogenous hypoglycemia syndrome
   C. Dumping syndrome
   D. Increased insulin sensitivity
   E. Postbariatric hypoglycemia

56 A 57-year-old man with type 2 diabetes mellitus is hospitalized with a new diagnosis of congestive heart failure (ejection fraction <10%). His cardiac status is now stabilized with inotropic support. He is being evaluated for advanced heart failure therapies, and he will most likely be hospitalized for another 5 to 7 days. You are consulted for glycemic management.

He is eating well and does not report any gastrointestinal disturbances. His is receiving subcutaneous injections of insulin glargine, 10 units each morning, plus a low-dose supplemental insulin scale when his blood glucose is greater than 180 mg/dL (>10.0 mmol/L). His estimated glomerular filtration rate is 42 mL/min per 1.73 m².

His point-of-care blood glucose values over the past 24 hours are as follows:

Day	Time	Blood glucose	Insulin lispro correction dose
Yesterday	10:45 PM	244 mg/dL (SI: 13.5 mmol/L)	2 units
Today	07:18 AM	166 mg/dL (SI: 9.2 mmol/L)	–
Today	11:58 AM	212 mg/dL (SI: 11.8 mmol/L)	4 units
Today	05:18 PM	203 mg/dL (SI: 11.3 mmol/L)	4 units

Which of the following evidence-based therapies should be recommended as an addition to his hospital glycemic control regimen?

    A. Sitagliptin
    B. Metformin
    C. Pioglitazone
    D. Canagliflozin

Female Reproduction Board Review

Kathryn A. Martin, MD

1 A 27-year-old pregnant woman sees her obstetrician for her 25-week visit. She was in good health before she conceived. She is very concerned about new symptoms that began 5 weeks ago and are rapidly progressing, including excess hair, deepening of her voice, and clitoral enlargement. Her only medications include prenatal vitamins and some dietary supplements. Her husband is in good health and takes no medication.

On physical examination, her blood pressure is 105/60 mm Hg. She has facial acne. There are terminal hairs on her upper lip, chin, neck, midsternum, and upper and lower back. A modified Ferriman-Gallwey score is 12 (score >8 = hirsutism). She has clitoromegaly (8×5 mm = 40 mm^2 [upper limit of normal = 35 mm^2]), and her voice is deep. There is no increased supraclavicular fullness or dorsocervical fat accumulation. She has lightly pigmented, narrow striae on her lower abdomen and hips.

Total testosterone = 953 ng/dL (8-60 ng/dL)
   (SI: 8.7 nmol/L [0.3-2.1 nmol/L])
DHEA-S = 200 µg/dL (44-332 µg/dL)
   (SI: 5.42 µmol/L [1.19-9.00 µmol/L])
LH = 5.0 mIU/mL (SI: 5.0 IU/L)
FSH = 2.5 mIU/mL (SI: 2.5 IU/L)

Pelvic ultrasonography shows polycystic ovary morphology and bilateral, solid ovarian masses. The left ovary has a 2×7-cm nodular mass with no cystic components, and the right ovary has a 3×5-cm nodular mass with no cystic components. A normal-appearing female fetus for 25 weeks' gestation is visualized.

Which of the following is the most likely cause of her virilization?
   A. Theca lutein cysts
   B. Polycystic ovary syndrome
   C. Luteomas of pregnancy
   D. Dietary supplements
   E. Nonclassic congenital adrenal hyperplasia due to 21-hydroxylase deficiency

2 A 50-year-old perimenopausal woman presents for follow-up regarding menopausal hormone therapy. At her initial visit 4 months ago, she described irregular menses occurring every 45 to 60 days, hot flashes during the day, and night sweats that were disrupting sleep. Menopausal hormone therapy (transdermal estradiol, 0.0375 mg, with micronized progesterone, 200 mg daily, for 12 days a month) was prescribed for relief of her vasomotor symptoms. Although her night sweats have resolved, she continues to have trouble sleeping (difficulty falling asleep, midcycle awakenings). Her only other medication is metformin, 1000 mg daily, with dinner, which was prescribed by her family physician for weight loss.

Which of the following is the most likely contributor to her unresolved sleep disturbance?
   A. Normal aging
   B. Anxiety and depression
   C. Restless leg syndrome
   D. Progestin therapy
   E. Metformin therapy

3 A 19-year-old woman seeks evaluation because she has still not had a period. She experienced normal growth and development, similar to that of her peers. She recalls developing axillary and pubic hair at about age 10 years and breast development at age 12 years. She has never been sexually active and has no other medical problems. She sometimes experiences cyclic mood changes, but she has never had pelvic pain. She has had minimal facial acne in the past and no hirsutism. A physical examination done by her pediatrician documented normal external genitalia, normal axillary and pubic hair, and Tanner stage 5 breast development. Her height is 69 in (175.3 cm), and weight is 135 lb (61.2 kg) (BMI = 19.9 kg/m²).

Laboratory test results:
LH = 6.0 mIU/mL (SI: 6.0 IU/L)
FSH = 7.0 mIU/mL (SI: 7.0 IU/L)
Estradiol = 55 pg/mL (SI: 202 pmol/L)
Prolactin = 14 ng/mL (4-30 ng/mL)
    (SI: 0.61 nmol/L [0.17-1.30 nmol/L])
Testosterone = 30 ng/dL (8-60 ng/dL)
    (SI: 1.0 nmol/L [0.3-2.1 nmol/L])

After 10 days of micronized progesterone, 200 mg daily, she has no withdrawal bleed. A course of estrogen followed by progestin still does not result in a withdrawal bleed. Pelvic ultrasonography is ordered.

Which of the following is the most likely finding on pelvic ultrasonography?
   A. Absent uterus
   B. Streak ovaries
   C. Intrauterine adhesions
   D. Absent uterus and ovaries
   E. Transverse vaginal septum

4 A 38-year-old woman with a history of premenstrual mood changes and polycystic ovary syndrome (polycystic ovaries on ultrasonography, acne, and mild-moderate hirsutism) presents for evaluation. Her menstrual cycles are usually regular (every 28-34 days). She is currently using topical agents for acne and local measures for hirsutism. She recalls taking a combined estrogen-progestin oral contraceptive briefly as a teenager for acne, but she stopped it during the first cycle because of nausea. You discuss using a low-dosage continuous regimen of a combined oral contraceptive (ethinyl estradiol,

20 mcg/norethindrone 1 mg), which should benefit her premenstrual mood changes, hirsutism, and acne. She is willing to try it again, as it has been more than 20 years since she last tried it. However, she remains very concerned about adverse effects.

On physical examination, her BMI is 29 kg/m², she has moderate facial acne, and a modified Ferriman-Gallwey score is 9.

Which of the following symptoms is this patient most likely to experience during the first few months of continuous combined oral contraceptive use?
   A. Weight gain
   B. Sexual dysfunction
   C. Depression
   D. Unscheduled bleeding (breakthrough bleeding)
   E. Hypertension

5 A 46-year-old woman seeks evaluation for irregular and sometimes heavy bleeding (occurring every 21 to 50 days), hot flashes during the day, frequent night sweats, and migraines. She has always had perimenstrual migraines, but they are now frequent and persist for several weeks after a period. She has never had auras. Endometrial biopsy performed by her gynecologist because of concerns about the bleeding was benign (proliferative endometrium). She is very eager to try some kind of hormone therapy for her hot flashes and she wonders whether it could also help her migraines.

Which of the following initial therapies should be suggested?
   A. Combined oral contraceptive: ethinyl estradiol, 20 mcg/norethindrone, 1 mg
   B. Oral 17β-estradiol, 2 mg daily with micronized progesterone, 200 mg on days 1 to 12
   C. Transdermal 17β-estradiol, 0.025 mg twice weekly, with micronized progesterone, 100 mg daily
   D. Levonorgestrel-releasing intrauterine device
   E. Gabapentin, 300 mg every night at bedtime

6 A 43-year-old transgender man attends an appointment to start gender-affirming hormone therapy. At his last visit, you reviewed the criteria, potential regimens, adverse effects, and need for regular monitoring. He has decided to start with parenteral testosterone (testosterone enanthate, 200 mg every 2 weeks), rather than the gel formulation. He is concerned about possible complications, such as heart attacks and blood clots, so he asks you to remind him about the most common adverse effects with injectable testosterone.

Which of the following is the most common adverse effect with testosterone therapy?
   A. Venous thromboembolism
   B. Prostate cancer
   C. Erythrocytosis
   D. Myocardial infarction
   E. Type 2 diabetes mellitus

7 A 35-year-old woman with polycystic ovary syndrome presents for follow-up. She has a history of oligomenorrhea with heavy bleeding, severe hirsutism, and obesity. She has been on a combined estrogen-progestin oral contraceptive containing 35 mcg ethinyl estradiol. During a ski trip 3 months ago, she sustained a traumatic femur fracture that required surgical repair. Her recovery was complicated by a deep venous thrombosis. Her combined oral contraceptive was discontinued during hospitalization, and she notes that her facial hair has become much worse, which she finds very distressing. She has no family history of deep venous thrombosis, pulmonary embolism, or stroke. A hypercoagulability panel done during hospitalization showed no evidence of a thrombophilia. She would like to restart the combined oral contraceptive because it keeps her periods regular, controls her hirsutism, and is her preferred contraceptive method.

On physical examination, her BMI is 30 kg/m². She has moderate to severe facial hirsutism. Her modified Ferriman-Gallwey score is 16 (hirsutism defined by a score >8).

Which of the following regimens would be best for managing her irregular menses and hirsutism and providing contraception?
   A. Switch to estrogen-progestin contraceptive patch
   B. Recommend nonhormonal form of contraception and metformin
   C. Continue oral contraceptive, but decrease the ethinyl estradiol dose to 20 mcg
   D. Recommend progestin intrauterine device and spironolactone
   E. Recommend oral progestin-only contraceptive

8 A 60-year-old woman presents with worsening hirsutism since menopause 5 years earlier. Her menarche was at age 12 years, and she always had regular menses. She had 2 uncomplicated pregnancies. She has gained weight over the years, and her BMI is now 35 kg/m². She has noticed increasing hair growth since menopause. More recently, she has noticed some deepening of her voice and enlargement of her clitoris.

On physical examination, she has increased facial hair and hair on her upper abdomen, midsternal area, and upper back (modified Ferriman-Gallwey score is 12 [>8 = hirsutism]). She has female-pattern balding and clitoromegaly (clitoral index 8 × 5 mm = 40 mm² [upper limit of normal = 35 mm²]). Acanthosis nigricans is seen on her elbows, axillae, and neck.

Laboratory test results:
   LH = 28.0 mIU/mL (>30.0 mIU/mL
      [postmenopausal]) (SI: 28.0 IU/L [>30.0 IU/L])
   FSH = 32.0 mIU/mL (>30.0 mIU/mL
      [postmenopausal]) (SI: 32.0 IU/L [>30.0 IU/L])
   Testosterone = 300 ng/dL (8-60 ng/dL)
      (SI: 10.4 nmol/L [0.3-2.1 nmol/L])
   DHEA-S = 280 µg/dL (15-157 µg/dL)
      (SI: 7.59 µmol/L [0.41-4.25 µmol/L])

Which of the following is this patient's most likely diagnosis?

   A. Adrenal virilizing tumor

   B. Ovarian hyperthecosis

   C. Granulosa tumor of the ovary

   D. Obesity-induced hyperandrogenism

   E. Sertoli-Leydig–cell tumor of the ovary

9 A 32-year-old woman is referred for anovulatory infertility. She has a history of irregular periods, acne, hirsutism, and obesity. Polycystic ovary syndrome was diagnosed at age 16 years. Her blood pressure is 130/80 mm Hg. She continues to have irregular cycles (25 to 50 days), but she has been trying to conceive for the past 6 months. Metformin was started 3 months ago to induce ovulation, and she has had 2 periods since then but has not conceived. Serum hCG is negative.

On physical examination, her BMI is 32 kg/m^2.

In this patient's case, which of the following treatments would most effectively induce ovulation and result in a live birth?

   A. Clomiphene citrate

   B. Progesterone suppositories

   C. Continue metformin

   D. Letrozole

   E. Gonadotropin therapy with recombinant FSH

10 A 32-year-old woman presents with a 6-month history of amenorrhea. She has been in excellent health except for a history of type 1 diabetes mellitus diagnosed at age 28 years. Her glycemic control has been good, with a hemoglobin A$_{1c}$ value of 7.0% (53 mmol/mol).

Recently, she has experienced hot flashes and night sweats. Both her mother and maternal aunt had early menopause at age 39 years and 40 years, respectively. The patient has a 19-year-old brother with intellectual disability.

Laboratory test results:

   FSH = 90.0 mIU/mL (2.0-12.0 mIU/mL)
     (SI: 90.0 IU/L [2.0-12.0 IU/L])
   Estradiol = <20 pg/mL (10-180 pg/mL)
     (SI: <73.4 pmol/L [36.7-660.8 pmol/L])

TSH = 3.0 mIU/L (0.5-5.0 mIU/L)
Prolactin = 7 ng/mL (4-30 ng/mL)
   (SI: 0.30 nmol/L [0.17-1.30 nmol/L])

Which of the following tests is most likely to identify her diagnosis?

   A. Karyotype analysis

   B. *FMR1* genetic testing

   C. 21-Hydroxylase antibody measurement

   D. TPO antibody measurement

   E. Antimullerian hormone measurement

11 A 28-year-old transgender man seeks gender-affirming hormone therapy (testosterone). The patient meets the criteria for gender-affirming hormone therapy, and findings from baseline evaluation, including complete blood cell count and Pap smear, are normal. You review his treatment options, expected results and potential risks, plans for future fertility, and the importance of regular monitoring.

After starting hormone therapy, which of the following should be done during the first year of treatment?

   A. Measurement of serum total testosterone immediately before a testosterone enanthate/cypionate injection or immediately before application of testosterone gel, every 3 months

   B. Hemoglobin A$_{1c}$ measurement every 6 months

   C. Hematocrit or hemoglobin measurement every 3 months

   D. Measurement of bone density at 1 year

   E. Pap smear at 1 year

12 A 25-year-old woman with polycystic ovary syndrome presents to discuss treatment options. Menarche was at age 11 years, and her menses have always been irregular. She had onset of hirsutism and acne at age 12 years. She was on oral contraceptives briefly as a teenager. Six months ago, she started metformin, 500 mg twice daily, for hirsutism and to regulate her menstrual cycles. Her cycles have become more regular, but she feels as if her hirsutism has not improved.

On physical examination, her BMI is 27 kg/m^2 and blood pressure is 110/70 mm Hg.

She wants to modify her regimen to improve her hirsutism. She is currently using barrier methods for contraception.

Which of the following treatment options would be best for this patient?
    A. Levonorgestrel-releasing intrauterine device and a higher metformin dosage
    B. Addition of spironolactone
    C. Combination estrogen-progestin oral contraceptive
    D. Addition of finasteride
    E. Addition of flutamide

13 A 46-year-old woman seeks advice for irregular menstrual cycles. She previously had 30- to 32-day cycles, but for the past 18 months, her menstrual periods have become unpredictable, occurring every 21 to 60 days. Her last menstrual period was 50 days ago. She has gained weight over the past 2 to 3 years, and current BMI is 31 kg/m². She has been having difficulty sleeping and wakes frequently at night. She is very worried and would like an evaluation to determine the etiology of her symptoms.

Laboratory test results from blood samples drawn on cycle day 50:
    LH = 15.0 mIU/mL (1.0-18.0 mIU/mL [follicular])
        (SI: 15.0 IU/L [1.0-18.0 IU/L])
    FSH = 24.0 mIU/mL (2.0-12.0 mIU/mL [follicular])
        (SI: 24.0 IU/L [2.0-12.0 IU/L])
    Estradiol = 180 pg/mL (10-180 pg/mL [follicular])
        (SI: 660.8 pmol/L [36.7-660.8 pmol/L])
    Progesterone = <1.0 ng/mL (2.0-20.0 ng/mL)
        (SI: 3.2 nmol/L [6.4-63.6 nmol/L])

Which of the following is the most likely cause of her clinical picture?
    A. Menopausal transition (perimenopause)
    B. Pregnancy
    C. Obesity
    D. Estradiol-secreting granulosa-cell tumor
    E. Polycystic ovary syndrome

14 A 28-year-old woman presents to discuss options to treat severe premenstrual dysphoria. Menarche was at age 12 years, and she has regular menses every 28 days. Since her mid-20s, she has been experiencing mood symptoms the week before her menses. Recently, she has been unable to work 1 to 2 days per month because of her mood swings, irritability, and sense of hopelessness during this time. She feels better once her period starts. Her family history is notable for hypertension, diabetes mellitus, and depression.

On physical examination, her BMI is 28 kg/m², and the rest of the findings are normal.

Which of the following is the best option for treating her premenstrual syndrome?
    A. Refer her for psychotherapy
    B. Start a selective serotonin reuptake inhibitor
    C. Start a tricyclic antidepressant
    D. Start a cyclic regimen of an estrogen-progestin oral contraceptive
    E. Start alprazolam

15 A 23-year-old woman presents with irregular menses followed by amenorrhea. Menarche was at age 14 years; her periods were irregular for 18 months, then regular every 28 days. About 2 years ago, her cycle length shortened to 25 days and then to 22 days. She has not had a period in 4 months. She is stressed in her new job. She runs 2 miles 3 times a week. Her BMI is 20 kg/m². She has no evidence of hirsutism or acne.

A pregnancy test is negative. Her TSH value is 2.1 mIU/L (0.5-5.0 mIU/L).

Which of the following are the best laboratory tests to order now?
    A. FSH, LH, testosterone, and DHEA-S
    B. FSH, estradiol, and prolactin
    C. FSH, estradiol, and 17-hydroxyprogesterone
    D. FSH, estradiol, and progesterone
    E. FSH, ACTH, and cortisol

16 A 28-year-old woman presents with infertility. She had menarche at age 13 years and had regular menses during high school and college except for amenorrhea when she ran cross-country. She took an oral contraceptive pill from age 22 to 27 years but stopped 18 months ago to try and conceive. She has Hashimoto thyroiditis and takes a stable dosage of levothyroxine. She is currently having menses every 24 to 25 days. She exercises 3 times per week for 1.5 hours each session. She has mild acne, no hot flashes, and no galactorrhea. Her BMI is 20 kg/m^2.

Laboratory test results from blood samples drawn on cycle day 3:
  FSH = 20.0 mIU/mL (2.0-12.0 mIU/mL)
    (SI: 20.0 IU/L [2.0-12.0 IU/L])
  LH = 10.0 mIU/mL (1.0-18.0 mIU/mL)
    (SI: 10.0 IU/L [1.0-18.0 IU/L])
  Estradiol = 28 pg/mL (10-180 pg/mL)
    (SI: 102.8 pmol/L [36.7-660.8 pmol/L])
  Antimullerian hormone = 0.5 ng/mL
    (0.9-9.5 ng/mL) (SI: 3.6 pmol/L
    [6.4-67.9 pmol/L])
  TSH = 2.1 mIU/L (0.5-5.0 mIU/L)

Which of the following is the most likely diagnosis?
  A. Polycystic ovary syndrome
  B. FSH-secreting pituitary adenoma
  C. Functional hypothalamic amenorrhea
  D. Primary ovarian insufficiency
  E. Autoimmune oophoritis

17 A 20-year-old woman with Turner syndrome is transitioning care from her pediatrician to an adult provider. She has a history of primary amenorrhea and short stature.
  On physical examination, her blood pressure is 140/90 mm Hg. Her height is 56 in (142.2 cm) (BMI = 28 kg/m^2). She has absent breast development and scant pubic and axillary hair. She is on a combined estrogen-progestin regimen and has been seeing her pediatrician yearly. Last year, cardiac MRI showed no evidence of aortic dilatation and no significant cardiovascular anomalies.

Past laboratory test results:
  FSH = 35.0 mIU/mL (2.0-12.0 mIU/mL)
    (SI: 35.0 IU/L [2.0-12.0 IU/L])
  LH = 28.0 mIU/mL (1.0-18.0 mIU/mL)
    (SI: 28.0 IU/L [1.0-18.0 IU/L])
  Estradiol = <10 pg/mL (10-180 pg/mL)
    (SI: <36.7 pmol/L [36.7-660.8 pmol/L])
  Karyotype = 45,X

Which of the following tests should be ordered today (and at each yearly visit)?
  A. Hemoglobin A$_{1c}$ measurement, kidney ultrasonography, liver enzymes
  B. Thyroid function tests, hemoglobin A$_{1c}$ measurement, liver enzymes
  C. Electrocardiography, celiac disease screening, hemoglobin A$_{1c}$ measurement
  D. Complete blood cell count, thyroid function tests, echocardiography
  E. Antimullerian hormone measurement, transvaginal ultrasonography

18 A 32-year-old woman with polycystic ovary syndrome presents to discuss the health risks associated with her diagnosis. She had menarche at age 11 years and has had hirsutism and acne since age 13 years. She gained weight in her 20s (from 120 lb [54.5 kg] to 190 lb [86.4 kg]). She is currently on a combined estrogen-progestin oral contraceptive for hyperandrogenism and cycle management. She has been trying to lose weight, and she started an exercise program to improve her chances for later fertility.

In addition to a cardiometabolic risk assessment (blood pressure, BMI, lipid profile, and oral glucose tolerance test), for which comorbidities should the patient be screened at her initial visit?
  A. Celiac disease
  B. Coronary heart disease
  C. Autoimmune thyroid disease
  D. Depression and anxiety
  E. Endometrial cancer

Male Reproduction Board Review

Frances J. Hayes, MB BCh, BAO

1 A 21-year-old man with hypogonadism secondary to Klinefelter syndrome returns for follow-up. He has stopped injections of testosterone enanthate (prescribed at the last visit), as he found them too painful. Since stopping treatment, he has noticed increasing tiredness and decreasing sex drive. He has a history of obstructive sleep apnea and is not consistent about the use of continuous positive airway pressure. He has seen a commercial for a new testosterone product (testosterone undecanoate) that can be taken by mouth and asks if he can try it.

On physical examination, his BMI is 33 kg/m^2 and blood pressure is 135/90 mm Hg.

If treatment with oral testosterone undecanoate were initiated in this patient, which of the following parameters should be monitored closely after initiation?

A. PSA
B. Blood pressure
C. Liver function
D. TSH

2 A 48-year-old White man is referred to discuss initiation of testosterone replacement therapy. His primary care physician had diagnosed hypogonadism following a workup for fatigue, decreased libido, and erectile dysfunction. He is quite symptomatic, and he is eager to start therapy. On review of symptoms, he has no headache, vision problems, or lower urinary tract symptoms. His family history is negative for prostate cancer.

On physical examination, his BMI is 31 kg/m^2. He appears healthy, is well virilized, and has normal testes. His prostate feels normal on rectal examination.

Laboratory test results:

Total testosterone (8 AM) = 190 ng/dL (300-900 ng/dL) (SI: 6.6 nmol/L [10.4-31.2 nmol/L]) (repeated value = 205 ng/dL [SI: 7.1 nmol/L])
Free testosterone = 6.0 ng/dL (9.0-30.0 ng/dL) (SI: 0.21 nmol/L [0.31-1.04 nmol/L])
LH = 5.9 mIU/mL (1.0-9.0 mIU/mL) (SI: 5.9 IU/L [1.0-9.0 IU/L])
FSH = 6.2 mIU/mL (1.0-13.0 mIU/mL) (SI: 6.2 IU/L [1.0-13.0 IU/L])
Prolactin = 9.2 ng/mL (4-18 ng/mL) (SI: 0.40 nmol/L [0.17-0.78 nmol/L])
Free T_4 = 1.4 ng/dL (0.8-1.8 ng/dL) (SI: 18.0 pmol/L [10.30-23.17 pmol/L])
Cortisol = 18.5 μg/dL (5-25 μg/dL) (SI: 510.4 nmol/L [137.9-689.7 nmol/L])
Hematocrit = 45% (41%-50%) (SI: 0.45 [0.41-0.50])

Which of the following is the best next step in this patient's management?

A. Start testosterone replacement therapy
B. Start a phosphodiesterase inhibitor
C. Measure PSA
D. Perform pituitary MRI

3 A 66-year-old man returns for follow-up of hypogonadism. After an initial discussion of the different treatment options, he opted for a gel delivery system and has been applying 40.5 mg of a 1.62% testosterone gel every morning. At his last evaluation on this testosterone dosage 6 months ago, his total testosterone concentration was 450 ng/dL (15.6 nmol/L) and hematocrit was 47% (0.47). He feels well on this regimen, and his pretreatment symptoms of fatigue and low libido have now resolved.

Current laboratory test results (sample drawn at 7 AM yesterday):

Total testosterone = 1005 ng/dL (300-900 ng/dL)
(SI: 34.9 nmol/L [10.4-31.2 nmol/L])
Hematocrit = 47.2% (41%-50%)
(SI: 0.472 [0.41-0.50])
PSA = 1.5 ng/mL (<3.8 ng/mL)
(SI: 1.5 µg/L [<3.8 µg/L])

Which of the following is the best next step in this patient's management?

A. Reduce the dosage of his 1.62% testosterone gel to 20.25 mg daily
B. Measure testosterone 2 to 8 hours after the gel has been applied
C. Switch to intramuscular injections of testosterone enanthate
D. Switch to 40.5 mg of 1.62% testosterone gel on alternate days

4 A 55-year-old man presents for evaluation of a 3-month history of fatigue. His history is notable for migraine headaches for which he has been prescribed topiramate, 50 mg twice daily. He drinks 2 to 3 beers daily. He is not currently sexually active, but he has had unprotected intercourse with a number of partners in the past.

On physical examination, his BMI is 24.5 kg/m². He is well virilized. His thyroid is firm to palpation. He has no stigmata of chronic liver disease.

Laboratory test results:

Testosterone = 350 ng/dL (300-900 ng/dL)
(SI: 12.1 nmol/L [10.4-31.2 nmol/L])
SHBG = 1.8 µg/mL (1.1-6.7 µg/mL)
(SI: 16 nmol/L [10-60 nmol/L])
TSH = 45 mIU/mL (0.5-5.0 mIU/L)
Free T$_4$ = 0.5 ng/mL (0.8-1.8 ng/dL)
(SI: 6.44 pmol/L [10.30-23.17 pmol/L])
AST = 60 U/L (20-48 U/L)
(SI: 1.00 µkat/L [0.33-0.80 µkat/L])
ALT = 58 U/L (10-40 U/L)
(SI: 0.97 µkat/L [0.17-0.67 µkat/L])

Which of the following is the most likely cause of this patient's SHBG level?

A. Topiramate
B. Liver disease
C. Hypothyroidism
D. HIV infection
E. Age

5 A 71-year-old man returns to clinic for follow-up of hypogonadism 12 months after starting testosterone therapy. At the time of diagnosis, findings on prostate examination were normal and his PSA level was 1.5 ng/mL (1.5 µg/L). Following treatment with a 1.62% testosterone gel, 40.5 mg daily, his testosterone level is 490 ng/dL (17.0 nmol/L). The patient reports a significant improvement in energy levels, mood, and libido since starting treatment, and he has no lower urinary tract symptoms.

On physical examination, his prostate examination findings are unchanged.

His current PSA concentration is 3.5 ng/mL (<5.3 ng/mL) (SI: 3.5 µg/L [<5.3 µg/L]).

Which of the following is the best next step in this patient's management?

A. Discontinue testosterone therapy
B. Reduce the dose of the 1.62% testosterone gel to 20.25 mg
C. Refer for prostate biopsy
D. Recheck his PSA level
E. Start a 5α-reductase inhibitor

6 A 19-year-old college freshman is referred because of a decrease in sex drive and difficulty getting and sustaining an erection. He reports going through puberty at the same time as his peers. He had been feeling depressed due to academic pressures and the death of his father and was prescribed escitalopram, 10 mg daily. He finds that exercising up to 2 hours per day helps to alleviate his stress. He eats what he reports to be a very healthy, largely vegetarian diet.

On physical examination, he is a fit, muscular man with a BMI of 21 kg/m². He is normally virilized and has no gynecomastia. Examination shows testicular volume of 15 mL bilaterally with a right-sided hydrocele.

Laboratory test results:

Testosterone = 125 ng/dL (300-900 ng/dL)
(SI: 4.3 nmol/L [10.4-31.2 nmol/L])

LH = 1.7 mIU/mL (1.0-9.0 mIU/mL)
(SI: 1.7 IU/L [1.0-9.0 IU/L])

FSH = 3.0 mIU/mL (1.0-13.0 mIU/mL)
(SI: 3.0 IU/L [1.0-13.0 IU/L])

Prolactin = 10 ng/mL (4-23 ng/mL)
(SI: 0.43 nmol/L [0.17-1.00 nmol/L])

Hemoglobin = 12.8 g/dL (13.8-17.2 g/dL)
(SI: 128 g/L [138-172 g/L])

Hematocrit = 40.8% (41%-50%)
(SI: 0.408 [0.41-0.51])

Leptin = <0.6 ng/mL (0.7-5.3 ng/mL)

Findings on pituitary MRI are normal.

Which of the following is the most likely cause of this patient's hypogonadism?

A. Congenital leptin deficiency
B. Kallmann syndrome
C. Functional hypogonadotropic hypogonadism
D. Hydrocele
E. Anabolic steroid use

7 A 19-year-old man is referred for evaluation following a new diagnosis of Kallmann syndrome based on his inability to smell, lack of any secondary sex characteristics, and hypogonadotropic hypogonadism. His family history is notable for a 10-year-old brother who is also anosmic and a maternal uncle with Kallmann syndrome. Genetic testing identifies a pathogenic variant in the *ANOS1* gene (formerly known as *KAL1*).

Which of the following features is most likely to be present on this patient's physical examination?

A. Syndactyly
B. Synkinesia
C. Coloboma
D. Axillary freckling
E. Short fourth metacarpal

8 An 18-year-old high school senior is referred because of lack of secondary sex characteristics and small testes. He followed the 50th percentile for growth throughout childhood but did not experience a growth spurt in his teenage years. His height is now at the 25th percentile. He has a normal sense of smell. He does not take any prescribed medications. His father, who accompanies him, reports that he himself was also a "late bloomer," but then developed fully and had no problems with fertility.

On physical examination, his height is 66 in (168 cm), arm span is 68.9 in (175 cm), and BMI is 22 kg/m². He has slight axillary hair and Tanner stage 2 pubic hair but no facial or chest hair. He has no gynecomastia. His testes measure 2 mL bilaterally. His visual fields are full to confrontation.

Laboratory test results (sample drawn at 8 AM):

Total testosterone = 50 ng/dL (300-900 ng/dL)
(SI: 1.7 nmol/L [10.4-31.2 nmol/L])

Free T$_4$ = 1.3 ng/dL (0.8-1.8 ng/dL)
(SI: 16.7 pmol/L [10.30-23.17 pmol/L])

LH = <0.2 mIU/mL (1.0-9.0 mIU/mL)
(SI: <0.2 IU/L [1.0-9.0 IU/L])

FSH = 0.3 mIU/mL (1.0-13.0 mIU/mL)
(SI: 0.3 IU/L [1.0-13.0 IU/L])

Prolactin = 10 ng/mL (4-18 ng/mL)
(SI: 0.43 nmol/L [0.17-0.78 nmol/L])

Cortisol (8 AM) = 20.0 µg/dL (5-25 µg/dL)
(SI: 551.8 nmol/L [137.9-689.7 nmol/L])

IGF-1, low-normal for age and sex

Which of the following is the most likely diagnosis?

A. Constitutional delay of growth and puberty
B. Congenital hypogonadotropic hypogonadism
C. Pathogenic variant in the *PROP1* gene
D. Pathogenic variant in the *POU1F1* gene

9 A 45-year-old man is referred because of fatigue, low sex drive, and lack of spontaneous erections. On review of systems, he also describes pain in the small joints of his hands. He takes no medications. His mother has psoriatic arthropathy.

On physical examination, his BMI is 25 kg/m² and blood pressure is 130/80 mm Hg. He has normal secondary sexual characteristics and no gynecomastia. He has no striae, bruises, joint swelling, or rashes and has no difficulty rising from a squatting position. Testicular volume is 20 mL bilaterally.

Laboratory test results:
    Total testosterone = 185 ng/dL (300-900 ng/dL)
        (SI: 6.4 nmol/L [10.4-31.2 nmol/L])
    Serum prolactin = 20 ng/mL (4-18 ng/mL)
        (SI: 0.87 nmol/L [0.17-0.78 nmol/L])
    FSH = 3.5 mIU/mL (1.0-13.0 mIU/mL)
        (SI: 3.5 IU/L [1.0-13.0 IU/L])
    LH = 2.9 mIU/mL (1.0-9.0 mIU/mL)
        (SI: 2.9 IU/L [1.0-9.0 IU/L])

Pituitary MRI shows a 5-mm hypoenhancing lesion.

Which of the following conditions most likely explains this patient's presentation?
    A. Hyperprolactinemia with hook effect
    B. Hereditary hemochromatosis
    C. Opioid abuse
    D. Cushing disease
    E. Psoriatic arthropathy

10 A 39-year-old man with a 20-year history of type 1 diabetes mellitus presents for routine diabetes follow-up. On review of systems, he reports normal libido but some difficulty getting and sustaining an erection. He has also noticed that he produces less semen when he ejaculates. He wishes to start a family and has been having regular, unprotected intercourse with his 36-year-old wife for the past 9 months without success.

Laboratory test results:
    Testosterone = 280 ng/dL (300-900 ng/dL)
        (SI: 9.7 nmol/L [10.4-31.2 nmol/L])
    LH = 3.5 mIU/mL (1.0-9.0 mIU/mL)
        (SI: 3.5 IU/L [1.0-9.0 IU/L])
    FSH = 6.9 mIU/mL (1.0-13.0 mIU/mL)
        (SI: 6.9 IU/L [1.0-13.0 IU/L])
    Hemoglobin A$_{1c}$ = 9.5% (4.0%-5.6%)
        (80 mmol/mol [20-38 mmol/mol])

Semen analysis shows a volume of 0.5 mL (normal >1.5 mL) and sperm concentration of 9 million/mL. A similar pattern is seen on repeated testing.

Which of the following is the most appropriate next step in this patient's management?
    A. Start hCG injections
    B. Perform a postejaculatory urine analysis for semen
    C. Refer to urology for microdissection testicular sperm extraction
    D. Start testosterone therapy
    E. Start an α-adrenergic blocker

11 A 33-year-old man with Kallmann syndrome is referred by a colleague for a second opinion on fertility management. He has been treated with hCG, 1000 IU by subcutaneous injection every other day for 9 months. On this regimen, his testes increased in size from 2 to 4 mL in the first 6 months and have now reached a plateau.

Hormone profile checked on the day his injection is due:
    Testosterone = 350 ng/dL (300-900 ng/dL)
        (SI: 8.7 nmol/L [10.4-31.2 nmol/L])
    Estradiol = 40 pg/mL (10-40 pg/mL)
        (SI: 146.8 pmol/L [36.7-146.8 pmol/L])
    LH = 0.6 mIU/mL (1.0-9.0 mIU/mL)
        (SI: 0.6 IU/L [1.0-9.0 IU/L])
    FSH = 1.0 mIU/mL (1.0-13.0 mIU/mL)
        (SI: 1.0 IU/L [1.0-13.0 IU/L])

Semen analysis shows azoospermia.

Which of the following would be most helpful in improving this patient's fertility?
    A. Switch from hCG to recombinant LH injections
    B. Increase the dosage of hCG to 1500 IU every other day
    C. Switch his current hCG regimen from every other day to daily
    D. Add FSH, 75 IU daily
    E. Switch to clomiphene citrate, 50 mg daily

12 A 32-year-old man is referred for evaluation of azoospermia noted during workup for primary infertility. He and his wife have had unprotected intercourse for the past 2 years without a confirmed pregnancy. The patient underwent normal puberty and reports normal libido and erections. His wife is 30 years old and her infertility workup is normal.

On physical examination, his BMI is 25.5 kg/m². He is well virilized and has no gynecomastia. His testes are 15 mL bilaterally.

Laboratory test results:
   Total testosterone = 500 ng/dL (300-900 ng/dL)
      (SI: 17.4 nmol/L [10.4-31.2 nmol/L])
   FSH = 21.5 mIU/mL (1.0-13.0 mIU/mL)
      (SI: 21.5 IU/L [1.0-13.0 IU/L])
   LH = 5.0 mIU/mL (1.0-9.0 mIU/mL)
      (SI: 5.0 IU/L [1.0-9.0 IU/L])
   Karyotype = 46,XY

A second semen analysis documents a pH of 7.5 (normal >7.2) and volume of 3 mL (normal ≥1.5 mL) and confirms azoospermia.

Which of the following genetic conditions does this patient most likely have?
   A. Y-Chromosome microdeletion
   B. Retrograde ejaculation
   C. Kallmann syndrome
   D. Mosaic Klinefelter syndrome
   E. Congenital bilateral absence of the vas deferens

13 A 25-year-old man is referred by his oncologist after a semen analysis showed azoospermia. He has completed chemotherapy with cyclophosphamide for Hodgkin lymphoma and is in remission. He reports normal energy levels and libido and has no difficulty getting or sustaining an erection.

Which of the following hormone profiles is most likely in this patient?

Answer	Testosterone	LH	FSH
A.	Normal	Normal	Normal
B.	Normal	Normal/high	High
C.	Low	Low	Low
D.	Low	Low	High

14 A 21-year-old transgender woman calls to discuss her hormone regimen for gender dysphoria, which was started 6 months earlier. She is currently being treated with monthly injections of the GnRH agonist leuprolide, 3.75 mg intramuscularly, and a 17β-estradiol patch, 0.1 mg twice weekly. Her estrogen dosage was increased from 0.075 mg 6 weeks ago. Her estradiol concentration is now 150 pg/mL (551 pmol/L) with a testosterone concentration of 22 ng/dL (0.76 nmol/L). She has noticed a significant decrease in facial and body hair but would like to see more breast development. At her last physical examination, her BMI was 30 kg/m² and she had Tanner stage 3 breast development.

Which of the following is the best next step in this patient's management?
   A. Continue leuprolide but increase the dosage of estradiol patch to 0.2 mg twice weekly
   B. Continue leuprolide but switch from the estradiol patch to an oral contraceptive pill containing 35 mcg of ethinyl estradiol
   C. Continue current regimen
   D. Continue current regimen and add spironolactone, 50 mg twice daily
   E. Refer for breast augmentation

15 You are asked to consult on a 35-year-old transgender woman admitted to the hospital with acute pancreatitis. Hypertriglyceridemia was diagnosed when she was in her late teens. She was prescribed rosuvastatin and fenofibrate, but she has not taken her medications consistently. She has been treated with conjugated equine estrogens, 1.25 mg daily, and spironolactone, 100 mg twice daily, since age 18 years when she started living as a woman. In her late 20s, she had breast augmentation and facial feminization surgery. She does not smoke cigarettes.

Laboratory test results (sample drawn while fasting):

Total testosterone = 125 ng/dL (8-60 ng/dL) (SI: 4.3 nmol/L [0.3-2.1 nmol/L])

Estradiol = 25 pg/mL (SI: 91.8 pmol/L)

Triglycerides = 1050 mg/dL (<150 mg/dL [optimal]) (SI: 11.87 mmol/L [<1.70 mmol/L])

Glucose = 90 mg/dL (70-99 mg/dL) (SI: 5.0 mmol/L [3.9-5.5 mmol/L])

Lipase = 640 IU/L (<160 IU/L)

Following discontinuation of hormone therapy, her triglyceride level decreased to 380 mg/dL (4.29 mmol/L). During the consultation, the patient expresses a keen desire to resume gender-affirming hormone therapy.

Which of the following is the most appropriate management option for this patient's gender dysphoria following discharge from the hospital?

A. Resume spironolactone but remain off conjugated equine estrogen

B. Switch her regimen to a GnRH agonist with a 0.05-mg estradiol patch

C. Tell the patient that she is not a candidate for any further hormone therapy

D. Resume spironolactone and switch her estrogen regimen to ethinyl estradiol

E. Resume spironolactone and add finasteride, 5 mg

16 You are asked to evaluate gynecomastia in a 55-year-old man who was admitted to the medicine service with an asthma exacerbation. His medical history is notable for a left orchidopexy at age 7 years, as well as hypothyroidism treated with levothyroxine, 112 mcg daily.

On physical examination, he has diminished facial and axillary hair, bilateral nontender breast enlargement, microphallus, hypospadias, and testes measuring 3 mL bilaterally.

Laboratory test results:

Total testosterone = 805 ng/dL (300-900 ng/dL) (SI: 27.9 nmol/L [10.4-31.2 nmol/L])

LH = 26.2 mIU/mL (1.0-13.0 mIU/mL) (SI: 26.2 IU/L [1.0-13.0 IU/L])

FSH = 19.0 mIU/mL (1.0-9.0 mIU/mL) (SI: 19.0 IU/L [1.0-9.0 IU/L])

TSH = 3.5 mIU/L (0.5-5.0 mIU/L)

Which of the following is the most likely diagnosis?

A. Congenital adrenal hyperplasia due to 21-hydroxylase deficiency

B. Klinefelter syndrome with concomitant testosterone therapy

C. 5α-Reductase deficiency

D. Polyglandular autoimmune syndrome type 2

E. Partial androgen insensitivity syndrome

17 A 32-year-old man presents for evaluation of a 3-month history of tender gynecomastia. On questioning, he also endorses fatigue and decreased libido, although he can still get and sustain an erection. He has been taking finasteride for male-pattern balding.

On physical examination, his BMI is 22 kg/m² and pulse rate is 90 beats/min. His thyroid gland is normal in size with no palpable nodules. He has normal facial, axillary, and pubic hair. He has bilateral gynecomastia, which is tender to palpation. His phallus is normal, and testes are 15 mL bilaterally with no palpable masses.

Laboratory test results:

Total testosterone = 100 ng/dL (300-900 ng/dL) (SI: 3.5 nmol/L [10.4-31.2 nmol/L])

Estradiol = 140 pg/mL (10-40 pg/mL) (SI: 513.9 pmol/L [36.7-146.8 pmol/L])

FSH = 1.0 mIU/mL (1.0-13.0 mIU/mL) (SI: 1.0 IU/L [1.0-13.0 IU/L])

LH = 0.5 mIU/mL (1.0-9.0 mIU/mL) (SI: 0.5 IU/L [1.0-9.0 IU/L])

Prolactin = 25 ng/mL (4-23 ng/mL) (SI: 1.09 nmol/L [0.17-1.00 nmol/L])

Which of the following most likely explains his hormone profile?
- A. Hyperprolactinemia
- B. Decreased 5α-reductase activity due to finasteride
- C. Estrogen-secreting testicular tumor
- D. Hyperthyroidism

18 A 28-year-old man presents for evaluation of a 3-month history of tender gynecomastia. He is otherwise well with normal energy levels and sexual function. His medical history is remarkable for hepatitis C and premature male-pattern balding for which he takes finasteride, 1 mg daily.

On physical examination, his BMI is 22 kg/m² and pulse rate is 80 beats/min. His thyroid gland is not enlarged. He has tender bilateral gynecomastia. His phallus is normal, and testes are 15 mL bilaterally with no masses palpable.

Laboratory test results:
Total testosterone = 930 ng/dL (300-900 ng/dL)
(SI: 32.3 nmol/L [10.4-31.2 nmol/L])
Free testosterone (calculated) = 40 ng/dL
(9.0-30.0 ng/dL) (SI: 1.39 nmol/L
[0.31-1.04 nmol/L])
Estradiol = 90 pg/mL (10-40 pg/mL)
(SI: 330.4 pmol/L [36.7-146.8 pmol/L])
FSH = 0.5 mIU/mL (1.0-13.0 mIU/mL)
(SI: 0.5 IU/L [1.0-13.0 IU/L])
LH = 0.5 mIU/mL (1.0-9.0 mIU/mL)
(SI: 0.5 IU/L [1.0-9.0 IU/L])

Which of the following most likely explains this patient's hormone profile?
- A. Elevated SHBG due to hepatitis C
- B. Estrogen-secreting testicular tumor
- C. Decreased 5α-reductase activity due to finasteride
- D. Testosterone abuse
- E. Hyperthyroidism

Obesity and Lipids Board Review

Sangeeta R. Kashyap, MD

1 A 40-year-old woman with a longstanding history of class 2 obesity complicated by polycystic ovary syndrome and metabolic syndrome presents for follow-up. Over the past decade, she has made multiple unsuccessful attempts at weight loss with lifestyle modification. Two years ago, she underwent gastric bypass surgery and lost more than 60% of her excess body weight. At today's appointment, she describes experiencing afternoon fatigue, headache, and memory fog. On self-monitoring of blood glucose, she noted a value of 47 mg/dL (2.6 mmol/L), which resolved when she drank juice. She currently takes a multivitamin, calcium citrate, vitamin D, iron, and sublingual vitamin B_{12}. She states that her symptoms are worse after eating simple carbohydrates. She has no reflux or diarrhea. Her fasting glucose concentration is 98 mg/dL (5.4 mmol/L).

Which of the following strategies is the best next step in this patient's evaluation and management?
A. Advise her on appropriate dietary modification to manage dumping syndrome
B. Begin supplementation with pancreatic enzymes to treat symptoms of nutrient malabsorption
C. Begin treatment with a GLP-1 receptor agonist for neuroglycopenia related to postprandial hypoglycemia
D. Perform a mixed-meal tolerance test to diagnose hyperinsulinemic hypoglycemia after gastric bypass

2 On the basis of the clinical characteristics shown in the table, which of the listed patients with type 2 diabetes and a BMI of 44 kg/m² would be expected to achieve remission of diabetes (hemoglobin A_{1c} <5.7% [<39 mmol/mol] without the need for any diabetes medication) following bariatric surgery (see table)?

Answer	Patient age	Current hemoglobin A$_{1c}$	Duration of diabetes	Diabetes medication	Type of bariatric procedure
A.	68 years	8.2% (66 mmol/mol)	11 years	Basal insulin, 70 units; sitagliptin; metformin	Roux-en-Y gastric bypass
B.	48 years	7.0% (53 mmol/mol)	4 years	Metformin	Roux-en-Y gastric bypass
C.	55 years	6.2% (44 mmol/mol)	10 years	Basal insulin, 20 units	Sleeve gastrectomy
D.	32 years	7.0% (53 mmol/mol)	8 years	Metformin, glimepiride	Laparoscopic gastric banding

3 A 35-year-old woman with class 1 obesity (BMI = 31 kg/m²) and obstructive sleep apnea has lost 20 lb (9.1 kg) in 4 months by adhering to a Mediterranean meal plan of 1800 calories per day with 15% saturated fat intake and regular cardio training 5 times per week.

However, her weight has now plateaued, and in the past 2 weeks she has started to regain weight despite no changes to her caloric intake (which she monitors with an app) or exercise program.

In addition to reduced satiety and increased hunger, which of the following metabolic adaptations are present with diet-induced weight loss that promote weight regain?

Answer	Total daily expenditure	Resting metabolic rate	Exercise energy expenditure
A.	Reduced	Reduced	Reduced
B.	Increased	Reduced	Increased
C.	Stable	Reduced	Increased
D.	Reduced	Increased	Increased

4 A 32-year-old woman with class 1 obesity (BMI = 34 kg/m^2) complicated by hypertriglyceridemia and hypertension presents for a follow-up appointment. She has been adhering to a regimen of alternate-day fasting. She consumes only 25% of her calories on fast days and 125% of her calories on feast days. After 6 months following this meal plan, the patient has lost 6% of her total body weight.

Which of the following patterns of cardiometabolic benefits is expected following alternate-day fasting compared with daily caloric restriction?

Answer	Dietary adherence	Weight loss	Triglycerides	Blood pressure
A.	Improved	Increased	Decreased	Decreased
B.	Worsened	No difference	No difference	No difference
C.	Improved	No difference	No difference	No difference
D.	Improved	No difference	Increased	Decreased

5 A 48-year-old woman presents with dyslipidemia and elevated LDL-cholesterol concentrations. She has a history of diet-controlled hypertension, myocardial infarction, and ischemic stroke and no history of diabetes. Her fasting glucose concentration is 115 mg/dL (6.4 mmol/L), and hemoglobin A$_{1c}$ level is 5.9% (41 mmol/mol). There is a family history of coronary artery disease on her paternal side. Her primary care physician wants to initiate a statin, but the patient is worried that her blood glucose will get worse.

Which of the following is the best next step in this patient's management?
A. Start pravastatin, 10 mg daily, and reevaluate in 3 months
B. Start rosuvastatin, 10 mg daily, and reevaluate in 3 months
C. Start metformin and in 3 months add rosuvastatin, 10 mg daily
D. Start both metformin and pravastatin

6 A 54-year-old woman with class 1 obesity (BMI = 32 kg/m^2) and type 2 diabetes mellitus is interested in pursuing an intensive lifestyle modification program with meal replacement shakes and regular exercise training for weight loss to lower her cardiovascular risk. She has a history of metabolic syndrome with elevated triglyceride levels and hypertension and is taking atorvastatin and losartan. Her father had a myocardial infarction at age 60 years.

Based on data from randomized controlled trials evaluating the effect of intensive lifestyle modification vs standard care on cardiovascular risk in patients with type 2 diabetes, which of the following benefits can this patient expect over time?
A. Significant reduction in cardiovascular disease mortality
B. Significant reduction in physical fitness levels
C. Significant improvement in quality of life, depression, and sleep apnea
D. Substantial weight loss that peaks within the first year and is durable over 5 years
E. No change in hemoglobin A$_{1c}$ levels with weight loss

7 A 32-year-old man with a positive family history of cardiovascular disease but no known cardiovascular risk factors (normal fasting blood glucose, LDL cholesterol <130 mg/dL [<3.37 mmol/L], normal blood pressure, BMI = 26 kg/m^2) would like advice on which dietary factors have been shown to have favorable benefits on cardiovascular risk reduction.

Which of the following dietary factors have been shown in epidemiologic studies to have a neutral effect (ie, not protective) on cardiovascular risk?

A. Omega-3 fatty acids
B. Fiber
C. Plant stanols and sterols
D. Moderate alcohol consumption
E. Antioxidant supplements (ie, vitamins C and E) and folic acid

8 A 44-year-old woman with dyslipidemia and class 3 obesity (BMI = 42 kg/m²) is diagnosed with nonalcoholic fatty liver disease based on elevated liver transaminase levels and liver ultrasonography that shows steatosis. Transient elastography of the liver shows some evidence of fibrosis, and a subsequent liver biopsy demonstrates ballooning and lobular inflammation. Her hemoglobin A_{1c} level is 5.2% (33 mmol/mol), and her fasting plasma glucose concentration is 88 mg/dL (4.9 mmol/L).

Which of the following therapies would be best for managing this patient's nonalcoholic steatohepatitis?

A. Vitamin D, 4000 IU daily
B. Vitamin E, 800 IU daily
C. Pioglitazone, 30 mg daily
D. Atorvastatin, 40 mg daily
E. Metformin, 1500 mg daily

9 A 55-year-old man is referred for management of hyperlipidemia. He has type 2 diabetes mellitus (hemoglobin A_{1c} = 6.6% [49 mmol/mol]), hypertension, and coronary heart disease. He had a non–ST-elevation myocardial infarction 2 years ago. He most likely has heterozygous familial hyperlipidemia given his peak total cholesterol concentration of 382 mg/dL (9.89 mmol/L) and LDL-cholesterol concentration of 293 mg/dL (7.59 mmol/L). He had myalgias while taking atorvastatin, rosuvastatin, and simvastatin. He is currently tolerating pravastatin, 20 mg daily; ezetimibe, 10 mg daily; and niacin, 500 mg daily. He is very concerned about preventing a second cardiovascular disease event.

Laboratory test results:
Total cholesterol = 284 mg/dL (<200 mg/dL [optimal]) (SI: 7.36 mmol/L [<5.18 mmol/L])
LDL cholesterol = 200 mg/dL (<100 mg/dL [optimal]) (SI: 5.18 mmol/L [<2.59 mmol/L])
HDL cholesterol = 55 mg/dL (>60 mg/dL [optimal]) (SI: 1.42 mmol/L [>1.55 mmol/L])
Triglycerides = 300 mg/dL (<150 mg/dL [optimal]) (SI: 3.39 mmol/L [<1.70 mmol/L])

Which of the following should be recommended as the best next step in this patient's management?

A. Increase the niacin dosage to 1 g daily
B. Add alirocumab
C. Add fenofibrate
D. Perform lipopheresis
E. Increase the pravastatin dosage to 80 mg daily

10 A man with HIV infection who is currently treated with a protease inhibitor and antiviral medications is referred for mild lipoatrophy and results of a recent lipid panel.

Laboratory test results:
Total cholesterol = 280 mg/dL (<200 mg/dL [optimal]) (SI: 7.25 mmol/L [<5.18 mmol/L])
LDL cholesterol = 180 mg/dL (<100 mg/dL [optimal]) (SI: 4.66 mmol/L [<2.59 mmol/L])
HDL cholesterol = 30 mg/dL (>60 mg/dL [optimal]) (SI: 0.78 mmol/L [>1.55 mmol/L])
Triglycerides = 350 mg/dL (<150 mg/dL [optimal]) (SI: 3.96 mmol/L [<1.70 mmol/L])
Hemoglobin A_{1c} = 6.2% (4.0%-5.5%) (44 mmol/mol [20-38 mmol/mol])

Atorvastatin, 10 mg daily, is initiated, and his LDL-cholesterol concentration decreases to 120 mg/dL (3.11 mmol/L).

Which of the following is most likely to occur and prevent the use of a higher statin dosage in this patient?

A. Diabetes mellitus
B. Myositis
C. Inhibition of antiviral agents
D. Worsening of lipoatrophy
E. Hepatitis

11 A 30-year-old woman with systemic lupus erythematosus is referred for dyslipidemia. Her current medications include prednisone, 20 mg daily; hydrochlorothiazide; lisinopril; metoprolol; and infliximab.

Laboratory test results:
   Total cholesterol = 300 mg/dL (<200 mg/dL [optimal]) (SI: 7.77 mmol/L [<5.18 mmol/L])
   HDL cholesterol = 30 mg/dL (>60 mg/dL [optimal]) (SI: 0.78 mmol/L [>1.55 mmol/L])
   Triglycerides = 760 mg/dL (<150 mg/dL [optimal]) (SI: 8.59 mmol/L [<1.70 mmol/L])
   LDL cholesterol cannot be estimated

You are concerned that medications could be contributing to her dyslipidemia. Which of the following adjustments should be recommended?
   A. Switch prednisone to dexamethasone
   B. Switch lisinopril to losartan
   C. Switch hydrochlorothiazide to a loop diuretic
   D. Switch metoprolol to amlodipine

12 A 68-year-old woman is referred for further treatment of hypercholesterolemia. She had a myocardial infarction 1 year ago and was discharged from the hospital on an atorvastatin dosage of 80 mg daily, which was decreased to 40 mg daily 3 months later due to myalgias. She subsequently tried varying dosages of rosuvastatin, simvastatin, and lovastatin, all of which caused myalgias. She is currently taking ezetimibe, 10 mg daily, and her cardiologist wants to add the PCSK9 inhibitor evolocumab to reduce her cardiovascular risk, but she is concerned about potential adverse effects.

Which of the following is the most likely adverse effect she would experience with PCSK9 inhibitor therapy?
   A. Cognitive dysfunction
   B. Elevation of liver enzymes
   C. Myalgias
   D. Skin irritation/rash

13 A 42-year-old man with a peak lifetime BMI of 48 kg/m² had laparoscopic gastric bypass in another state 2 years ago, after which he lost 60 lb (27.3 kg). Eight months after his surgery, his employer transferred him to a location out of the country, so he was unable to follow-up with his bariatric surgeon over the last year. He is home on vacation, and he comes to clinic for a check-up. He takes no medications and relates that he was taking his vitamin supplements postoperatively, but he ran out more than 6 months ago. He has developed numbness and tingling in his feet and hands. He also thinks he has a middle ear problem after the long flight home because he feels off-balance. Routine bloodwork indicates mild anemia.

Which of the following deficiencies does this patient most likely have?
   A. Vitamin B_{12}
   B. Folate
   C. Thiamine
   D. Zinc
   E. Copper

14 A 19-year-old woman accompanied by her parents seeks help managing severe obesity that began in the first year of life. Her growth rate was faster than that of other children her age, and she always appeared to have "big bones." She underwent normal puberty. Her school performance has been normal, although she struggles with depression. Her current BMI is 48 kg/m².

Which of the following genetic syndromes of obesity does she most likely have?
   A. Prader-Willi syndrome
   B. Melanocortin 4 receptor (*MC4R*) pathogenic variant
   C. Leptin deficiency
   D. Leptin receptor deficiency

15 A 46-year-old woman presents for medically supervised weight loss with a meal replacement program. She has migraines, hypertension, metabolic syndrome, hyperlipidemia, depression, and kidney stones. She has had a cholecystectomy for cholelithiasis.

On physical examination, her height is 65 in (165.1 cm) and weight is 205 lb (93.2 kg) (BMI = 34.1 kg/m²).

She begins a 500-kcal, low-fat, high-fiber diet and regular exercise (walking 10,000 steps daily). She loses 12 lb (5.5 kg) in 3 months, 6 lb (2.7 kg) in the following 3 months, and then plateaus at 190 lb (86.4 kg).

Current medications are lisinopril, metformin, atorvastatin, escitalopram, and norethindrone.

Her current weight is 187 lb (85 kg) (BMI = 31.1 kg/m²), and waist circumference is 38 in (96.5 cm). Her blood pressure is 160/84 mm Hg, and pulse rate is 72 beats/min.

Given her medical problems and current medications, which of the following weight-loss medications would be best?

A. Orlistat
B. Liraglutide
C. Phentermine/topiramate
D. Topiramate
E. Naltrexone/bupropion

16 A 43-year-old man seeks help to address high cholesterol. After experiencing an episode of angina, he had a positive treadmill stress test.

On physical examination, he has a firm papulonodular rash on both elbows and orange-yellow linear xanthomas of his palmar creases.

Fasting lipid panel:
  Total cholesterol = 325 mg/dL (<200 mg/dL [optimal]) (SI: 8.42 mmol/L [<5.18 mmol/L])
  LDL cholesterol = 227 mg/dL (<100 mg/dL [optimal]) (SI: 5.88 mmol/L [<2.59 mmol/L])
  HDL cholesterol = 30 mg/dL (>60 mg/dL [optimal]) (SI: 0.78 mmol/L [>1.55 mmol/L])
  Triglycerides = 340 mg/dL (<150 mg/dL [optimal]) (SI: 3.84 mmol/L [<1.70 mmol/L])

Which of the following abnormalities does this man most likely have?

A. ABCA1 deficiency
B. LDL-receptor deficiency
C. Apolipoprotein E2/E2
D. Apolipoprotein C2 deficiency
E. Overproduction of apolipoprotein B

17 A 55-year-old man is anxious about his cardiovascular risk. He exercises regularly, has a blood pressure of 115/65 mm Hg, and avoids high-fat, high-cholesterol foods. His father smoked 2 packs of cigarettes daily until having a myocardial infarction at age 62 years.

Laboratory test results:
  Total cholesterol = 190 mg/dL (<200 mg/dL [optimal]) (SI: 4.92 mmol/L [<5.18 mmol/L])
  LDL cholesterol = 105 mg/dL (<100 mg/dL [optimal]) (SI: 2.72 mmol/L [<2.59 mmol/L])
  HDL cholesterol = 70 mg/dL (>60 mg/dL [optimal]) (SI: 1.81 mmol/L [>1.55 mmol/L])
  Triglycerides = 75 mg/dL (<150 mg/dL [optimal]) (SI: 0.85 mmol/L [<1.70 mmol/L])

Which additional test could be ordered to best assess this man's cardiovascular disease risk?

A. Coronary artery calcium score
B. LDL particle size distribution
C. Apolipoprotein B
D. Apolipoprotein A1 levels
E. HOMA-IR (homeostatic model assessment for insulin resistance)

18 A 45-year-old woman with rheumatoid arthritis is referred for hypercholesterolemia and statin-induced myalgias. Creatine kinase has never been documented to be elevated. Her physician has tried treating her with daily simvastatin, atorvastatin, and rosuvastatin.

Laboratory test results:
  Total cholesterol = 250 mg/dL (<200 mg/dL [optimal]) (SI: 6.48 mmol/L [<5.18 mmol/L])
  LDL cholesterol = 160 mg/dL (<100 mg/dL [optimal]) (SI: 4.14 mmol/L [<2.59 mmol/L])
  HDL cholesterol = 35 mg/dL (>60 mg/dL [optimal]) (SI: 0.91 mmol/L [>1.55 mmol/L])
  Triglycerides = 250 mg/dL (<150 mg/dL [optimal]) (SI: 2.83 mmol/L [<1.70 mmol/L])

Which of the following is the best next step in this patient's care?

A. Start atorvastatin plus coenzyme Q10

B. Start rosuvastatin once weekly

C. Start red yeast rice

D. Start fish oil

E. Measure creatine phosphokinase

19 A 30-year-old woman seeks assistance with weight loss. Her height is 62 in (157.5 cm), and weight is 174 lb (79.1 kg) (BMI = 31.8 kg/m²). She is otherwise healthy and takes no medications. She has recently started going to the gym 3 times a week for a combination of aerobic exercise and resistance training. Many people at the gym are following a ketogenic diet and she would like to know what to expect if she tries this diet.

Which of the following is a potential adverse effect of a ketogenic diet?

A. Cataract formation

B. Glucosuria

C. Eruptive xanthoma

D. Kidney stones

20 A 39-year-old man seeks help treating elevated cholesterol. His father died of a myocardial infarction at age 29 years and his brother developed angina at age 32 years. The patient has intermittent chest pain that is consistent with angina, but he has not had any diagnostic testing. He takes atorvastatin, 80 mg daily, and on this medication his fasting LDL-cholesterol concentration is 245 mg/dL (6.35 mmol/L).

On physical examination, he has thickened Achilles tendons and nodules on the extensor tendons of his hands and corneal arcus.

Which of the following medications should be added to his regimen as the best next step?

A. Ezetimibe

B. Fenofibrate

C. Evolocumab

D. Niacin

21 A 45-year-old man with hyperlipidemia seeks advice for secondary prevention of cardiovascular disease. He had a myocardial infarction 6 months ago complicated by a stroke. He does not smoke cigarettes. He started exercising, and initiated a high-intensity statin (atorvastatin, 80 mg daily). His LDL-cholesterol concentration decreased from 174 mg/dL (4.51 mmol/L) to less than 100 mg/dL (<2.59 mmol/L). Despite aggressive risk factor modification, he had a second heart attack 3 months ago. He had a twin brother who died suddenly of a myocardial infarction last year at age 44 years.

On physical examination, his blood pressure is 126/74 mm Hg and pulse rate is 72 beats/min. BMI is 27 kg/m², and waist circumference is 36 in (91.4 cm).

Laboratory test results:
Total cholesterol = 155 mg/dL (<200 mg/dL [optimal]) (SI: 4.01 mmol/L [<5.18 mmol/L])
LDL cholesterol = 85 mg/dL (<100 mg/dL [optimal]) (SI: 2.20 mmol/L [<2.59 mmol/L])
HDL cholesterol = 44 mg/dL (>60 mg/dL [optimal]) (SI: 1.14 mmol/L [>1.55 mmol/L])
Triglycerides = 128 mg/dL (<150 mg/dL [optimal]) (SI: 1.45 mmol/L [<1.70 mmol/L])
Hemoglobin A_{1c} = 5.3% (4.0%-5.6%) (34 mmol/mol [20-38 mmol/mol])
TSH = 2.24 mIU/L (0.5-5.0 mIU/L)
ALT = 24 U/L (10-40 U/L) (SI: 0.40 μkat/L [0.17-0.67 μkat/L])

Which of the following most likely explains his high cardiovascular disease risk despite good response to statin therapy?

A. Apolipoprotein A1 deficiency

B. Elevated apolipoprotein B

C. ABCA1 deficiency

D. Elevated lipoprotein (a)

22 A 52-year-old man presents for aggressive treatment of dyslipidemia. There is a strong history of cardiovascular disease in male family members (in their 50s). His brother had a myocardial infarction at age 56 years, and his father died of a myocardial infarction at age

52 years. The patient has had type 2 diabetes for 15 years and takes metformin, once-daily insulin glargine, and once-weekly semaglutide. He also has hypertension, but his blood pressure is well controlled on lisinopril. His BMI is 38 kg/m².

He has been on atorvastatin, 80 mg daily, for the last 7 years and added ezetimibe, 10 mg daily, 3 years ago.

Current laboratory test results:
Hemoglobin A_{1c} = 7.4% (4.0%-5.6%) (57 mmol/mol [20-38 mmol/mol])
Total cholesterol = 179 mg/dL (<200 mg/dL [optimal]) (SI: 4.64 mmol/L [<5.18 mmol/L])
LDL cholesterol = 86 mg/dL (<100 mg/dL [optimal]) (SI: 2.23 mmol/L [<2.59 mmol/L])
HDL cholesterol = 39 mg/dL (>60 mg/dL [optimal]) (SI: 1.01 mmol/L [>1.55 mmol/L])
Triglycerides = 270 mg/dL (<150 mg/dL [optimal]) (SI: 3.05 mmol/L [<1.70 mmol/L])
ALT = 52 U/L (10-40 U/L) (SI: 0.87 μkat/L [0.17-0.67 μkat/L])

Which of the following is the best next step to further reduce this patient's risk of cardiovascular disease?
A. No change in current therapy
B. Gemfibrozil, 600 mg twice daily
C. Icosapent ethyl, 2 g twice daily
D. Fenofibrate, 160 mg daily
E. Niacin ER, 3 g daily

23 A 52-year-old man presents with class 3 obesity, BMI of 48 kg/m², type 2 diabetes mellitus (hemoglobin A_{1c} = 8.2% [66 mmol/mol]), and nonalcoholic fatty liver disease. His American Heart Association 10-year risk of cardiovascular disease is 16%. His primary care physician recommended starting atorvastatin, 40 mg daily. His liver transaminase levels (ALT, AST) are chronically elevated because of fatty liver disease. He is concerned about taking atorvastatin, as he has read that statins can cause liver injury.

Laboratory test results (sample drawn while fasting):
LDL cholesterol = 164 mg/dL (<100 mg/dL [optimal]) (SI: 4.25 mmol/L [<2.59 mmol/L])
Triglycerides = 242 mg/dL (<150 mg/dL [optimal]) (SI: 2.73 mmol/L [<1.70 mmol/L])
ALT = 88 U/L (10-40 U/L) (SI: 1.47 μkat/L [0.17-0.67 μkat/L])
AST = 76 U/L (20-48 U/L) (SI: 1.27 μkat/L [0.33-0.80 μkat/L])

In addition to dietary counseling, which of the following treatments is the best approach to this patient's management?
A. Atorvastatin
B. Omega-3 fatty acids
C. Fenofibrate
D. Ezetimibe
E. Niacin

24 A 32-year-old woman with hypertriglyceridemia is planning to have a second child. She had gestational diabetes mellitus during her first pregnancy with subsequent progression to type 2 diabetes after delivery. She has been on a regimen of metformin, sitagliptin, and gemfibrozil, which has maintained her triglyceride concentration around 300 mg/dL (3.39 mmol/L). She is seeking guidance regarding her lipid medication.

Laboratory test results (drawn while patient is off medications):
Total cholesterol = 300 mg/dL (<200 mg/dL [optimal]) (SI: 7.77 mmol/L [<5.18 mmol/L])
Triglycerides = 315 mg/dL (<150 mg/dL [optimal]) (SI: 3.56 mmol/L [<1.70 mmol/L])
HDL cholesterol = 31 mg/dL (>60 mg/dL [optimal]) (SI: 0.80 mmol/L [>1.55 mmol/L])
Fasting glucose = 105 mg/dL (70-99 mg/dL) (SI: 5.8 mmol/L [3.9-5.5 mmol/L])
Hemoglobin A_{1c} = 7.0% (4.0%-5.6%) (53 mmol/mol [20-38 mmol/mol])

Which of the following is the most reasonable strategy now?
   A. Continue gemfibrozil
   B. Change gemfibrozil to fenofibrate
   C. Stop gemfibrozil
   D. Change gemfibrozil to a statin

25 A 46-year-old woman presents for medically supervised weight loss with a meal replacement program. She has migraines, hypertension, type 2 diabetes mellitus, hyperlipidemia, depression, and kidney stones. She has had a cholecystectomy for cholelithiasis. Current medications are lisinopril, metoprolol, metformin, atorvastatin, escitalopram, and norethindrone.

On physical examination, her height is 65 in (165.1 cm) and weight is 205 lb (93.2 kg) (BMI = 34.1 kg/m^2). Her blood pressure is 162/88 mm Hg, and pulse rate is 76 beats/min. Waist circumference is 40 in (101.5 cm).

Of the patient's medications, which of the following is considered weight promoting?
   A. Lisinopril
   B. Metformin
   C. Metoprolol
   D. Atorvastatin
   E. Escitalopram

26 A 67-year-old woman presents for help with weight loss. After retiring last year, she focused on improving her health. Her medical history is notable for prediabetes, nonalcoholic fatty liver disease, migraines, and glaucoma. Her peak weight was 270 lb (122.7 kg) (BMI = 43 kg/m^2). She lost 25 lb (11.4 kg) by increasing physical activity (30 minutes walking daily) and participating in an app-based weight-loss program. She was able to lower her BMI to 39.5 kg/m^2. She then regained 10 lb (4.5 kg), which prompted her primary care physician to prescribe phentermine; she then lost 15 lb (6.8 kg) over 6 months. She is interested in combination therapy with topiramate, which she has heard is even more effective when used with phentermine.

Which of her current medications would preclude her from starting combination therapy with topiramate?
   A. Metoprolol
   B. Travoprost ophthalmic solution
   C. Pioglitazone
   D. Metformin

27 A 36-year-old man with obesity (BMI = 38 kg/m^2), dyslipidemia, and type 2 diabetes mellitus (hemoglobin A$_{1c}$ = 7.4% [57 mmol/mol]) has been referred to a hepatologist because of chronically elevated liver transaminase concentrations (ALT = 120 U/L [2.00 μkat/L], AST = 90 U/L [1.50 μkat/L]). He has an appointment in endocrinology after a liver biopsy diagnoses nonalcoholic steatohepatitis (NASH) with stage 3 fibrosis. He has been informed that he is at high risk for cirrhosis and is very distressed. He wants to know what he should do to avoid liver cirrhosis. The hepatologist prescribed pioglitazone.

Which of the following treatments offers the greatest chance of NASH regression over the next year?
   A. Lifestyle modification to achieve 10% weight loss
   B. Exenatide, 10 mg daily
   C. Canagliflozin, 100 mg daily
   D. Metformin, 500 mg twice daily

28 A 48-year-old man with obesity seeks advice about his diet. He has a family history of obesity, premature coronary disease, and type 2 diabetes mellitus. He wants to know which diet would be best for him.

Which of the following dietary approaches has been shown in randomized controlled trials to reduce the risk of cardiovascular disease?
   A. Fat-restricted, balanced calorie-deficit diet
   B. Mediterranean diet
   C. Low-carbohydrate diet
   D. High-protein diet
   E. No specific dietary pattern has been shown to be superior to others in long-term studies

Pituitary Board Review

Laurence Katznelson, MD

1 A 37-year-old woman with ACTH-dependent Cushing syndrome has an MRI finding of a 4-mm left-sided sellar lesion, adjacent to the cavernous sinus. The ACTH concentration is 58 pg/mL (12.8 pmol/L). Inferior petrosal sinus catheterization shows central ACTH hypersecretion, and there is lateralization to the left side. The patient undergoes transsphenoidal surgery, and the left-sided lesion is determined to be an adenoma, subsequently staining positive for ACTH. The adjacent dura has tumor involvement as well. Postoperatively, the serum cortisol fails to normalize. Reoperation with left hemihypophysectomy does not result in further cortisol lowering, and no tumor is detected.

Laboratory test results:
Hemoglobin A_{1c} = 7.5% (4.0%-5.6%)
(58 mmol/mol [20-38 mmol/mol])
Fasting ACTH = 28 pg/mL (10-60 pg/mL)
(SI: 6.2 pmol/L [2.2-13.2 pmol/L])
Cortisol = 26.4 µg/dL (5-25 µg/dL)
(SI: 728.3 nmol/L [137.9-689.7 nmol/L])

Medical therapy is initiated, and over the subsequent weeks her cushingoid features improve and her plasma glucose level normalizes. Her current plasma ACTH concentration is 42 pg/mL (9.2 pmol/L) and morning cortisol concentration is 11.5 µg/dL (317.3 mmol/L). However, a few months later she notes bothersome hair growth on her face and periareolar areas.

Which of the following medications is she most likely receiving?
A. Mifepristone
B. Ketoconazole
C. Pasireotide
D. Osilodrostat
E. Mitotane

2 A 39-year-old man presents with acromegaly. He previously underwent transsphenoidal surgery for a macroadenoma, and he has residual disease in the left cavernous sinus. His postoperative IGF-1 concentration was 932 ng/mL (106-277 ng/mL) (SI: 122.1 nmol/L [13.9-36.3 nmol/L]). He was started on lanreotide depot, 90 mg monthly, which normalized his IGF-1 level. He asks whether he may be a candidate for the oral octreotide capsule.

Which of the following outcomes is expected if he switches to the oral octreotide capsule?
A. Increased gastrointestinal complaints
B. Increased GH levels
C. Increased glucose levels
D. Maintenance of normal IGF-1 levels (in most patients)
E. Increased IGF-1 levels (in most patients)

3 A 43-year-old woman presents with weight loss, tremor, palpitations, and sweating. She has had mild frontal headaches and describes normal vision.

Laboratory test results:
Free T_4 = 2.8 ng/dL (0.8-1.8 ng/dL)
(SI: 36.0 pmol/L [10.30-23.17 pmol/L])
Total T_3 = 413 ng/dL (70-200 ng/dL)
(SI: 6.36 nmol/L [1.08-3.08 nmol/L])

TSH = 1.9 mIU/L (0.5-5.0 mIU/L)
Prolactin = 28 ng/mL (4-30 ng/mL)
(SI: 1.22 nmol/L [0.17-1.30 nmol/L])

A radioiodine scan reveals 50% uptake in a homogeneous pattern in the thyroid gland. Brain MRI reveals a 2.1-cm pituitary adenoma invading the cavernous sinus.

Which of the following is the best next step in this patient's evaluation?
   A. Serum α-subunit measurement
   B. Somatostatin receptor scintography with a DOTATATE scan
   C. Genetic testing for pathogenic variants in the thyroid hormone receptor gene
   D. Assessment for heterophile antibodies to TSH
   E. Thyroid-stimulating immunoglobulin measurement

4 A 35-year-old man with a history of hypopituitarism after surgical removal of a nonfunctioning pituitary tumor is interested in fertility. He has a 7-year-old son. A 1.7-cm nonsecretory pituitary macroadenoma was detected incidentally at age 32 years, and he underwent transsphenoidal surgery. He has panhypopituitarism and currently takes hormone replacement with levothyroxine, hydrocortisone, GH, and intramuscular testosterone ester. He was taking injectable testosterone esters, although he discontinued them 3 months ago. He feels well and states he has normal libido and erectile function.

On physical examination, he is well virilized. Testes are 8-mL bilaterally and have normal consistency. Two semen analyses have documented azoospermia.

Laboratory test results:
   Serum testosterone = 78 ng/dL (300-900 ng/dL)
   (SI: 2.71 nmol/L [10.4-31.2 nmol/L])
   LH = 0.9 mIU/mL (1.0-9.0 mIU/L)
   (SI: 0.9 IU/L [1.0-9.0 IU/L])
   FSH = 1.1 mIU/mL (1.0-13.0 mIU/L)
   (SI: 1.1 IU/L [1.0-13.0 IU/L])

Which of the following is the best next step in this patient's management?
   A. Start hCG injections, 3 times weekly
   B. Start hCG injections, 3 times weekly, and FSH injections, twice weekly
   C. Refer for microdissection testicular sperm extraction
   D. Start clomiphene citrate
   E. Suggest he consider adoption

5 A 19-year-old man presents with delay in puberty and frontal headaches. In retrospect, he has had poor energy, frequent urination, increased thirst, and a 46-lb (20.9-kg) weight gain over the past 2 years. Testing reveals a prolactin concentration of 42.7 ng/mL (1.9 nmol/L) (similar on dilution), panhypopituitarism, and diabetes insipidus. He is found to have a 2.3-cm cystic sellar mass with suprasellar extension, abutting the optic chiasm. An ophthalmologist identifies bilateral homonymous hemianopsia.

Which of the following is the most likely diagnosis?
   A. Gonadotroph adenoma
   B. Prolactinoma
   C. Craniopharyngioma
   D. Silent corticotroph adenoma
   E. Langerhans cell histiocytosis

6 An internist refers a 26-year-old man for suspected diabetes insipidus. He reports a constant sense of thirst, and he believes he drinks more fluids and urinates more often than other people.

Laboratory test results:
   Serum sodium = 138 mEq/L (136-142 mEq/L)
   (SI: 138 mmol/L [136-142 mmol/L])
   Serum osmolality = 270 mOsm/kg
   (275-295 mOsm/kg) (SI: 270 mmol/kg
   [275-295 mmol/kg])
   Plasma glucose (fasting) = 89 mg/dL (70-99 mg/dL)
   (SI: 4.9 mmol/L [3.9-5.5 mmol/L])
   24-Hour urine total volume = 3.5 L/24 h
   Urine osmolality = 70 mOsm/kg
   (150-1150 mOsm/kg) (SI: 70 mmol/kg
   [150-1150 mmol/kg])

A fluid-deprivation test over 4 hours results in a rise in serum sodium from to 141 mEq/L to 145 mEq/L and no change in serum osmolality. The osmolality of urine collections over this period increases from 70 mOsm/kg to 525 mOsm/kg.

On the basis of these results, which of the following would be the most effective therapy for this patient?
  A. Amiloride
  B. Thiazide diuretic
  C. Indomethacin
  D. Referral for psychiatric evaluation
  E. DDAVP (desmopressin)

7 Cushing disease is diagnosed in a 33-year-old woman. MRI shows a 4-mm pituitary lesion. Following transsphenoidal surgery, her morning cortisol concentration is 1.2 µg/dL (33.1 nmol/L), and she is discharged home on glucocorticoids, which are weaned over 4 months. She loses weight, and her cushingoid appearance resolves over the next 6 months. Approximately 18 months after surgery, she returns for a clinic visit, as she is concerned that the Cushing syndrome has recurred. Her blood pressure is 133/88 mm Hg. She has modest moon facies, facial plethora, and modest supraclavicular fat.

She undergoes a 1-mg overnight dexamethasone-suppression test, and the morning cortisol concentration is 1.2 µg/dL (5-25 µg/dL) (SI: 33.1 nmol/L [137.9-689.7 nmol/L]). Other laboratory values:
  Morning ACTH = 35 pg/mL (10-60 pg/mL)
    (SI: 7.7 pmol/L [2.2-13.2 pmol/L])
  Free T_4 = 1.4 ng/dL (0.8-1.8 ng/dL)
    (SI: 18.0 pmol/L [10.30-23.17 pmol/L])

Which of the following is the next test to perform to evaluate for Cushing syndrome?
  A. Late-night salivary cortisol measurement
  B. Pituitary MRI
  C. Morning serum cortisol measurement in 6 months
  D. 24-Hour urinary free cortisol excretion
  E. Another ACTH measurement

8 A 53-year-old woman has a classic history and examination findings of Cushing syndrome. Her urinary free cortisol excretion is 3-fold above the reference range, and her ACTH and morning cortisol concentrations are 2-fold above their respective reference ranges. On MRI, her pituitary is of normal size, and there is no focal lesion. Inferior petrosal sinus sampling using corticotropin-releasing hormone stimulation shows a 1.5-fold central step-up in ACTH levels compared with peripheral levels, but no clear lateralization.

Which of the following should be performed as the next management step?
  A. Corticotropin-releasing hormone test
  B. Dexamethasone corticotropin-releasing hormone test
  C. Chest CT
  D. Another inferior petrosal sinus sampling
  E. High-dose dexamethasone-suppression test

9 A 33-year-old woman has developed Cushing syndrome during her second month of pregnancy. She has hypertension, diabetes mellitus, hirsutism, and wide, purple striae on her abdomen.

Laboratory test results:
  Serum cortisol (8 AM) = 37 µg/dL (5-25 µg/dL)
    (SI: 1020.8 nmol/L [137-39-689.7 nmol/L])
  ACTH = 129 pg/mL (10-60 pg/mL)
    (SI: 28.4 pmol/L [2.2-13.2 pmol/L])
  Urinary free cortisol = 475 µg/24 h (4-50 µg/24 h)
    (SI: 1311 nmol/d [11-138 nmol/d])

MRI shows a 6-mm pituitary adenoma.

Which of the following treatment options is absolutely contraindicated?
  A. Mifepristone
  B. Metyrapone
  C. Transsphenoidal surgery in the second trimester
  D. Pasireotide
  E. Cabergoline

10 A 44-year-old man is evaluated for persistent fatigue. He was previously diagnosed with a seizure disorder and craniopharyngioma, and he underwent transsphenoidal surgery followed by fractionated radiation therapy 7 years ago. He developed hypopituitarism, and he has been taking levothyroxine, 88 mcg orally daily; hydrocortisone, 25 mg orally daily; transdermal testosterone, 5 g daily; and desmopressin, 0.3 mg orally twice daily. He notes difficulty with short-term memory and has been unable to function at work due to poor attention span. Family history and personal medical history are unremarkable (aside from his craniopharyngioma).

On physical examination, he appears fatigued and slightly depressed. His blood pressure is 115/84 mm Hg, pulse rate is 84 beats/min, and BMI is 29 kg/m². He has increased abdominal girth, but examination findings are otherwise normal.

Laboratory test results:
Free T_4 = 1.6 ng/dL (0.8-1.8 ng/dL)
  (SI: 20.6 pmol/L [10.30-23.17 pmol/L])
Prolactin = 7.6 ng/mL (4-23 ng/mL)
  (SI: 0.33 nmol/L [0.17-1.00 nmol/L])
Testosterone = 320 ng/dL (300-900 ng/dL)
  (SI: 11.1 nmol/L [10.4-31.2 nmol/L])
IGF-1 = 115 ng/dL (98-261 ng/mL)
  (SI: 15.1 nmol/L [12.8-34.2 nmol/L])
Comprehensive chemistry panel, normal
Complete blood cell count, normal

Which of the following is the best next step in his endocrine management?
A. Refer to a psychiatrist for management of depression
B. Perform a macimorelin-stimulation test to assess GH levels
C. Measure random GH level
D. Perform an insulin tolerance test

11 An 18-year-old girl had a craniopharyngioma resected at age 15 years with resultant panhypopituitarism. She has been treated with levothyroxine, hydrocortisone, and GH. An oral contraceptive was recently started for estrogen and progesterone replacement. Over the past year, she has only grown 1 cm and her height is now 64 in (162.6 cm). A recent hand and wrist film shows almost complete epiphyseal closure. After 1 month off GH therapy, her IGF-1 concentration is −2.7 standard deviations.

If she does not continue GH treatment, which of the following is most likely?
A. Significant weight gain
B. Glucose intolerance
C. Reduced mortality rate
D. Increased lean body mass
E. Decreased peak bone mass

12 A 52-year-old woman presents with acromegaly. Her IGF-1 concentration is 1226 ng/mL (84-233 ng/mL) (SI: 160.6 nmol/L [11.0-30.5 nmol/L]), and she has a 2.5-cm pituitary macroadenoma with invasion of the left cavernous sinus. She undergoes transsphenoidal surgery, and her 12-week postoperative IGF-1 concentration is 968 ng/mL (126.8 nmol/L). MRI shows 7.5-mm residual disease in the cavernous sinus. She has persistent headaches, arthralgias, and sweating. She is postmenopausal. Octreotide LAR is initiated with a dosage increase to 30 mg intramuscular monthly. On this dosage, her IGF-1 concentration is 770 ng/mL (100.9 nmol/L). Her symptoms persist. MRI findings remain unchanged.

Which of the following options would be most effective in controlling her acromegaly within the next 6 months?
A. Increase the octreotide LAR dosage to 40 mg every 28 days
B. Stop octreotide LAR and switch to cabergoline
C. Add pegvisomant
D. Proceed with radiation therapy
E. Refer for reoperation

13 A 52-year-old woman has had hypopituitarism for 10 years after resection of a nonfunctioning pituitary adenoma. She has been treated with levothyroxine, hydrocortisone, a low-dosage oral contraceptive pill, and daily GH injections. Because her sister recently developed breast cancer, the patient has decided to stop her oral contraceptive. During the next month, she notices progressive joint aches and sweating.

Which of the following is the best next step for management to relieve these new symptoms?

A. Increase the levothyroxine dosage
B. Decrease the GH dosage
C. Increase the GH dosage
D. Increase the hydrocortisone dosage
E. Decrease the hydrocortisone dosage

14 A 29-year-old man is referred to restart GH replacement therapy. He states that he received GH injections for many years as a child and stopped when he completed growth at age 18 years. He has also taken thyroid hormone replacement since age 12 years. During his 20s, he has noted persistent fatigue, and he has had difficulty losing weight. He had a concussion at age 16 years while playing football.

On physical examination, he has increased abdominal girth, normal virilization, and 25-mL testes bilaterally.

Laboratory testing reveals a serum IGF-1 concentration of 60 ng/mL (117-321 ng/mL) (SI: 7.9 nmol/L [15.3-42.1 nmol/L]). Following a glucagon-stimulation test, the peak GH value is 0.8 ng/mL (0.8 µg/L).

MRI is shown (*see image*).

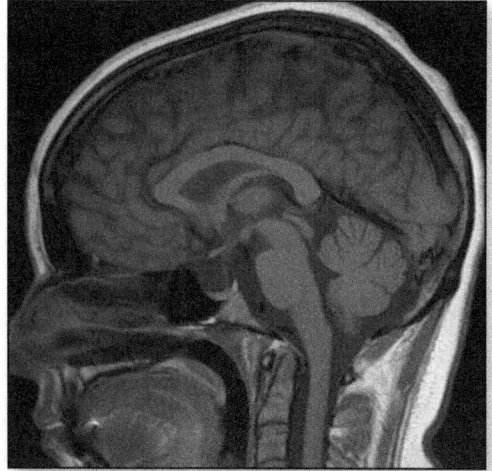

Which of the following is the most likely cause of these biochemical findings?

A. Pathogenic variant in the *PROP1* gene
B. Trauma-induced pituitary infarction
C. Pathogenic variant in the *TBX19* gene (*TPIT*)
D. Langerhans cell histiocytosis
E. Hemochromatosis

15 A 37-year-old woman presents with a sellar mass and headache. She is G2,P2 and had an uneventful pregnancy until her complicated delivery 3 days ago. During the delivery, she had a massive hemorrhage and received 4 units of packed red blood cells. She had hypotension, treated with saline infusion. Headache prompted an urgent MRI, which revealed large, heterogeneous sellar contents without chiasmal compression.

On physical examination, she appears uncomfortable. Her vital signs are stable. Examination findings, including those from neurologic examination, are normal.

Which of the following is the first manifestation of this disorder?

A. Inability to lactate
B. Low free T_4 concentration
C. Weight gain
D. Absent menses

16 A 44-year-old woman is diagnosed with a 3.2-cm clinically nonfunctioning pituitary macroadenoma that is causing chiasmal compression. Her preoperative evaluation reveals no evidence of acromegaly, Cushing disease, or salt and water imbalance. Her laboratory testing shows normal pituitary function. She undergoes transsphenoidal surgery, which is uneventful. On postoperative day 1, she develops polyuria and polydipsia, and the following laboratory values are documented:

Serum sodium = 152 mEq/L (136-142 mEq/L)
 (SI: 152 mmol/L [136-142 mmol/L])
Urine osmolality = 110 mOsm/kg
 (150-1150 mOsm/kg) (SI: 110 mmol/kg
 [150-1150 mmol/kg])

She is treated with DDAVP, 0.1 mg orally as needed, and symptoms resolve by postoperative day 3, so DDAVP is discontinued. She presents to the emergency department on postoperative day 7 and describes nausea and marked fatigue. She is admitted to the intensive care unit due to the following laboratory test results:

> Serum sodium = 121 mEq/L (SI: 121 mmol/L)
> Urine osmolality = 373 mOsm/kg
>   (SI: 373 mmol/kg)

On physical examination, she appears uncomfortable. Her blood pressure is 104/72 mm Hg. Her weight is 130 lb (59 kg).

Which of the following will correct her serum sodium most effectively?

   A. Restrict free water intake to less than 1500 mL/24 h
   B. Start demeclocycline
   C. Start tolvaptan
   D. Start intravenous furosemide
   E. Start hypertonic saline at a rate of 5 mL/h

17 A 23-year-old woman was previously well and had regular menses. After discontinuing barrier contraception, she became pregnant within 2 months. Her pregnancy went well, but during her third trimester she developed headaches and mild weakness.

On physical examination, she is an ill-appearing woman. Her blood pressure is 96/68 mm Hg, and pulse rate is 74 beats/min. Her uterus is appropriately sized for 36 weeks' gestation.

Laboratory test results:

> Free T$_4$ = 0.9 ng/dL (0.8-1.8 ng/dL)
>   (SI: 11.6 pmol/L [10.3-23.2 pmol/L])
> TSH = 1.3 mIU/L (0.5-5.0 mIU/L)
> Prolactin = 198 ng/mL (4-30 ng/mL)
>   (SI: 8.61 nmol/L [0.17-1.30 nmol/L])

Noncontrast MRI shows diffusely enlarged sellar contents extending above the sella and impinging the optic chiasm (*see image*). A Goldmann visual field examination shows a small degree of bilateral superior and temporal visual field defects.

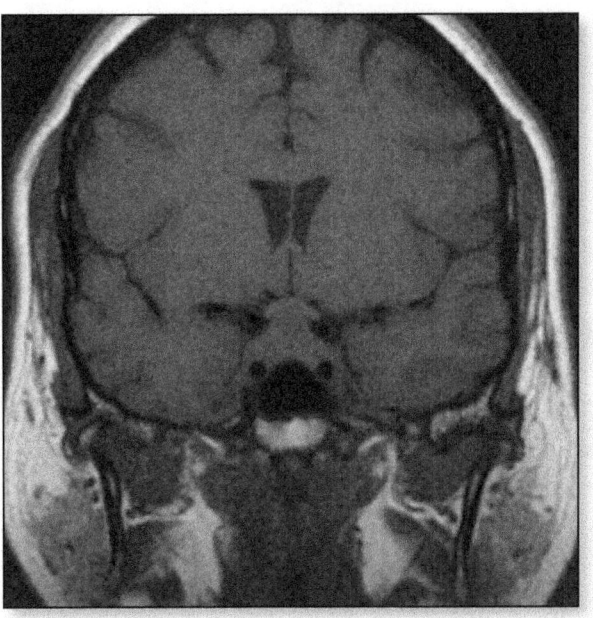

Which of the following is the most likely diagnosis?

   A. Prolactinoma
   B. Clinically nonfunctioning pituitary adenoma
   C. Craniopharyngioma
   D. Lymphocytic hypophysitis
   E. Pituitary apoplexy

18 A 53-year-old woman has a medical history of stage 2 breast cancer diagnosed 4 years ago, status post mastectomy, local radiation therapy, and adjuvant chemotherapy. She is currently in remission. She recently slipped and struck her head, without loss of consciousness. However, given persistent headaches, she underwent head CT, which revealed a 1.5-cm sellar mass with suprasellar extension. In retrospect, she noted abrupt onset of frequent urination and increased thirst in the previous 3 weeks. MRI is performed 4 weeks later and shows that the mass is now 2 cm.

On physical examination, she appears tired. Her blood pressure is 98/66 mm Hg, pulse rate is 92 beats/min, and BMI is 21.1 kg/m^2.

Laboratory test results:

> Serum sodium = 152 mEq/L (136-142 mEq/L)
>   (SI: 152 mmol/L [136-142 mmol/L])
> Prolactin = 122 ng/mL (4-30 ng/mL)
>   (SI: 5.30 nmol/L [0.17-1.30 nmol/L])

FSH = 15.0 mIU/mL (>30 mIU/mL
   [postmenopausal]) (SI: 15.0 IU/L [>30 IU/L])
LH = 12.0 mIU/mL (>30 mIU/mL
   [postmenopausal]) (SI: 12.0 IU/L [>30 IU/L])
Plasma glucose = 89 mg/dL (70-99 mg/dL)
   (SI: 4.9 mmol/L [3.9-5.5 mmol/L])

Chest CT shows no evidence of lesion or adenopathy.

Which of the following is this patient's most likely diagnosis?
   A. Clinically nonfunctioning pituitary adenoma
   B. Prolactinoma
   C. Craniopharyngioma
   D. Metastasis
   E. Neurosarcoidosis

19 A 46-year-old man presents with loss of libido and erectile dysfunction. His primary care physician documented his testosterone level to be 180 ng/dL (6.2 nmol/L) and referred him for further evaluation.

Laboratory test results (sample drawn at 8 AM):
   Repeated testosterone = 171 ng/dL
      (300-900 ng/dL) (SI: 5.9 nmol/L
      [10.4-31.2 nmol/L])
   LH = 0.9 mIU/mL (1.0-9.0 mIU/L) (SI: 0.9 IU/L
      [1.0-9.0 IU/L])
   FSH = 1.1 mIU/mL (1.0-13.0 mIU/L) (SI: 1.1 IU/L
      [1.0-13.0 IU/L])
   Prolactin = 2513 ng/mL (4-23 ng/mL)
      (SI: 109.3 nmol/L [0.17-1.00 nmol/L])
   TSH, normal
   Cortisol, normal

MRI shows a 1.7-cm adenoma with substantial extension into the left cavernous sinus.

At a cabergoline dosage of 1.0 mg twice weekly, his prolactin level normalizes, his tumor greatly reduces in size, his testosterone level increases to 602 ng/dL (20.9 nmol/L), and his erectile function returns. However, his wife complains that he has recently become obsessed with sexuality, to the point that it is hindering their relationship.

Which of the following is the most likely explanation for his current behavior?
   A. The normalized testosterone level
   B. Hypothalamic damage from the tumor
   C. An adverse effect of cabergoline
   D. Behavior change unrelated to his tumor
      or treatment

20 A 35-year-old woman develops bothersome headaches. Despite longstanding normal menstrual cycles, she has had amenorrhea for the past 6 months. Her prolactin concentration is 188 ng/mL (4-30 ng/mL) (SI: 8.2 nmol/L [0.17-1.30 nmol/L]) and is unchanged on dilution. Head MRI shows a 2.8 × 2.8 × 2.2-cm hypoenhancing sellar and suprasellar mass, which abuts the optic chiasm. Her visual field tests show minor temporal-superior deficits. The rest of her physical examination findings are unremarkable.

Laboratory test results:
   Free T$_4$ = 0.9 ng/dL (0.8-1.8 ng/dL)
      (SI: 11.6 pmol/L [10.30-23.17 pmol/L])
   Cortisol (8 AM) = 7.1 µg/dL (5-25 µg/dL)
      (SI: 195.9 nmol/L [137.9-689.7 nmol/L])
   Estradiol = 22 pg/mL (10-180 pg/mL)
      (SI: 81 pmol/L [36.7-660.8 pmol/L])
   IGF-1 = 122 ng/mL (113-297 ng/mL)
      (SI: 16.0 nmol/L [14.8-38.9 nmol/L])

On the basis of the presented information, which of the following treatments should be recommended?
   A. Start bromocriptine, 5 mg orally 3 times daily
   B. Start octreotide LAR, 20 mg intramuscularly
      monthly
   C. Perform transsphenoidal surgery
   D. Start cabergoline, 1.0 mg orally twice weekly
   E. Perform stereotactic radiosurgery

21 A 48-year-old man is referred after head MRI performed for evaluation of headache showed a pituitary mass—a 0.9-cm right-sided pituitary adenoma without parasellar extension (*see image*). He has been feeling well. He has no vision symptoms.

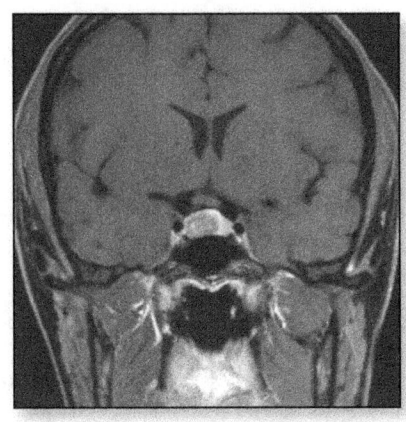

On physical examination, his blood pressure is 136/70 mm Hg and pulse rate is 74 beats/min. His skin has normal texture, and his reflexes are normal. He saw a local neurosurgeon who recommended surgery.

Laboratory test results (8 AM):
Testosterone = 325 ng/dL (300-900 ng/dL)
(SI: 11.3 nmol/L [10.4-31.2 nmol/L])
LH = 2.3 mIU/mL (1.0-9.0 mIU/L)
(SI: 2.3 IU/L [1.0-9.0 IU/L])
FSH = 1.4 mIU/mL (1.0-13.0 mIU/L)
(SI: 1.4 IU/L [1.0-13.0 IU/L])
Cortisol (8 AM) = 15.7 μg/dL (5-25 μg/dL)
(SI: 433.1 nmol/L [137-39-689.7 nmol/L])
Prolactin = 5.7 ng/mL (4-23 ng/mL)
(SI: 0.2 nmol/L [0.17-1.00 nmol/L])
Free T$_4$ = 1.2 ng/dL (0.8-1.8 ng/dL)
(SI: 15.4 pmol/L [10.3-23.2 pmol/L])
Serum sodium = 143 mEq/L (136-142 mEq/L)
(SI: 143 mmol/L [136-142 mmol/L])

Which of the following is the best next step in this patient's management?
A. Visual field testing
B. Transsphenoidal surgery
C. Another MRI in 12 months
D. Radiotherapy

22 A 75-year-old man is referred because a pituitary incidentaloma was identified on CT performed after he fell on the ice and struck his head. Subsequent MRI confirmed a 1.3-cm, T1-hypoenhancing mass that appeared to be a pituitary adenoma, with no suprasellar extension. He states that he has been feeling well, but generally has been slowing down. He attributes this to aging. He has no headaches or vision symptoms. He had a myocardial infarction 10 years ago and subsequent 3-vessel coronary bypass surgery. He has hypertension. His only medications are a statin, a daily baby aspirin, and lisinopril.

On physical examination, he appears his stated age. His blood pressure is 136/70 mm Hg, and pulse rate is 74 beats/min. His skin has normal texture, and his reflexes are normal. Testes are 10 mL bilaterally.

Laboratory test results (sample drawn at 8 AM):
LH = 2.3 mIU/mL (1.0-9.0 mIU/L)
(SI: 2.3 IU/L [1.0-9.0 IU/L])
FSH = 1.4 mIU/mL (1.0-13.0 mIU/L)
(SI: 1.4 IU/L [1.0-13.0 IU/L])
Cortisol = 17 μg/dL (5-25 μg/dL) (SI: 469.0 nmol/L [137.9-689.7 nmol/L])
Testosterone = 295 ng/dL (300-900 ng/dL)
(SI: 10.2 nmol/L [10.4-31.2 nmol/L])
Free T$_4$ = 1.1 ng/dL (0.8-1.8 ng/dL)
(SI: 14.2 pmol/L [10.30-23.17 pmol/L])
Prolactin = 112 ng/mL (4-23 ng/mL)
(SI: 4.87 nmol/L [0.17-1.00 nmol/L])
Creatinine = 1.5 mg/dL (0.7-1.3 mg/dL)
(SI: 132.6 μmol/L [61.9-114.9 μmol/L])
IGF-1 = 135 ng/dL (98-261 ng/mL)
(SI: 17.7 nmol/L [12.8-34.2 nmol/L])

Which of the following is the best next step in this patient's management?
A. Perform visual field testing
B. Refer to an experienced pituitary surgeon
C. Refer for stereotactic radiosurgery
D. Start dopamine agonist
E. Repeat the MRI in 6 months

Thyroid Board Review

Jacqueline Jonklaas, MD, PhD, MPH

1 A 36-year-old woman presents for ongoing management of thyroid cancer. She underwent total thyroidectomy to treat papillary thyroid cancer 2 months ago. The pathology report described a 2.4-cm focus of classic papillary thyroid cancer with 2 additional foci of 1.5 and 0.7 cm, extension of the tumor into perithyroidal soft tissue, and close proximity of the tumor to the resection margin (0.1 cm). Twenty-one of 24 central compartment lymph nodes contained thyroid cancer. The patient takes her levothyroxine regularly. Her medical history includes end-stage kidney disease due to glomerulonephritis for which she undergoes hemodialysis. Physical examination and postoperative ultrasonography do not show any abnormal lateral cervical nodes.

Based on her pathology findings, you recommend that she consider ablation with radioactive iodine in order to decrease her risk of thyroid cancer recurrence. You suggest a diagnostic scan and then selection of an appropriate ^{131}I activity.

Given the additional consideration of end-stage kidney disease, which of the following is the best approach for the patient?
   A. Do not administer ^{131}I
   B. Only administer ^{123}I
   C. Administer standard ^{131}I activity after 4 weeks of a low-iodine diet
   D. Administer ^{131}I activity that is 10% of standard activity
   E. Administer ^{131}I activity that is 50% of standard activity

2 A 64-year-old man is found to have a T3 N1b papillary thyroid cancer following thyroidectomy and lateral and central compartment lymph node dissection. Radioactive iodine remnant ablation is planned for approximately 7 weeks after surgery. Two weeks after surgery, he develops swelling and pain in his left neck in the area where the Jackson-Pratt drain had been located. He becomes febrile and is evaluated in the emergency department, where he undergoes neck CT with intravenous contrast. He is treated for an abscess with incision, drainage, and antibiotics and recovers uneventfully.

He is seen in consultation by his nuclear medicine physician 2 weeks later, and he provides the history of the neck imaging that was performed in the emergency department. As the patient's endocrinologist, you are asked whether any modifications are required to the patient's instructions and schedule for radioactive iodine treatment. His ablation is scheduled in 3 weeks, and he has been instructed to start a low-iodine diet in 1 week.

Which of the following is the most appropriate modification of the patient's instructions and schedule?
   A. Ask the patient to increase his fluid intake, take daily furosemide, and maintain his schedule
   B. Ask the patient to start his low-iodine diet now and maintain his schedule
   C. Maintain current instructions and schedule
   D. Defer radioactive iodine for at least 3 months
   E. Delay his schedule by 1 week

3 A 39-year-old woman develops shortness of breath, fatigue, and anosmia and is subsequently diagnosed with COVID-19 infection. Initially, she does well at home and her respiratory symptoms seem to be resolving. She then develops acute onset of neck pain radiating to her jaw and left ear. Shortly afterwards, she has onset of fever, tachycardia, weight loss, and dysphagia. Dyspnea returns, along with worsening palpitations. She presents to the emergency department and is found to be in atrial fibrillation.

Physical examination findings are notable for an irregular heart rate of 130 beats/min, a firm, exquisitely tender, and slightly enlarged thyroid gland, and a hand tremor. During evaluation, she spontaneously converts to normal sinus rhythm.

Laboratory test results:
    White blood cell count = 9000/μL (4500-11,000/μL)
        (SI: 9.0×10^9/L [4.5-11.0×10^9/L])
    Erythrocyte sedimentation rate = 110 mm/h
        (0-20 mm/h)
    TSH <0.02 mIU/L (0.5-5.0 mIU/L)
    Free T_4 = 3.0 ng/dL (0.8-1.8 ng/dL)
        (SI: 38.6 pmol/L [10.30-23.17 pmol/L])
    Total T_3 = 288 ng/dL (70-200 ng/dL)
        (SI: 4.44 nmol/L [1.08-3.08 nmol/L])

An ^{123}I thyroid scan and uptake are performed. The patient responds well to treatment with β-adrenergic blockers and prednisone and remains in normal sinus rhythm. She is discharged from the hospital with instructions to have thyroid testing repeated in 2 weeks.

Which of the following patterns and degree of ^{123}I uptake would have been anticipated on her thyroid scan and uptake?
    A. Elevated uptake in a homogeneous pattern
    B. Elevated uptake in a heterogeneous pattern
    C. A "hot nodule" in the left lobe
    D. Minimal uptake throughout both lobes of the thyroid
    E. Normal uptake

4 A 63-year-old man is transferred from a local hospital for treatment of a left middle cerebral artery cerebrovascular accident. Upon arrival, only part of his medical records can be located, and the list of medications administered at the previous hospital cannot be found. You are consulted about the management of his thyroid condition and are provided the currently available thyroid test results.

On physical examination, he has mild conjunctival irritation and a diffusely enlarged thyroid gland. His blood pressure is 135/80 mm Hg, and pulse rate is 60 beats/min. He is unable to provide a history or details of his medical therapy.

Thyroid function test results (*see table*).

After reviewing these records, which of the following is the most likely explanation for these series of laboratory results?
    A. Amiodarone was started on day 1
    B. Methimazole was stopped on day 1
    C. Levothyroxine therapy was started on day 1
    D. Liothyronine was started on day 5
    E. Levothyroxine therapy was started on day 5

5 A 29-year-old woman presents to the emergency department at 10 weeks' gestation because of 3 weeks of unremitting nausea and vomiting that have not responded to antiemetic agents. A previous pregnancy was uneventful. She has lost 20 lb (9.1 kg) since the start of the current pregnancy. She has noted weakness, fatigue, constipation, and palpitations.

On physical examination, her blood pressure is 102/64 mm Hg, pulse rate is 133 beats/min, and respiratory rate is 30 breaths/min. Her thyroid gland is of normal size and without a bruit. She is tremulous but has no hyperreflexia.

Pelvic ultrasonography shows a viable singleton pregnancy.

Analyte	Day 1	Day 5	Day 11	Day 18
TSH	178 mIU/L	155 mIU/L	0.819 mIU/L	0.179 mIU/L
Free T_4	<0.10 ng/dL (SI: 1.3 pmol/L)	0.13 ng/dL (SI: 1.7 pmol/L)	0.43 ng/dL (SI: 5.5 pmol/L)	0.85 ng/dL (SI: 10.9 pmol/L)
Total T_3	32 ng/dL (SI: 0.49 nmol/L)	212 ng/dL (SI: 3.26 nmol/L)	574 ng/dL (SI: 8.84 nmol/L)	627 ng/dL (SI: 9.66 nmol/L)

Reference ranges: TSH, 0.5-5.0 mIU/L; free T_4, 0.8-1.8 ng/dL (SI: 10.30-23.17 pmol/L); total T_3, 70-200 ng/dL (SI: 1.08-3.08 nmol/L).

Initial laboratory test results:

β-hCG = 298,506 IU/L (~288,000 IU/L at 9-12 weeks' gestation)

TSH = <0.005 mIU/L (0.5-5.0 mIU/L)

Total T$_4$ = 75 µg/dL (5.5-12.5 µg/dL) (SI: 965.3 nmol/L [94.02-213.68 nmol/L])

Total T$_3$ = 774 ng/dL (70-200 ng/dL) (SI: 11.9 nmol/L [1.08-3.08 nmol/L])

Free T$_4$ = >8.0 ng/dL (0.8-1.8 ng/dL) (SI: >103.0 pmol/L [10.30-23.17 pmol/L])

Sodium = 130 mEq/L (136-142 mEq/L) (SI: 130 mmol/L [136-142 mmol/L])

Potassium = 2.7 mEq/L (3.5-5.0 mEq/L) (SI: 2.7 mmol/L [3.5-5.0 mmol/L])

Creatinine = 1.08 (0.6-1.1 mg/dL) (SI: 95.5 µmol/L [53.0-97.2 µmol/L])

AST = 220 U/L (20-48 U/L) (SI: 3.67 µkat/L [0.33-0.80 µkat/L])

ALT = 269 U/L (10-40 U/L) (SI: 4.49 µkat/L [0.33-0.80 µkat/L])

The patient develops ventricular fibrillation and cardiac arrest but has subsequent return of spontaneous circulation. She is admitted to the intensive care unit and treated with propylthiouracil, hydrocortisone, and an esmolol drip. Thyroid antibodies (thyroid-stimulating immunoglobulin, TPO, and TRAb) are negative. Ultrasonography shows a normal-sized thyroid gland with diffusely increased vascularity. The patient's vital signs and laboratory parameters rapidly improve. She is discharged from the hospital on a regimen of propylthiouracil, 50 mg twice daily.

Subsequent thyroid function and treatment are shown (see table).

Analyte	13 weeks' gestation	After delivery
TSH	0.007 mIU/L	3.14 mIU/L
Free T$_4$	1.04 ng/dL (SI: 13.4 pmol/L)	1.04 ng/dL (SI: 13.4 pmol/L)
Total T$_3$	140 ng/dL (SI: 2.2 nmol/L)	...
Medication	Propylthiouracil, 50 mg twice daily (discontinued)	None

Which of the following diagnoses is the most likely explanation for this patient's hyperthyroidism?

A. Choriocarcinoma
B. Familial gestational hyperthyroidism
C. Hyperemesis gravidarum
D. Hydatidiform mole
E. Twin pregnancy

6 A 49-year-old man is incidentally found to have a 2.6-cm thyroid nodule. The patient has no compressive symptoms, is clinically and biochemically euthyroid, and has no family history of thyroid disorders. Thyroid ultrasonography shows that the nodule is isoechoic with regular margins and without calcifications (*see images, arrows*). No abnormal lymph nodes are seen in the lateral neck.

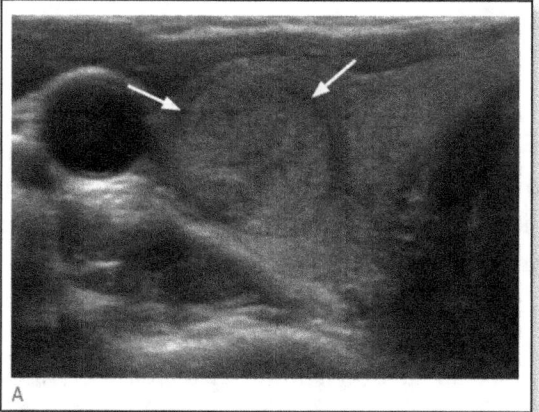

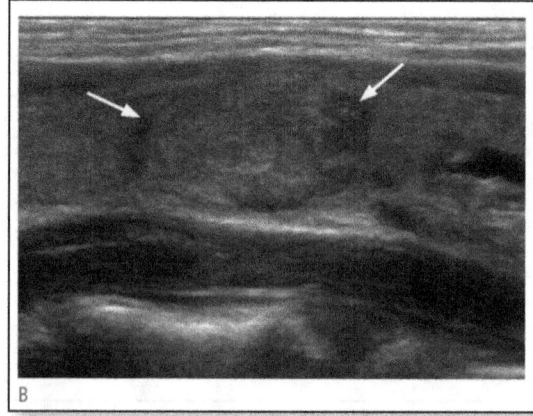

A = transverse view, B = longitudinal view.

The patient elects to observe the nodule, but follow-up ultrasonography performed 18 months later shows that the nodule has increased to 3.4 cm.

A nodule biopsy is performed, and the cytology is reported as Bethesda III, follicular lesion of undetermined significance. The cytologic material is sent for molecular testing, and an *NRAS* pathogenic variant is identified as the sole mutation.

Which of the following is most likely to be found if the patient undergoes surgery?
- A. Tall cell variant of papillary thyroid cancer
- B. Diffuse sclerosing variant of papillary thyroid cancer
- C. Benign follicular adenoma
- D. Hobnail variant of papillary thyroid cancer
- E. Columnar variant of papillary thyroid cancer

7 A 50-year-old woman undergoes hysterectomy and oophorectomy because of a history of uterine fibroids and ovarian cysts. Following surgery, the patient develops multiple symptoms of estrogen deficiency, including vasomotor symptoms, insomnia, and vaginal dryness. She requests hormone therapy for her menopausal symptoms. The patient also had a diagnosis of Hashimoto hypothyroidism for which she has taken levothyroxine for several years. She takes her levothyroxine regularly in the morning, and she has been biochemically and clinically euthyroid on this therapy.

Thyroid function test results:
    TSH = 1.9 mIU/L (0.5-5.0 mIU/L)
    Total T$_4$ = 8.9 µg/dL (5.5-12.5 µg/dL)
        (SI: 114.5 nmol/L [94.02-213.68 nmol/L])
    Thyroxine-binding globulin = 17.1 µg/mL
        (13-39 µg/mL)

The patient initially begins treatment with oral estrogen (1-mg estradiol tablet daily). Later she chooses to switch to transdermal estrogen (1-mg estradiol gel daily).

Which of the following patterns best depicts the thyroid parameter profiles associated with oral estrogen and then transdermal estrogen?

	Oral estrogen			Transdermal estrogen		
Answer	TSH	T$_4$	TBG	TSH	T$_4$	TBG
A.	↔	↑	↑	↔	↑	↑
B.	↑	↑↑	↑↑	↔	↔	↔
C.	↑	↔	↔	↑	↑↑	↑↑
D.	↑	↓	↓	↔	↔	↔
E.	↔	↔	↔	↔	↔	↔

8 A 39-year-old man with papillary thyroid cancer presents for follow-up. He had a good response to treatment with radioactive iodine 2 years ago and was doing well at his last visit. At today's visit, however, he states he is not doing well. He feels tired and has gained weight. He has stopped regular exercise due to his fatigue. He states that he is taking his prescribed dosage of levothyroxine (225 mcg) regularly each morning, which he achieves by taking one 200-mcg tablet and one 25-mcg tablet. He has filled all his levothyroxine prescriptions regularly and has 1 refill remaining. He keeps his levothyroxine in his bedroom and puts 2 tablets of levothyroxine per day into a weekly pill dispenser.

On physical examination, his vital signs are unremarkable and there is no palpable tissue in the thyroid bed or palpable lymph nodes. He appears fatigued and seems to have difficulty concentrating.

Laboratory test results:

Analyte	Current visit	Last visit
TSH	73.0 mIU/L	1.43 mIU/L
Free T$_4$	0.13 ng/dL (SI: 1.67 pmol/L)	1.33 ng/dL (SI: 17.12 pmol/L)
Thyroglobulin	0.6 ng/mL (SI: 0.6 µg/L)	<0.1 ng/mL (SI: <0.1 µg/L)

Reference ranges: TSH, 0.5-5.0 mIU/L; free T$_4$, 0.8-1.8 ng/dL (SI: 10.30-23.17 pmol/L); thyroglobulin, <1.0 ng/mL (SI: <1.0 µg/L).

Based on the available information, which of the following is the most likely explanation for this patient's current thyroid function test results?

    A. Heterophilic antibodies causing false elevation of TSH

    B. MacroTSH

    C. Patient is now taking large doses of biotin

    D. Patient error in taking levothyroxine

    E. Deterioration of levothyroxine due to improper storage

9 A 65-year-old woman presents for follow-up. She underwent total thyroidectomy 5 years ago for papillary thyroid carcinoma. Pathology showed a 4.3-cm left-sided tumor, tall cell variant, without extrathyroidal extension or vascular invasion. Six of 11 unilateral lymph nodes were involved. Her tumor was stage II (T3N1bM0). She was subsequently treated with radioactive iodine, with a posttreatment scan that showed uptake in the thyroid bed and in a left-sided cervical node. Follow-up whole-body scan 1 year after the ablation was negative. She currently feels well.

Laboratory test results:

    TSH = 0.01 mIU/L

    Free T_4 = 2.1 ng/dL (0.8-1.8 mg/dL)

      (SI: 27.0 pmol/L [10.30-23.17 pmol/L])

    Thyroglobulin = <0.1 ng/mL (SI: <0.1 µg/L)

    Thyroglobulin antibodies, negative

Recent neck ultrasonography shows 2 left-sided level IV lymph nodes and no thyroid remnant tissue. Both lymph nodes are oblong with visible hila, regular margins, and no microcalcifications and measure 0.5 cm and 0.4 cm.

Which of the following is the most appropriate next step?

    A. Continue current levothyroxine, schedule PET scan

    B. Continue current levothyroxine, schedule radioactive iodine whole-body scan

    C. Increase levothyroxine dosage, schedule ultrasonography in 6 months

    D. Decrease levothyroxine dosage, schedule repeated TSH measurement in 6 to 8 weeks

    E. Decrease levothyroxine dosage, schedule radioactive iodine whole-body scan

10 A 72-year-old man underwent total thyroidectomy for medullary thyroid cancer 5 years ago. He has recently moved from out of state and would like to reestablish care. His history is notable for several comorbidities, including stage III chronic kidney disease, gastroesophageal reflux disease, and primary hyperparathyroidism. Recent CT and PET imaging show extensive local disease in his neck, as well as liver metastases. The calcitonin concentration measured by immunochemiluminometric assay in the office of his previous endocrinologist was greater than 2000 pg/mL (>584 pmol/L) 3 months ago. However, the calcitonin concentration is only 198 pg/mL (57.8 pmol/L) when measured with immunoradiometric assay today. His serum carcinoembryonic antigen concentration is elevated at 140 µg/L (0-5 µg/L).

Which of the following is the most likely explanation for the lower serum calcitonin level?

    A. Chronic kidney disease

    B. Omeprazole use

    C. Hook effect

    D. Heterophilic antibodies to calcitonin

    E. Procalcitonin cross-reactivity

11 A 32-year-old man with widely invasive follicular thyroid cancer undergoes total thyroidectomy followed by radioiodine remnant ablation with 150 mCi [131]I. He subsequently develops lung metastases and is treated with an additional 200 mCi, with an objective decrease in the size of the lung metastases and reduction in serum thyroglobulin levels.

Which of the following is the most likely adverse effect from this patient's radioiodine therapy?

    A. Permanent loss of taste

    B. Excessive dental caries

    C. Azoospermia

    D. Leukemia

    E. Hypoparathyroidism

12 A 47-year-old man starts a regimen of interferon alfa for chronic hepatitis C. Three months later, he reports palpitations and a 5-lb (2.3-kg) weight loss. He has no eye discomfort, vision problems, or neck pain. On physical examination, his pulse rate is 95 beats/min, and his thyroid gland is 25 g without tenderness, nodules, or bruit.

Laboratory test results:
TSH = <0.01 mIU/L (0.5-5.0 mIU/L)
Free T$_4$ = 2.4 ng/dL (0.8-1.8 ng/dL)
(SI: 30.9 pmol/L [10.30-23.17 pmol/L])
TPO antibody titer = 230 IU/mL (<2.0 IU/mL)
(SI: 180 kIU/L [<2.0 kIU/L])
Radioactive iodine uptake at 24 hours = 0.4%

His hepatologist stops the interferon alfa.

Which of the following should be recommended now?
A. Methimazole
B. Prednisone
C. Intravenous immunoglobulin
D. Atenolol
E. Propylthiouracil

13 A 63-year-old man with refractory atrial fibrillation is prescribed amiodarone. Baseline thyroid function is normal. One month later, the patient is asymptomatic, but is noted to have the following laboratory findings:
Total T$_4$ = 13.4 µg/dL (5.5-12.5 µg/dL)
(SI: 172.5 nmol/L [94.02-213.68 nmol/L])
Free T$_4$ = 1.91 ng/dL (0.8-1.8 ng/dL)
(SI: 24.6 pmol/L [10.30-23.17 pmol/L])
Total T$_3$ = 65 ng/dL (70-200 ng/dL) (SI: 1.0 nmol/L
[1.08-3.08 nmol/L])
TSH = 4.1 mIU/L (0.5-5.0 mIU/L)

Which of the following is the most likely explanation for these findings?
A. Type 1 amiodarone-induced thyrotoxicosis
B. Type 2 amiodarone-induced thyrotoxicosis
C. Expected changes in euthyroid patients on amiodarone
D. Assay interference by amiodarone metabolites
E. Euthyroid sick syndrome

14 A 62-year-old woman with hypothyroidism is admitted to the surgical intensive care unit with acute necrotizing pancreatitis. Her serum TSH concentration 1 month before admission was 1.8 mIU/L. Her outpatient levothyroxine dosage is 100 mcg daily, which she has been taking in the morning on an empty stomach. Her surgical team is concerned about poor levothyroxine absorption due to bowel edema and would like to change to parenteral thyroid hormone therapy.

Which of the following regimens would be most appropriate?
A. Levothyroxine, 150 mcg intravenously once daily
B. Levothyroxine, 100 mcg intravenously once daily
C. Levothyroxine, 1000 mcg intramuscularly once weekly
D. Levothyroxine, 70 mcg intravenously once daily
E. Liothyronine, 25 mcg intravenously twice daily

15 A 23-year-old woman in her 12th week of pregnancy is found to have a 1.9-cm thyroid nodule. She has no associated adenopathy in the neck.

Laboratory test results:
Serum TSH = 0.1 mIU/L (0.5-5.0 mIU/L)
Free T$_4$ = 1.2 ng/dL (0.8-1.8 ng/dL)
(SI: 15.4 pmol/L [10.30-23.17 pmol/L])

Thyroid ultrasonography shows that the nodule is solid and hypoechoic and has irregular margins.

Which of the following should be the next step in this patient's management?
A. Fine-needle aspiration
B. Technetium thyroid scan
C. Thyroid lobectomy
D. Initiation of methimazole
E. Initiation of propylthiouracil

16 An 18-year-old man has severe intellectual disability and congenital hypotonia that has progressed to spasticity. He does not speak or ambulate and has been unable to maintain his weight. He has 3 similarly affected male family members in 2 generations.

On physical examination, his pulse rate is 88 beats/min, and he has a normal thyroid gland.

Laboratory test results:
Free T_4 = 0.8 ng/dL (0.8-1.8 ng/dL)
(SI: 10.3 pmol/L [10.30-23.17 pmol/L])
Free T_3 = 6.5 pg/mL (2.3-4.2 pg/mL)
(SI: 10.0 pmol/L [3.53-6.45 pmol/L])
Total T_3 = 360 ng/dL (70-200 ng/dL)
(SI: 5.5 nmol/L [1.08-3.08 nmol/L])
TSH = 2.9 mIU/L (0.5-5.0 mIU/L)

Which of the following genetic etiologies is most likely responsible?
A. Activating pathogenic variant in the type 3 deiodinase (D3) gene
B. Pathogenic variant in the thyroid hormone receptor β gene
C. Thyroid hormone transporter defect
D. Inactivating pathogenic variant in the thyrotropin receptor gene
E. Pathogenic variant in the thyrotropin-releasing hormone receptor gene

17 A 25-year-old woman who has followed a vegan diet for the last 6 years is planning pregnancy sometime in the next 6 months. She has no history of thyroid disease.

On physical examination, her pulse rate is 80 beats/min and blood pressure is 132/78 mm Hg. She has slight thyroid enlargement without palpable nodules. Her serum TSH concentration is 2.1 mIU/L.

Which of the following is the best recommendation now?
A. Change to a diet containing animal products
B. Add twice-weekly kelp to current diet
C. Start a daily prenatal multivitamin containing 150 mcg iodine
D. Start supersaturated potassium iodide (SSKI), 1 drop twice daily
E. Change from iodized table salt to sea salt

18 A 27-year-old woman with Graves hyperthyroidism has been treated with methimazole, 10 mg daily, for 14 months. On palpation, her thyroid gland is at the upper limit of normal size. There is no bruit. She does not smoke cigarettes. She is interested in stopping methimazole.

Current laboratory test results:
TSH = 0.7 mIU/L (0.5-5.0 mIU/L)
Total T_3 = 166 ng/dL (70-200 ng/dL)
(SI: 2.56 nmol/L [1.08-3.08 nmol/L])
Free T_4 = 1.6 ng/dL (0.8-1.8 ng/dL)
(SI: 20.59 pmol/L [10.30-23.17 pmol/L])
TPO antibodies = 594 IU/mL (<2.0 IU/mL)
(SI: 594 kIU/L [<2.0 kIU/L])
Thyroid-stimulating immunoglobulin = 396%
(≤120% of basal activity)

Which of the following characteristics of this patient predicts a greater likelihood that her Graves hyperthyroidism will recur if methimazole is stopped?
A. Age
B. TPO antibody titer
C. Thyroid-stimulating immunoglobulin level
D. Thyroid size
E. Cigarette smoking status

19 A 35-year-old woman with Hashimoto thyroiditis and vitamin D deficiency is referred for advice regarding levothyroxine dosing. Two years ago, her condition was well controlled on 100 mcg daily of levothyroxine, but in order to maintain a normal TSH value, her physician has repeatedly increased her dosage, and she currently takes 300 mcg daily. The patient uses a pill sorter to take her prescription each morning on an empty stomach. She waits until lunch before taking a multivitamin with iron and a calcium supplement. Her weight is stable at 145.2 lb (66 kg), and she has no diarrhea or abdominal pain. Physical examination reveals a small, firm goiter but is otherwise unremarkable.

Laboratory test results:
Serum TSH = 11.6 mIU/L (0.5-5.0 mIU/L)
Free T_4 = 1.0 ng/dL (0.8-1.8 ng/dL)
(SI: 12.9 pmol/L [10.3-23.2 pmol/L])

Which of the following should be the next step in the evaluation of this patient's increasing levothyroxine dosage requirement?

A. Move the timing of when she takes the calcium tablets and multivitamins to just before the evening meal
B. Screen for occult celiac disease
C. Measure TSH with a different assay
D. Change to T_4/T_3 combination therapy
E. Measure vitamin B_{12}

20 A 52-year-old woman is referred for evaluation of a neck mass. The patient notes dysphagia with solid foods and positional dyspnea when lying on her right side. Medical history is noncontributory.

On physical examination, she has a large goiter extending below the clavicle on the left side. Her serum TSH concentration is 0.5 mIU/L, and radioiodine uptake is 13% at 24 hours. Ultrasonography shows a multinodular goiter with confluent isoechoic nodules throughout. Results from FNA biopsy of the largest nodule are benign. Noncontrast CT of the neck is shown (*see image*).

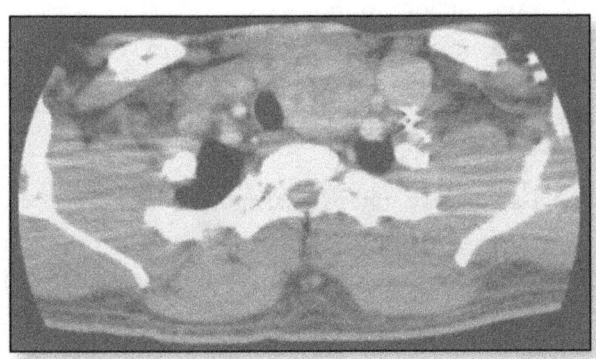

Which of the following is the best next step in this patient's management?

A. Levothyroxine suppressive therapy
B. Radioiodine therapy using recombinant human TSH
C. Thermal ablation therapy
D. Thyroidectomy from collar incision
E. No intervention until symptoms progress

21 A 47-year-old man undergoes thyroidectomy for a 4.0-cm papillary thyroid cancer with microscopic extrathyroidal extension. After discussion of the benefits and risks associated with radioiodine remnant ablation, he elects to proceed. The patient strongly prefers to not miss work, but he will do whatever is advised to maximize the success of remnant ablation. He requests an opinion regarding whether he should use thyroid hormone withdrawal or recombinant human TSH–stimulated radioiodine remnant ablation, as well as the best dose to receive.

Which of the following regimens would be preferred for this patient?

A. Thyroid hormone withdrawal, using 30 mCi ^{131}I
B. Thyroid hormone withdrawal, using 100 mCi ^{131}I
C. Recombinant human TSH, using 30 mCi ^{131}I
D. Recombinant human TSH, using 100 mCi ^{131}I
E. Thyroid hormone withdrawal and recombinant human TSH, using 100 mCi ^{131}I

22 A 63-year-old man with metastatic renal cell carcinoma is prescribed sunitinib therapy. The patient has no history of thyroid dysfunction, and baseline thyroid function is normal.

Which of the following thyroid abnormalities is most likely to occur in this patient after starting sunitinib?

A. Primary hypothyroidism
B. Secondary hypothyroidism
C. Primary hyperthyroidism
D. Secondary hyperthyroidism
E. "Euthyroid sick" syndrome

23 A 52-year-old man presents with palpitations. His weight has recently decreased from 237 to 211 lb (107.7 to 95.9 kg). He has otherwise been healthy and has had no recent illnesses. He states that he takes no medications or supplements.

On physical examination, his thyroid is nontender and there is no goiter. He has a fine tremor of his outstretched hands, and his pulse rate is 97 beats/min. He has no stigmata of Graves disease.

Laboratory test results:
    TSH = <0.01 mIU/L (0.5-5.0 mIU/L)
    Free T$_4$ = 4.3 ng/dL (0.8-1.8 ng/dL)
        (SI: 55.35 pmol/L [10.30-23.17 pmol/L])
    Total T$_3$ = 290 ng/dL (70-200 ng/dL)
        (SI: 4.47 nmol/L [1.08-3.08 nmol/L])
    Radioactive iodine uptake = <1% at 24 hours
        (15%-30%)

A spot urinary iodine concentration on the day of the radioactive iodine uptake test is not elevated.

Which of the following tests is most likely to reveal the diagnosis?
    A. Radioactive iodine uptake/scan after a low-iodine diet
    B. Serum thyroglobulin measurement
    C. Assessment of serum erythrocyte sedimentation rate
    D. Thyroid ultrasonography with color Doppler
    E. Thyroid-stimulating immunoglobulin measurement

24 A 79-year-old woman reports a 2-week history of left-sided neck pain and palpitations. Physical examination reveals firm enlargement (about 1.5 times normal size) and tenderness over the right thyroid lobe. Laboratory testing shows an elevated free T$_4$ level and suppressed TSH level. Thyroid-stimulating immunoglobulin is normal. She is prescribed prednisone.

Three weeks later, the patient notes persistent pain, now accompanied by dysphagia, and a further increase in size of the right thyroid lobe (now 3 times normal size). Thyroid function test results are essentially unchanged. Ultrasonography reveals an enlarged and heterogeneous right thyroid lobe with increased vascularity.

Which of the following should be the next step in this patient's management?
    A. Perform FNA biopsy
    B. Start methimazole
    C. Change prednisone to intravenous methylprednisolone
    D. Perform contrast CT of the neck
    E. Refer for thyroidectomy

25 A thyroid nodule is found in a 42-year-old woman with a history of hypothyroidism. Ultrasound-guided FNA biopsy of the palpable nodule is interpreted as suspicious for papillary carcinoma. She undergoes total thyroidectomy without complications. Surgical pathology shows a 2.4-cm intrathyroidal, fully encapsulated papillary carcinoma with clear margins, no lymphovascular invasion, and no positive lymph nodes. Three months ago, her TSH concentration was 0.7 mIU/L on levothyroxine, 112 mcg daily. Her dosage was increased to 137 mcg daily at the time of her surgery.

Current laboratory test results 1 week postoperatively:
    TSH = 0.3 mIU/L (0.5-5.0 mIU/L)
    Thyroglobulin (measured using a radioimmunoassay) = 17 ng/mL (SI: 17 µg/L)
    Thyroglobulin antibodies = <4.0 IU/mL

Which of the following is the best next step?
    A. Repeated thyroglobulin measurement using an immunometric assay
    B. Repeated thyroglobulin and thyroglobulin antibody measurements in 6 weeks using the same radioimmunoassay
    C. Measurement of thyroglobulin in serially diluted sera
    D. Measurement of thyroglobulin by mass spectrometry
    E. Radioactive iodine ablation

26 A 75-year-old woman with longstanding subclinical hyperthyroidism takes methimazole, 7.5 mg daily. At the time of her diagnosis, she expressed concern about exposure to radioactive materials and desired to have medical therapy. She takes her current medications regularly. She has recently developed fatigue and is concerned about this symptom.

On physical examination, her pulse rate is 64 beats/min and her thyroid gland is enlarged and nodular.

Laboratory test results:
    TSH = 8.9 mIU/L (0.5-5.0 mIU/L)
    Free T$_4$ = 0.75 ng/dL (0.8-1.8 ng/dL)
        (SI: 9.7 pmol/L [10.30-23.17 pmol/L])

Thyroid scan from 2 years earlier is shown (*see image*).

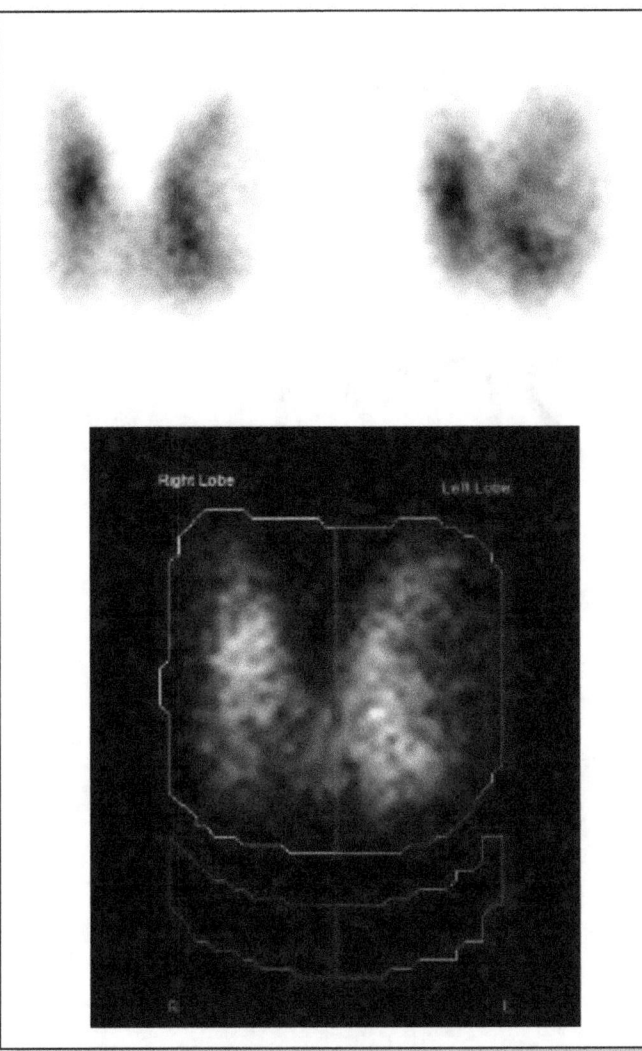

Which of the following is the most important next step in this patient's management?

A. Perform the thyroid scan again with radioactive iodine uptake
B. Reduce the methimazole dosage
C. Discontinue methimazole and start levothyroxine therapy
D. Discontinue methimazole
E. Treat the patient with ^{131}I based on the uptake from her prior scan

27 A 54-year-old woman with longstanding nontoxic multinodular goiter reports taking high doses of a nutritional supplement marketed for thyroid health for the last 4 months. Two months ago, she developed palpitations, tremor, heat intolerance, and weight loss.

Laboratory test results:
TSH = <0.01 mIU/L (0.5-5.0 mIU/L)
Total T$_3$ = 287 ng/dL (70-200 ng/dL)
(SI: 4.4 nmol/L [1.08-3.08 nmol/L])
Free T$_4$ = 3.9 ng/dL (0.8-1.8 ng/dL)
(SI: 50.2 pmol/L [10.30-23.17 pmol/L])
TPO antibodies = <2.0 IU/mL (<2.0 IU/mL)
(SI: <2.0 kIU/L [<2.0 kIU/L])
Serum thyroglobulin = 79 ng/mL (3-42 ng/mL)
(SI: 79 µg/L [3-42 µg/L])

Which of the following is most likely to be present in the supplements?

A. Adrenal extract
B. Iodine
C. Thyroid hormone extract
D. Perchlorate
E. Biotin

28 A 26-year-old woman is noted to have a 1.2-cm right thyroid nodule during the ninth week of pregnancy. The patient has no relevant medical history, and her family history is negative for thyroid cancer. Ultrasonography reveals no suspicious features and FNA biopsy is deferred. At 18 weeks' gestation, the nodule is noted to have a maximal diameter of 2.4 cm and is solid on ultrasonography.

On physical examination, in addition to the nodule, a 2-cm ipsilateral central compartment lymph node is noted. FNA biopsy confirms papillary thyroid cancer in both the nodule and lymph node. Her serum TSH concentration is 0.9 mIU/L (0.5-5.0 mIU/L).

Which of the following is the best next step in this patient's management?

A. Start levothyroxine suppressive therapy
B. Refer for immediate total thyroidectomy with neck dissection
C. Defer surgery until the third trimester
D. Recommend no intervention until after delivery
E. Perform ethanol ablation of the lymph node now; defer thyroidectomy until after delivery

ENDOCRINE
BOARD
REVIEW 2021

Adrenal Board Review

Tobias Else, MD

1 **ANSWER: D) Homocysteine and methylmalonic acid measurement**

Autoimmune polyendocrine syndromes (APS) can be grouped into APS type 1 and APS type 2. APS type 1 is an autosomal recessive disorder caused by pathogenic variants in the *AIRE* gene. The main manifestations are primary adrenal insufficiency, hypoparathyroidism, and mucocutaneous candidiasis, but other autoimmune endocrinopathies can also occur (eg, hypothyroidism [20%], pernicious anemia [15%]). This patient lacks the core manifestations of hypoparathyroidism and mucocutaneous candidiasis, but she most likely has 2 manifestations of APS type 2. The main manifestations of APS type 2 in patients with adrenal insufficiency are hypothyroidism (40%), type 1 diabetes mellitus (10%), vitamin B_{12} deficiency (10%), and vitiligo (10%).

Further evaluation for atrophic gastritis and vitamin B_{12} deficiency will most likely identify this reversible cause of the patient's neurologic symptoms. While values well below the lower limit of normal are often diagnostic for B_{12} deficiency, borderline levels (200-300 pg/mL) are best followed up by homocysteine and methylmalonic acid level measurement (Answer D). Methylmalonic acid is the most specific and sensitive marker for vitamin B_{12} deficiency. Treatment consists of vitamin B_{12} supplementation, either with initially intramuscular B_{12} or high oral doses. Atrophic gastritis and vitamin B_{12} deficiency can present with neurologic symptoms without any hematologic or gastrointestinal symptoms or signs.

Celiac disease is best diagnosed with esophagogastroduodenoscopy and deep duodenal biopsies (Answer C). Celiac disease coexists in about 5% of patients with APS type 2. Celiac disease is associated with a broad spectrum of neurologic manifestations, but other symptoms or signs are commonly present as well. Assessing for tissue transglutaminase-IgA antibodies (Answer E) is the screening of choice for celiac disease. IgA deficiency can lead to false-negative screening, but in this case tissue transglutaminase-IgG was also negative.

Diminished ankle reflexes, particularly with a delayed relaxation phase, are associated with hypothyroidism. However, there is no concern in this patient that the slightly increased/upper-limit TSH reflects current severe underreplaced hypothyroidism and no other hypothyroid symptoms are present. Thus, free T_4 measurement (Answer B) is not necessary.

Adrenoleukodystrophy (Answer A) is an X-linked recessive disorder and can initially present with adrenal insufficiency and later with myelopathy with the neurologic manifestations of sensory ataxia and neurogenic bladder dysfunction. Although female carriers can develop myelopathy, adrenal insufficiency in female carriers is exceedingly rare.

EDUCATIONAL OBJECTIVE

Identify atrophic gastritis as an autoimmune disorder that occurs with adrenal insufficiency.

REFERENCE(S)

Erichsen MM, Løvås K, Skinningsrud B, et al. Clinical, immunological, and genetic features of autoimmune primary adrenal insufficiency: observations from a Norwegian registry. *J Clin Endocrinol Metab.* 2009;94(12):4882-4890. PMID: 19858318

Bruserud O, Oftedal BE, Landegren N, et al. A longitudinal follow-up of autoimmune polyendocrine syndrome type 1. *J Clin Endocrinol Metab.* 2016;101(8):2975-2983. PMID: 27253668

Green R, Allen LH, Bjørke-Monsen A-L, et al. Vitamin B$_{12}$ deficiency. *Nat Rev Dis Primers.* 2017;3:17040. PMID: 28660890

Kemp S, Huffnagel IC, Linthorst GE, Wanders RJ, Engelen M. Adrenoleukodystrophy - neuroendocrine pathogenesis and redefinition of natural history. *Nat Rev Endocrinol.* 2016;12(10):606-615. PMID: 27312864

2 ANSWER: D) Measure plasma free metanephrines, calcitonin, and carcinoembryonic antigen

This patient has a germline pathogenic variant in the *RET* gene conferring an increased risk for manifestations related to multiple endocrine neoplasia (MEN) type 2A, such as primary hyperparathyroidism, medullary thyroid cancer, and pheochromocytoma. The p.V804M variant is associated with a moderate risk for medullary thyroid cancer (American Thyroid Association guidelines), and recent studies have shown a lower risk for medullary thyroid cancer than previously estimated. Therefore, the best initial screening and lifelong surveillance for this patient is annual biochemical screening with calcium (currently normal), metanephrines (plasma or urine), calcitonin, and carcinoembryonic antigen (CEA) (Answer D). Catecholamines, epinephrine, and norepinephrine should not be used for pheochromocytoma screening due to lack of sensitivity and specificity. Measurement of plasma or urinary metanephrines is the standard of care. Only in the case of elevated or increased levels of metanephrines or calcitonin/CEA would imaging be indicated to evaluate for a pheochromocytoma or medullary thyroid cancer, respectively.

Thyroidectomy (Answer A) should not be immediately recommended, but it is definitely indicated if there is evidence for disease. Preoperatively, pheochromocytoma must be excluded. Imaging (Answers B and E) is not part of regular screening for MEN 2A because all manifestations are best surveilled biochemically.

While PTH and 25-hydroxyvitamin D (Answer C) are often measured along with calcium, a calcium level is sufficient to screen for primary hyperparathyroidism.

EDUCATIONAL OBJECTIVE
Guide tumor surveillance for a patient with *RET*-related multiple endocrine neoplasia type 2A.

REFERENCE(S)
Loveday C, Josephs K, Chubb D, et al. p.Val804Met, the most frequent pathogenic mutation in RET, confers a very low lifetime risk of medullary thyroid cancer. *J Clin Endocrinol Metab.* 2018;103(11):4275-4282. PMID: 29590403

Wells SA Jr, Asa SL, Dralle H, et al; American Thyroid Association Guidelines Task Force on Medullary Thyroid Carcinoma. Revised American Thyroid Association guidelines for the management of medullary thyroid carcinoma. *Thyroid.* 2015;25(6):567-610. PMID: 25810047

3 ANSWER: D) Perform CT of the chest, abdomen, and pelvis

This patient has a 1.8-cm carotid body tumor. While carotid body tumors can produce catecholamines, the greater than 28-fold elevation of normetanephrine in this case is far out of proportion. Only a 2- to 3-fold elevation would be expected maximally. The same range of normetanephrine elevation can be seen with tricyclic antidepressants. However, holding them for a few days is usually enough time to obtain reliable plasma metanephrine values. Thus, holding cyclobenzaprine for at least 4 weeks (Answer A) is not necessary. Urinary metanephrines (Answer B) would most likely show the same result with frank elevation and this would not be helpful in further management. The significant increase in plasma normetanephrine suggests the coexistence of another functional paraganglioma or pheochromocytoma as part of a hereditary paraganglioma syndrome. Most of these tumors are discovered in the abdomen, and therefore cross-sectional imaging (Answer D) is the best next step. If no tumor is obvious on abdominal imaging, additional cross-sectional chest imaging should be considered. With a 28-fold elevation of normetanephrine, one would expect a tumor size of at least 4 cm, which would not be missed by any cross-sectional imaging. Functional imaging (Answer C) is not useful. Indeed, MIBG scans should only be conducted when ^{131}I-MIBG therapy is planned. Once a decision has been made to proceed with surgery, α-blockade (Answer E) is a reasonable approach. However, surgery should be considered for the most morbid lesion first, which, in this case, is probably an abdominal paraganglioma or pheochromocytoma.

EDUCATIONAL OBJECTIVE

Construct the differential diagnosis for a patient with elevated metanephrine levels.

REFERENCE(S)

Lenders JW, Duh Q-Y, Eisenhofer G, et al; Endocrine Society. Pheochromocytoma and paraganglioma: an Endocrine Society clinical practice guideline. *J Clin Endocrinol Metab.* 2014;99(6):1915-1942. PMID: 24893135

Rao D, van Berkel A, Piscaer I. Impact of 123 I-MIBG scintigraphy on clinical decision making in pheochromocytoma and paraganglioma. *J Clin Endocrinol Metab.* 2019:jc.2018-02355. PMID: 30822354

Eisenhofer G, Deutschbein T, Constantinescu G, et al. Plasma metanephrines and prospective prediction of tumor location, size and mutation type in patients with pheochromocytoma and paraganglioma. *Clin Chem Lab Med.* 2020;59(2):353-363. PMID: 33001846

4 ANSWER: C) *SDHD*

The presence of 4 paragangliomas and a pheochromocytoma in this family, as well as the patient's personal history of a paraganglioma and pheochromocytoma, is highly suggestive of a hereditary predisposition to paraganglioma/pheochromocytoma. Genes associated with paraganglioma and pheochromocytoma are shown in the table (*see following page*). The predominance of head and neck paragangliomas is more suggestive of a variant in *SDHD*, *SDHC*, or *SDHB*. Pathogenic variants in the *VHL* gene (Answer D) and *RET* gene (Answer E) (multiple endocrine neoplasia type 2) are mainly associated with adrenal pheochromocytomas and are less likely to be the etiology in this case. Pathogenic variants in *SDHC* (Answer A) have a much lower penetrance, rarely affect more than 1 or 2 family members, and rarely affect the adrenal glands. The inheritance of all of these genetic conditions is autosomal dominant. The risk of tumor development associated with *SDHD* pathogenic variants (Answer C), however, depends on the sex of the transmitting parent. Because of maternal imprinting, if the variant is inherited from the father, there is risk for paraganglioma and pheochromocytoma, while if the variant is inherited from the mother, the individual will be a carrier but is not at risk for tumor development. This is the inheritance pattern observed in this patient's family.

EDUCATIONAL OBJECTIVE

Identify the pattern of inheritance of pathogenic variants in the *SDHD* gene.

REFERENCE(S)

Benn DE, Robinson BG, Clifton-Bligh RJ. 15 years of paraganglioma: clinical manifestations of paraganglioma syndromes types 1-5. *Endocr Relat Cancer.* 2015;22(4):T91-T103. PMID: 26273102

Table. Genes Associated With Paraganglioma and Pheochromocytoma

Syndrome	Gene(s)	Tumor locations	Hormone products	Other features
Familial paraganglioma type 1	SDHD	Head and neck paraganglioma, multiple; mediastinal paraganglioma; rarely adrenal medulla	Normetanephrine, metanephrine, dopamine, or none	Clear cell renal cell carcinoma, gastrointestinal stromal tumor, pituitary adenoma
Familial paraganglioma type 2	SDHAF2	Head and neck paraganglioma, multiple; rarely adrenal medulla	Unknown	Unknown
Familial paraganglioma type 3	SDHC	Head and neck paraganglioma; mediastinal paraganglioma	Normetanephrine or none	Unknown
Familial paraganglioma type 4	SDHB	Abdominal and pelvic paraganglioma; mediastinal paraganglioma; rarely adrenal medulla	Normetanephrine, dopamine, or none	Often malignant paraganglioma; clear cell renal cell carcinoma, gastrointestinal stromal tumor, pituitary adenoma
Familial paraganglioma	SDHA	Head and neck or other paraganglioma; adrenal medulla	Unknown	Unknown
Multiple endocrine neoplasia type 2A and 2B	RET	Adrenal medulla, bilateral	Metanephrine >> normetanephrine	Medullary thyroid carcinoma, hyperparathyroidism; marfanoid habitus and mucosal ganglioneuromas (2B only)
Neurofibromatosis type 1	NF1	Adrenal medulla	Metanephrine or metanephrine and normetanephrine	Café-au-lait spots, neurofibromas, peripheral nerve sheath tumors
von Hippel–Lindau syndrome	VHL	Adrenal medulla, bilateral; rarely paraganglioma	Normetanephrine	Retinal and central nervous system hemangioblastomas, clear cell renal cell carcinoma, pancreatic islet-cell tumors, other
Familial pheochromocytoma	TMEM127	Adrenal medulla	Normetanephrine and metanephrine	Renal cell carcinoma
Familial pheochromocytoma	MAX	Adrenal medulla, bilateral	Normetanephrine and metanephrine	Unknown
Fumarate hydratase deficiency	FH	Head and neck paraganglioma; adrenal medulla	Normetanephrine	Papillary renal cell carcinoma, uterine fibroids, cutaneous leiomyoma

5 **ANSWER: C) Perform transesophageal echocardiography and blood cultures**

Cushing syndrome remains first and foremost a clinical diagnosis. This patient does not have any expected clinical features other than weakness, which can be seen as the only symptom with fast-progressing hypercortisolism. However, fast-progressing hypercortisolism usually occurs with either adrenocortical carcinoma (excluded by the normal abdominal CT in this vignette) or paraneoplastic ectopic ACTH. However, a fast-growing tumor as a source would be visible on a CT of the chest, abdomen, and pelvis. Weight loss would be very unusual with any kind of Cushing syndrome. Therefore, this patient most likely has another cause of hypercortisolism, such as infection, and the most likely source is endocarditis associated with the artificial heart valve. Thus, transesophageal echocardiography and blood cultures (Answer C) would be the best steps now.

In patients with severe illness, cortisol production becomes partially independent of ACTH, which therefore is normal or at least inadequately normal. Severe nonendocrine disease could also explain the other endocrine abnormalities, such as the thyroid and gonadal changes. With physiologic response of the hypothalamic-pituitary-adrenal axis to a stress stimulus (endocarditis and sepsis in this patient), there is no need for further evaluation such as salivary cortisol measurement (Answer B) or petrosal sinus sampling (Answer E) or even for treatment of hypercortisolism (Answer A). The abnormality on pituitary MRI is most likely a small Rathke cyst. Resuming testosterone replacement and starting thyroid hormone replacement (Answer D) would also not affect the underlying condition.

EDUCATIONAL OBJECTIVE
Identify physiologic and pathophysiologic causes of hypercortisolism.

REFERENCE(S)
Holub M, Džupová O, Růžková M, et al. Selected biomarkers correlate with the origin and severity of sepsis. *Mediators Inflamm.* 2018;2018:7028267. PMID: 29769838

Peeters B, Langouche L, Van den Berghe G. Adrenocortical stress response during the course of critical illness. *Compr Physiol.* 2017;8(1):283-298. PMID: 29357129

6 **ANSWER: C) Obtain measurements of 24-hour urinary cortisol and plasma ACTH and start spironolactone**

Osilodrostat is a recently approved medication for the treatment of Cushing disease that is either not curable by surgery or persists after surgery. When using medication to control hypercortisolism, it is important to consider its mechanism of action. Osilodrostat (like metyrapone) is an 11-hydroxylase inhibitor, which will decrease cortisol production but increase deoxycorticosterone production. It has mineralocorticoid activity, similar to the mechanism in 11-hydroxylase deficiency). Hypertension and hyperkalemia can occur, particularly in patients with quite elevated urine cortisol who also respond well to therapy. The best therapy is a mineralocorticoid receptor antagonist, such as spironolactone. While the mainstay of treatment evaluation is by clinical examination and evaluation, it would be helpful to also gauge the further effect of the drug and repeat the measurements of 24-hour urinary cortisol and plasma ACTH (Answer C).

Simply continuing therapy (Answer D) might be an option, but it would not address the hypokalemia and hypertension. These adverse effects are most likely occurring because the patient is responding to therapy, and a further dosage increase (Answer B) is not indicated. Therefore, there is also no reason to switch to an alternative agent, such as a glucocorticoid receptor antagonist (Answer E). It is important to note that with mifepristone therapy, cortisol levels cannot be used to monitor treatment effect, which should be mainly done by assessing clinical response and fasting glucose levels. Cortisol, and often ACTH, rises with mifepristone, as the drug also inhibits hypothalamic and pituitary feedback inhibition.

The other severe adverse effect of osilodrostat is adrenal insufficiency, which is unlikely in the setting of high blood pressure, and emergency measurements (Answer A) are not indicated. The patient's symptoms are most likely caused by steroid withdrawal due to drug effect.

EDUCATIONAL OBJECTIVE
Guide clinical surveillance in patients with Cushing syndrome who are treated with enzyme inhibitors.

REFERENCE(S)
Pivonello R, Fleseriu M, Newell-Price J, et al; LINC 3 Investigators. Efficacy and safety of osilodrostat in patients with Cushing's disease (LINC 3): a multicentre phase III study with a double-blind, randomised withdrawal phase. *Lancet Diabetes Endocrinol.* 2020;8(9):748-761. PMID: 32730798

Pivonello R, Ferrigno R, De Martino MC, et al. Medical treatment of Cushing's disease: an overview of the current and recent clinical trials. *Front Endocrinol (Lausanne)*. 2020;11:648. PMID: 33363514

7 ANSWER: B) Follicular-phase progesterone

Few women with classic 21-hydroxylase deficiency attempt to bear children (<25% of all and <10% of those with null *CYP21A2* alleles). For those who do attempt to have children, however, fecundity rates are close to that of the general population (>90%). Of the parameters that matter for achieving fertility, neither androgens nor the precursor 17-hydroxyprogesterone—which are characteristically elevated in this disease—are targets of therapy (thus, Answers A, C, D, and E are incorrect). Women with 21-hydroxylase deficiency can ovulate despite elevated adrenal-derived androgens. In contrast, high adrenal-derived progesterone in the follicular phase (Answer B) has the same effect as progestin-only contraceptives, making the cervical mucus unfavorable and thinning the endometrial lining, thus impairing sperm penetration and endometrial receptivity. The goal is a follicular-phase progesterone concentration less than 0.6 ng/mL (<2.0 nmol/L).

EDUCATIONAL OBJECTIVE
Titrate therapy for a woman with classic 21-hydroxylase deficiency who is attempting to bear children.

REFERENCE(S)
Auchus RJ, Arlt W. Approach to the patient: the adult with congenital adrenal hyperplasia. *J Clin Endocrinol Metab*. 2013;98(7):2645-2655. PMID: 23837188

Speiser PW, Arlt W, Auchus RJ, et al. Congenital adrenal hyperplasia due to steroid 21-hydroxylase deficiency: an Endocrine Society clinical practice guideline. *J Clin Endocrinol Metab*. 2018;103(11): 4043-4088. PMID: 30272171

Casteràs A, De Silva P, Rumsby G, Conway GS. Reassessing fecundity in women with classical congenital adrenal hyperplasia (CAH): normal pregnancy rate but reduced fertility rate. *Clin Endocrinol (Oxf)*. 2009;70(6):833-837. PMID: 19250265

8 ANSWER: E) Measure serum cortisol after 1 mg of dexamethasone

Because of hypertension and hypokalemia, this patient was evaluated for primary aldosteronism, and the screening aldosterone-to-renin ratio is positive, but only modestly so. Ordinarily, one would proceed to confirmatory testing, followed by CT, and then adrenal venous sampling to localize the source(s) of aldosterone. In this case, however, the weight gain, hyperglycemia, and dermal atrophy are suggestive of hypercortisolism as well. Proximal myopathy and striae are late manifestations in the development of Cushing syndrome and are insensitive findings. Because CT was performed, we know that she has a fairly large adrenal tumor—significantly larger than those that usually cause primary aldosteronism. Also, the contralateral (right) adrenal gland is somewhat atrophic, suggesting hypercortisolism from the left adrenal tumor. When the diameter of adrenal cortical tumors is greater than 2.4 cm, the risk of hypercortisolism rises, and if the tumor is removed without testing cortisol dynamics, adrenal crisis might occur postoperatively. In addition, the CT scan in this vignette was done only with contrast, so one cannot use density to determine whether the tumor is lipid-rich, which would exclude pheochromocytoma. However, plasma metanephrines would be elevated if a mass this large were a pheochromocytoma.

Spironolactone (Answer A) would treat the mineralocorticoid excess but not glucocorticoid manifestations, and this patient needs further evaluation before starting therapy. Left adrenalectomy or biopsy (Answers B and C) is incorrect because the possibilities of hypercortisolism (and pheochromocytoma) must be excluded before performing surgery or biopsy for a tumor of this size. Adrenal venous sampling (Answer D) is the gold standard for lateralizing aldosterone production in primary aldosteronism, but if the tumor is cosecreting cortisol—which is used to correct adrenal vein aldosterone concentrations for dilution with mixed venous blood—the suppression of cortisol from the contralateral adrenal will artifactually raise the aldosterone-to-cortisol ratio on the contralateral side. With the concern of hypercortisolism and the presence of a large adrenal tumor, performing a 1-mg overnight dexamethasone-suppression test (Answer E) before deciding whether referral for surgery or venous sampling is necessary is the correct next step.

In this case, the overnight dexamethasone-suppression test resulted in a cortisol concentration of 4.4 μg/dL (121 nmol/L). Subsequent test results:

ACTH = 6.0 pg/mL (10-60 pg/mL)
   (SI: 1.3 pmol/L [2.2-13.2 pmol/L])
DHEA-S = 22 μg/dL (18-244 μg/dL) (SI:
   0.60 μmol/L [0.49-6.61 μmol/L])
Urinary free cortisol, normal

Thus, the diagnosis of ACTH-independent hypercortisolism was established, which overrides the evaluation of primary aldosteronism and indicates that the large left adrenal tumor should be removed with perioperative glucocorticoid coverage. Coproduction of aldosterone and cortisol from adrenal cortical adenomas, particularly larger tumors, is well described. It is possible, although unlikely, that the primary aldosteronism is bilateral and unrelated to the adrenal tumor, so the patient should be rescreened for primary aldosteronism after adrenalectomy. If it persists, spironolactone would be an appropriate treatment. After adrenalectomy, this patient had resolution of hypercortisolemia, hyperaldosteronism, and hypertension.

EDUCATIONAL OBJECTIVE
Suspect cortisol coproduction in large aldosterone-producing adenomas.

REFERENCE(S)

Spath M, Korovkin S, Antke C, Anlauf M, Willenberg HS. Aldosterone- and cortisol-co-secreting adrenal tumors: the lost subtype of primary aldosteronism. *Eur J Endocrinol.* 2011;164(4):447-455. PMID: 21270113

Morelli V, Reimondo G, Giordano R, et al. Long-term follow-up in adrenal incidentalomas: an Italian multicenter study. *J Clin Endocrinol Metab.* 2014;99(3):827-834. PMID: 24423350

Fallo F, Bertello C, Tizzani D, et al. Concurrent primary aldosteronism and subclinical cortisol hypersecretion: a prospective study. *J Hypertens.* 2011;29(9):1773-1777. PMID: 21720261

9 **ANSWER: C) Normal serum potassium**
Mifepristone is a competitive antagonist for both the glucocorticoid receptor and the progesterone receptor, but it does not block cortisol action on the mineralocorticoid receptor. Mifepristone is used for the treatment of Cushing syndrome in patients with glucose intolerance or diabetes mellitus. Because mifepristone also antagonizes the feedback inhibition of cortisol on the adenoma, ACTH and cortisol production often rise in patients with Cushing disease on treatment, but not enough to offset the beneficial effects of glucocorticoid receptor blockade in peripheral tissues. Consequently, serum cortisol and plasma ACTH tend to rise and exert even greater effects on the mineralocorticoid receptor, which can cause hypokalemia and hypertension. For this reason, serum potassium must be corrected before starting mifepristone (thus, Answer C is correct and Answer E is incorrect).

Blood pressure occasionally rises, but it more commonly decreases after several weeks of treatment. This patient's degree of blood pressure control is acceptable for starting therapy (thus, Answer A is incorrect). When elevated, serum glucose decreases rapidly with mifepristone treatment, and the improved glycemic control is a reliable indicator of therapeutic effect. In fact, patients treated with insulin and hypoglycemic agents other than metformin should reduce their dosages before commencing mifepristone, and normalizing blood glucose with these agents before starting therapy can lead to dangerous hypoglycemia (thus, Answer B is incorrect). Plasma triglycerides also tend to improve slightly with mifepristone and do not worsen (thus, Answer D is incorrect).

Additional parameters to monitor as indications of therapeutic response include weight loss, improvement in cognition and depression (when present), and regression of cushingoid features, but these changes take much longer than the immediate reduction in glucose.

Because of potent progesterone receptor antagonism, menses cease and pregnancy is not possible during mifepristone therapy. Mifepristone causes abortion in pregnant women. Therefore, a negative pregnancy test was documented in this patient before starting therapy, but additional contraception is unnecessary. In addition, endometrial hypertrophy and vaginal bleeding can occur weeks to months after starting therapy and should be monitored.

EDUCATIONAL OBJECTIVE
Identify contraindications and precautions when using mifepristone therapy for Cushing disease.

REFERENCE(S)
Castinetti F, Fassnacht M, Johanssen S, et al. Merits and pitfalls of mifepristone in Cushing's syndrome. *Eur J Endocrinol.* 2009;160(6):1003-1010. PMID: 19289534

Fleseriu M, Biller BM, Findling JW, Molitch ME, Schteingart DE, Gross C; SEISMIC Study Investigators. Mifepristone, a glucocorticoid receptor antagonist, produces clinical and metabolic benefits in patients with Cushing's syndrome. *J Clin Endocrinol Metab.* 2012;97(6):2039-2049. PMID: 22466348

10 **ANSWER: C) Successful study: both adrenal glands are sources (bilateral hyperaldosteronism)**

For adrenal venous sampling, the cortisol concentrations in the adrenal vein samples are used to determine whether the adrenal veins were accessed and to correct for the fractional dilution of the adrenal vein blood with mixed venous blood.

This ratio of cortisol in the adrenal vein blood to the cortisol in the mixed venous blood is often called the selectivity index. The selectivity index on both sides should be greater than 2 if adrenal venous sampling is performed without cosyntropin infusion and greater than 4 if performed with cosyntropin. Otherwise, the sample does not contain sufficient adrenal vein blood to interpret the results. The study should not be interpreted unless both selectivity indices are greater than these minimum values, with the one exception discussed below. The right side, which is more difficult to access, more often fails the selectivity test than the left side. When access to the right side is successful, the steroids in the right-side sample are usually more concentrated than in the left-side sample due to the dilution of the left adrenal vein specimen from the inferior phrenic vein. In this case, the selectivity index on the right side is 37.5, and although the selectivity index on the left side is only 6, this value is sufficient for a valid study (thus, Answers A, D, and E are incorrect).

Although the absolute value of aldosterone in the right adrenal vein sample is much higher than in the left adrenal vein sample, the cortisol-corrected aldosterone (aldosterone-to-cortisol ratio) is well within a factor of 2 (4.0/3.8 = 1.05) (thus, Answer C is correct and Answer B is incorrect). If the aldosterone-to-cortisol ratio in one adrenal vein is much lower than in the mixed venous blood, which is called "contralateral suppression," aldosterone production can usually be confidently localized to the other adrenal, even if that implicated adrenal vein was not accessed adequately.

EDUCATIONAL OBJECTIVE
Interpret results of adrenal venous sampling.

REFERENCE(S)
Rossi GP, Auchus RJ, Brown M, et al. An expert consensus statement on the use of adrenal vein sampling for the subtyping of primary aldosteronism. *Hypertension.* 2014;63(1):151-160. PMID: 24218436

Funder JW, Carey RM, Mantero F, et al. The management of primary aldosteronism: case detection, diagnosis, and treatment: an Endocrine Society Clinical Practice Guideline. *J Clin Endocrinol Metab.* 2016;101(5):1889-1916. PMID: 26934393

Vaidya A, Malchoff CD, Auchus RJ; AACE Adrenal Scientific Committee. An individualized approach to the evaluation and management of primary aldosteronism. *Endocr Pract.* 2017;23(6):680-689. PMID: 28332881

11 ANSWER: C) Adrenocortical carcinoma

Functional benign adrenal adenomas generally produce a single major active hormone. Large cortisol-producing adenomas sometimes cosecrete aldosterone, but usually one hormone excess is dominant, while the second is mild. In contrast, overt, clinically manifested excess of more than one active steroid, such as androgen and mineralocorticoid, is characteristic of adrenocortical carcinomas (Answer C). Furthermore, the rapid progression of androgen excess alone, with very high testosterone and virilization (voice deepening), is worrisome for an adrenal or ovarian tumor. Coexistence of mineralocorticoid excess, disproportionate to the cortisol and aldosterone concentrations, suggests elevation of cortisol precursors, primarily corticosterone and 11-deoxycorticosterone. Adrenal carcinomas tend to be relatively deficient in 11β-hydroxylase activity, leading to elevation of 11-deoxycortisol and further upstream intermediates, which can account for the robust androgen and mineralocorticoid excess with normal or modestly elevated cortisol. 11-Deoxycortisol has emerged as one of the best markers for adrenal cancer, and it is clearly elevated in this case.

Macronodular adrenocortical hyperplasia (Answer A) typically manifests with pure cortisol excess, and the (apparent) mineralocorticoid excess is due to high cortisol and thus rises in parallel with cortisol production. DHEA-S is usually normal in hypercortisolemic patients with macronodular hyperplasia rather than suppressed as is often the case in hypercortisolemic patients with unilateral adrenal cortical adenomas, but this preservation of DHEA-S does not account for the profound androgen excess in this patient. While mild or nonclassic 11β-hydroxylase deficiency (Answer B) has been described, these patients have mild androgen excess and rarely have hypertension; the abrupt onset in adulthood as in this vignette is also inconsistent with a genetic etiology. While both Sertoli-Leydig–cell tumors (Answer E) and hyperthecosis (Answer D) can cause significant hyperandrogenemia and virilization, DHEA-S levels are not elevated in affected patients. Hyperthecosis usually has a slower onset, while Sertoli-Leydig–cell tumors lead to faster development of symptoms.

EDUCATIONAL OBJECTIVE
Suspect adrenal cortical carcinoma on the basis of clinical features.

REFERENCE(S)
Arlt W, Biehl M, Taylor AE, et al. Urine steroid metabolomics as a biomarker tool for detecting malignancy in adrenal tumors. *J Clin Endocrinol Metab.* 2011;96(12):3775- 3784. PMID: 21917861

Messer CK, Kirschenbaum A, New MI, Unger P, Gabrilove JL, Levine AC. Concomitant secretion of glucocorticoid, androgens, and mineralocorticoid by an adrenocortical carcinoma: case report and review of literature. *Endocr Pract.* 2007;13(4): 408-412. PMID: 17669719

12 ANSWER: E) Increase sodium intake

Chronic vasoconstriction in patients with pheochromocytoma induces a state of volume depletion. Often the hematocrit is slightly increased, and patients can be hypertensive but show orthostatic hypotension, especially with α-adrenergic blockade. After just a few doses of phenoxybenzamine, the patient was still hypertensive but now has an orthostatic rise in heart rate. Preoperative volume expansion via sodium loading (Answer E) is critical to mitigate postoperative hypotension. Often a β-adrenergic blocker is added once adequate α-blockade is established and volume expansion is completed, but the rise in heart rate with standing is maintaining the blood pressure with standing.

Adding metoprolol now (Answer A) could dangerously drop the patient's blood pressure. The phenoxybenzamine dosage will need to be increased later but not until his orthostasis improves (thus, Answer B is incorrect). Nicardipine (Answer C) is sometimes used as an alternative to α-adrenergic blockade, but phenoxybenzamine is effective in this patient; he simply needs time to allow volume expansion at the lower dose using either drug. The patient remains hypertensive and blood pressure is not at goal (<120/<80 mm Hg); therefore, blockade should be continued and the phenoxybenzamine dosage should be increased after volume repletion (thus, Answer D is incorrect).

EDUCATIONAL OBJECTIVE
Manage volume depletion in a patient with pheochromocytoma.

REFERENCE(S)
Lenders JW, Duh QY, Eisenhofer G, et al; Endocrine Society. Pheochromocytoma and paraganglioma: an Endocrine Society Clinical Practice Guideline. *J Clin Endocrinol Metab.* 2014;99(6):1915-1942. PMID: 24893135

Young WF Jr. Adrenal causes of hypertension: pheochromocytoma and primary aldosteronism. *Rev Endocr Metab Disord.* 2007;8(4):309-320. PMID: 17914676

13 ANSWER: C) Normal testosterone, high androstenedione, low LH

This patient has a history of adrenal insufficiency with bilateral testicular masses and medication nonadherence. This is an unfortunately common situation for young men with classic 21-hydroxylase deficiency who develop testicular adrenal rest tumors (TARTs). These are ACTH-responsive masses that are either ectopic adrenal tissue or reprogrammed steroidogenic stem cells in the testes that grow and produce a pattern of steroids similar to that of the adrenal cortex of these patients. The major clue is the bilateral nature of the tumors and their firm, irregular texture. In 21-hydroxylase deficiency, the adrenal produces abundant androstenedione and inefficiently converts this precursor to testosterone, so the major laboratory feature is elevated androstenedione, disproportionate to testosterone, which is typically "normal" but not derived from the normal testicular Leydig cells. The high adrenal androgen production suppresses LH. Initially, FSH is also low, but with time the masses compromise blood flow to the normal testis and cause irreversible damage to the Sertoli and germ cells, and FSH rises. Both the testicular mass and the suppressed gonadotropins cause infertility. TARTs and high FSH are poor prognostic factors for fertility in men with classic 21-hydroxylase deficiency. Intensification of glucocorticoid therapy can allow regression of the rests and restoration of fertility, but this can take many months. Surgical removal of TARTs often provides long-term control of the tumors, but it does not restore testicular function. The pattern of laboratory results expected in this patient is normal testosterone, high androstenedione, and low LH (Answer C).

The pattern depicted in Answer A implies LH-dependent androstenedione and testosterone production, which is incorrect. The pattern depicted in Answer B is typical of a Leydig-cell tumor producing estradiol but presents as a solitary, often small and round mass in one testis. The pattern in Answer D is typical of primary testicular failure and ignores the adrenal-derived androgens. The pattern in Answer E is typical of a nonfunctional testicular tumor such as a seminoma early in the disease course, and these cancers are also unilateral.

EDUCATIONAL OBJECTIVE
Diagnose testicular adrenal rest tumors in a man with 21-hydroxylase deficiency and predict patterns of laboratory test results.

REFERENCE(S)
Finkielstain GP, Chen W, Mehta SP, et al. Comprehensive genetic analysis of 182 unrelated families with congenital adrenal hyperplasia due to 21-hydroxylase deficiency. *J Clin Endocrinol Metab.* 2011;96(1):E161-E172. PMID: 20926536

Arlt W, Willis DS, Wild SH, et al; United Kingdom Congenital Adrenal Hyperplasia Adult Study Executive (CaHASE). Health status of adults with congenital adrenal hyperplasia: a cohort study of 203 patients. *J Clin Endocrinol Metab.* 2010;95(10):5110-5121. PMID: 20719839

Auchus RJ, Arlt W. Approach to the patient: the adult with congenital adrenal hyperplasia. *J Clin Endocrinol Metab.* 2013;98(7):2645-2655. PMID: 23837188

Reisch N, Rottenkolber M, Greifenstein A, et al. Testicular adrenal rest tumors develop independently of long-term disease control: a longitudinal analysis of 50 adult men with congenital adrenal hyperplasia due to classic 21-hydroxylase deficiency. *J Clin Endocrinol Metab.* 2013;98(11):E1820-E1826. PMID: 23969190

Claahsen-van der Grinten HL, Otten BJ, Takahashi S, et al. Testicular adrenal rest tumors in adult males with congenital adrenal hyperplasia: evaluation of pituitary-gonadal function before and after successful testis-sparing surgery in eight patients. *J Clin Endocrinol Metab.* 2007;92(2):612- 615. PMID: 17090637

King TF, Lee MC, Williamson EE, Conway GS. Experience in optimizing fertility outcomes in men with congenital adrenal hyperplasia due to 21 hydroxylase deficiency. *Clin Endocrinol (Oxf).* 2016;84(6):830-836. PMID: 26666213

14 ANSWER: B) Rescreen after correcting hypokalemia

Although many medications interact with the renin-angiotensin-aldosterone axis, most antihypertensive agents act by vasodilation or volume depletion, which tends to raise plasma renin activity. Thus, when the plasma renin activity is low (<1), the aldosterone-to-renin ratio (ARR) screen is generally valid. β-Adrenergic blockers can lower renin, but aldosterone falls as well. The ARR in this case is greater than 13, which is intermediate between a clearly positive screen (>20) (Answer E) and a normal screen (<4) (Answer A). During proper preparation for screening, however, it is important to first correct hypokalemia (Answer B), as low potassium impairs aldosterone production. Thus, in a setting of high

clinical suspicion and an unusual result with a very low potassium, the screen cannot be dismissed as normal and should be repeated after correcting the hypokalemia.

Candesartan and nifedipine are not significantly interfering with the screening since the plasma renin activity is less than 1 (thus, Answers C and D are incorrect). However, these drugs can cause false-negative screens if the renin is elevated.

EDUCATIONAL OBJECTIVE
Identify causes of false-negative screening for primary aldosteronism.

REFERENCE(S)
Raizman JE, Diamandis EP, Holmes D, Stowasser M, Auchus R, Cavalier E. A renin-ssance in primary aldosteronism testing: obstacles and opportunities for screening, diagnosis, and management. *Clin Chem.* 2015;61(8):1022-1027. PMID: 26106077

Funder JW, Carey RM, Mantero F, et al. The management of primary aldosteronism: case detection, diagnosis, and treatment: an Endocrine Society Clinical Practice Guideline. *J Clin Endocrinol Metab.* 2016;101(5):1889-1916. PMID: 26934393

15 ANSWER: C) Prolonged hyperkalemia

With sustained autonomous aldosterone excess, the normal zona glomerulosa can become suppressed. In this case, hyperkalemia can develop after adrenalectomy. Identified risk factors include older age, longer duration of hypertension, proteinuria, and most importantly, reduced renal function. This older man with longstanding hypertension, microalbuminuria, and elevated serum creatinine is therefore at significant risk for postoperative hyperkalemia (Answer C), which can be prolonged. Hyperkalemia can be treated with dietary potassium restriction, a thiazide diuretic, or fludrocortisone acetate, depending on the patient's blood pressure.

Patients with primary aldosteronism often have a slight rise in creatinine after adrenalectomy or upon addition of mineralocorticoid receptor antagonist therapy, but they rarely experience renal failure (Answer A). Unlike patients with pheochromocytoma who are receiving potent α1 receptor blockade, refractory hypotension (Answer B) does not develop postoperatively. Because the tumor was localized with adrenal venous sampling, recurrence of hyperaldosteronism (Answer D) is unlikely. Adrenal insufficiency (Answer E) can occur after removal of an aldosterone-secreting adenoma that is cosecreting cortisol, but these tumors tend to be larger than 3 cm, and cortisol withdrawal is very unlikely given the small size of the adenoma.

EDUCATIONAL OBJECTIVE
Identify risk factors for postadrenalectomy hyperkalemia in patients with primary aldosteronism.

REFERENCE(S)

Chiang WF, Cheng CJ, Wu ST, et al. Incidence and factors of post-adrenalectomy hyperkalemia in patients with aldosterone producing adenoma. *Clin Chim Acta.* 2013;424:114-118. PMID: 23727469

Fischer E, Hanslik G, Pallauf A, et al. Prolonged zona glomerulosa insufficiency causing hyperkalemia in primary aldosteronism after adrenalectomy. *J Clin Endocrinol Metab.* 2012;97(11):3965-3973. PMID: 22893716

Park KS, Kim JH, Ku EJ, et al. Clinical risk factors of postoperative hyperkalemia after adrenalectomy in patients with aldosterone-producing adenoma. *Eur J Endocrinol.* 2015;172(6):725-731. PMID: 25766046

16   ANSWER: D) Substitute prednisolone, 20 mg daily, for prednisone

Adrenal axis suppression from pharmacologic glucocorticoid dosing is common with dosages exceeding 5 mg daily of prednisone or its equivalent when given for 6 or more weeks. The duration of suppression is proportionate to both the dosage and duration of therapy. This woman is clinically cushingoid with laboratory data indicating a suppressed hypothalamic-pituitary-adrenal axis yet preserved renin and aldosterone. Ordinarily, as long as patients continue the same dosage of glucocorticoid, their physiology will not reflect glucocorticoid deficiency. In this case, however, the patient has developed acute hepatic injury and is taking prednisone, which is a prodrug that requires conversion by the liver to the active drug prednisolone (via 11β-hydroxysteroid dehydrogenase type 1). In a patient with severely compromised hepatocellular function, this conversion is impaired, and there is no exposure to active drug. Switching to an active form of glucocorticoid such as prednisolone (Answer D) will provide drug exposure. Any other active glucocorticoid such as hydrocortisone, methylprednisolone, or dexamethasone at appropriate dosages would also be correct.

Further testing (Answers A and E) is not necessary given the history, low ACTH and cortisol, and high renin and relatively high aldosterone (thus, Answers A and E are incorrect). Fludrocortisone at a dosage of 0.1 mg twice daily (Answer B) adds little to the aldosterone in her circulation and provides negligible glucocorticoid exposure. A higher prednisone dosage (Answer C) is not likely to help given the impaired liver function.

EDUCATIONAL OBJECTIVE
Choose glucocorticoid drugs in patients with liver failure.

REFERENCE(S)

Tomlinson JW, Walker EA, Bujalska IJ, et al. 11beta-hydroxysteroid dehydrogenase type 1: a tissue-specific regulator of glucocorticoid response. *Endocr Rev.* 2004;25(5):831-866. PMID: 15466942

Frey BM, Frey FJ. Clinical pharmacokinetics of prednisone and prednisolone. *Clin Pharmacokinet.* 1990;19(2):126-146. PMID: 2199128

Madsbad S, Bjerregaard B, Henriksen JH, Juhl E, Kehlet H. Impaired conversion of prednisone to prednisolone in patients with liver cirrhosis. *Gut.* 1980;21(1):52-56. PMID: 7364321

17   ANSWER: B) Late-night salivary cortisol measurement

The loss of cortisol diurnal rhythm is a defining feature of Cushing disease. Saliva is an ultrafiltrate of plasma, and salivary cortisol concentrations roughly reflect plasma free cortisol concentrations. At night, plasma cortisol concentrations fall, and salivary cortisol falls in parallel. Salivary cortisol testing has become routine and offers comparable diagnostic utility and greater convenience than late-night serum cortisol testing. In addition to its utility as a screening test for Cushing disease, late-night salivary cortisol testing is more sensitive than other conventional tests in detecting recurrent disease (thus, Answer B is correct). False-positive results with late-night salivary cortisol measurement occur in persons with gingival or tongue bleeding, with sleep disturbance, or who work night shifts. Also, contamination can influence test results, such as transfer of hydrocortisone cream from the hands to the device used to collect the saliva.

Twenty-four–hour urinary free cortisol measurement (Answer A) is quite variable and is a relatively insensitive test for detecting recurrent Cushing disease because only a small fraction (<1%) of cortisol is excreted unmetabolized, which only occurs when the cortisol concentration exceeds the binding capacity of plasma. Dexamethasone-suppression testing (Answers C and D) uses the attenuated feedback inhibition of the pituitary adenoma to dexamethasone compared with the normal pituitary, and cutoffs are empirically determined. This distinction is not as reliable as the loss of diurnal rhythm in early, recurrent Cushing disease. Inferior petrosal sinus sampling (Answer E) is only used to exclude ectopic ACTH syndrome *after* the diagnosis of ACTH-dependent hypercortisolism is established, and this test is not indicated in a patient with previous Cushing disease documented histologically as in this case.

EDUCATIONAL OBJECTIVE
Compare the diagnostic performance of different testing approaches for recurrent Cushing disease.

REFERENCE(S)
Carrasco CA, Coste J, Guignat L, et al. Midnight salivary cortisol determination for assessing the outcome of transsphenoidal surgery in Cushing's disease. *J Clin Endocrinol Metab.* 2008;93(12): 4728-4734. PMID: 18728161

Raff H, Auchus RJ, Findling JW, Niemann LK. Urine free cortisol in the diagnosis of Cushing's syndrome: is it worth doing and, if so, how? *J Clin Endocrinol Metab.* 2015;100(2):395-397. PMID: 25423573

Petersenn S, Newell-Price J, Findling JW, et al; Pasireotide B2305 Study Group. High variability in baseline urinary free cortisol values in patients with Cushing's disease. *Clin Endocrinol (Oxf).* 2014;80(2):261-269. PMID: 23746264

18 ANSWER: E) CT-guided percutaneous adrenal biopsy

The diagnosis of primary adrenal insufficiency may be suspected on the basis of many nonspecific signs and symptoms, volume depletion, hyponatremia, hyperkalemia, and, less commonly, incidentally discovered bilateral adrenal imaging abnormalities. This patient has many clinical features of adrenal insufficiency. Confirmation of primary adrenal insufficiency was secured with just basal biochemical studies. When ACTH levels exceed 80 to 100 pg/mL (17.6-22.0 pmol/L), maximum adrenocortical stimulation is achieved and cortisol levels greater than 18 µg/dL (>497 nmol/L) would be expected. This patient's markedly elevated ACTH level and his suboptimal cortisol response confirm the presence of primary adrenal insufficiency. Assessment of the renin-angiotensin-aldosterone system provides further confirmation, with a markedly elevated plasma renin activity and a low serum aldosterone. The differential diagnosis in this setting includes infiltrative and inflammatory processes, metastatic disease, bilateral adrenal hemorrhage, and primary adrenal lymphoma. The best option to establish the correct diagnosis in this patient is CT-guided percutaneous adrenal biopsy (Answer E). Pheochromocytoma should always be excluded before this procedure, but the trivial elevation of normetanephrine is inconsistent with functional tumors of that size and is due to volume depletion. Causes of false-positive elevations in plasma and urinary metanephrines include tricyclic antidepressants, serotonin norepinephrine reuptake inhibitors, clonidine withdrawal, and sleep apnea. In this patient, CT-guided percutaneous adrenal biopsy demonstrated findings consistent with histoplasmosis. He is from an area near the confluence of the Ohio and Mississippi Rivers, where histoplasmosis is endemic. Part of the biopsy should also be used for acid fast bacilli culture. An interferon-gamma release assay should also be done to test for tuberculosis, as this can present with the same clinical picture with adrenal insufficiency and increased adrenal gland size.

Patients with autoimmune adrenalitis have small rather than large adrenal glands, so 21-hydroxylase antibodies (Answer B), even if paradoxically positive, will not aid in the diagnosis. Urinary free cortisol (Answer A) is not used to diagnose cortisol deficiency. Because this patient clearly has primary adrenal insufficiency, a pituitary imaging study (Answer C) is unnecessary. Adrenal venous sampling (Answer D) is of no use in the evaluation of adrenal insufficiency.

Assessing for the presence of histoplasmosis antigen in the urine would be a reasonable alternative approach, but this was not listed as an answer option in this vignette.

EDUCATIONAL OBJECTIVE
Select the appropriate diagnostic test for the evaluation of adrenal insufficiency with bilateral adrenal gland enlargement.

REFERENCE(S)
Bornstein SR, Allolio B, Arlt W, et al. Diagnosis and treatment of primary adrenal insufficiency: an Endocrine Society Clinical Practice Guideline. *J Clin Endocrinol Metab.* 2016;101(2):364-389. PMID: 26760044

Kumar N, Singh S, Govil S. Adrenal histoplasmosis: clinical presentation and imaging features in nine cases. *Abdom Imaging.* 2003;28(5):703-708. PMID: 14628881

Zhou L, Peng W, Wang C, Liu X, Shen Y, Zhou K. Primary adrenal lymphoma: radiological; pathological, clinical correlation. *Eur J Radiol.* 2012;81(3):401-405. PMID: 21146945

Zieger MA, Siegelman SS, Hamrahian AH. Medical and surgical evaluation and treatment of adrenal incidentalomas. *J Clin Endocrinol Metab.* 2011;96(7):2004-2015. PMID: 21632813

19 ANSWER: B) Her risk of having a child with classic 21-OHD is >0.5%

The prevalence of classic and nonclassic 21-OHD in the general population is 1 in 16,000 and 1 in 1000, respectively. To have classic 21-OHD, an individual must either have no functional *CYP21A2* alleles or have less than 2% residual enzyme activity. Nearly all patients with classic 21-OHD are identified in infancy because of atypical genitalia, adrenal insufficiency, and/or abnormal newborn screening results (now available in many countries, including the United States). Most cases of nonclassic 21-OHD are never diagnosed, particularly when the affected individual is male. To have nonclassic 21-OHD, an individual must have at least 1 partially functional allele with 10% to 20% of residual enzyme activity and no wild-type allele. The other allele can be a classic 21-OHD pathogenic variant or deletion (0%-2% activity) or a second nonclassic 21-OHD allele. Studies have shown that about 70% of patients who are diagnosed with nonclassic 21-OHD are compound heterozygotes for a nonclassic allele and a classic allele. Furthermore, 4% of parents with children affected by classic 21-OHD actually have occult nonclassic 21-OHD, and they themselves are compound heterozygotes for classic and nonclassic 21-OHD alleles. Consequently, even without knowing this patient's genotype, we know she is at higher-than-average risk for having a child with classic 21-OHD.

In order to understand the calculations, one must know the carrier frequency of classic CAH alleles, which is approximately 2%. Therefore, the chance that the patient's partner carries a classic 21-OHD allele is 1 in 50. In the event that the partner carries a classic CAH allele, one-fourth of the couple's offspring will be homozygous for a classic CAH allele. Thus, without any genotype testing, the probability that this couple will have a child affected with classic CAH is 1 in 200 (0.5%) (1/50 × 1/4) (Answer B). The largest 2 studies of such patients documented the risk to be even a little higher than the theoretical risk, in the range of 1.5% to 2.5%.

Because the patient could be a compound heterozygote with 1 classic 21-OHD allele and

1 nonclassic allele, and her partner could possibly be a carrier of a classic CAH allele, she indeed could have a child with classic 21-OHD as outlined above (thus, Answer C is incorrect). The risk of 0.01% translates to the general population risk (1 in 16,000) (thus, Answer A is incorrect). If both the patient and her partner were to have a clinical diagnosis of nonclassic 21-OHD, it would be possible that both are homozygous for nonclassic 21-OHD alleles (and hence not at risk for having a child with classic 21-OHD). As discussed, this couple is at risk of having a child with classic 21-OHD if the patient has a classic CAH allele and her partner is simply a carrier of a classic CAH allele (not affected with 21-OHD) (thus, Answer D is incorrect). If she and her partner are both carriers of a classic CAH allele, then the probability of having a child affected with classic 21-OHD is 25% with each pregnancy. The diagram illustrates 2 of several possibilities.

EDUCATIONAL OBJECTIVE
Counsel a patient on the genetics of 21-hydroxylase deficiency and the frequencies of classic and nonclassic alleles.

REFERENCE(S)
Finkielstain GP, Chen W, Mehta SP, et al. Comprehensive genetic analysis of 182 unrelated families with congenital adrenal hyperplasia due to 21-hydroxylase deficiency. *J Clin Endocrinol Metab.* 2011;96(1):E161-E172. PMID: 20926536

Nandagopal R, Sinaii N, Avila NA, et al. Phenotypic profiling of parents with cryptic nonclassic congenital adrenal hyperplasia: findings in 145 unrelated families. *Eur J Endocrinol.* 2011;164(6): 977-984. PMID: 21444649

Moran C, Azziz R, Weintrob N, et al. Reproductive outcome of women with 21-hydroxylase-deficient nonclassic adrenal hyperplasia. *J Clin Endocrinol Metab.* 2006;91(9):3451-3456. PMID: 16822826

20 ANSWER: E) Antiresorptive therapy with a bisphosphonate or denosumab

This patient has evidence of metastatic pheochromocytoma at presentation by virtue of its presence in a thoracic vertebra and 2 suspicious pulmonary lesions. For the past 2 years, his condition has remained clinically stable with no evidence of biochemical progression and stable radiologic disease with the exception of intense

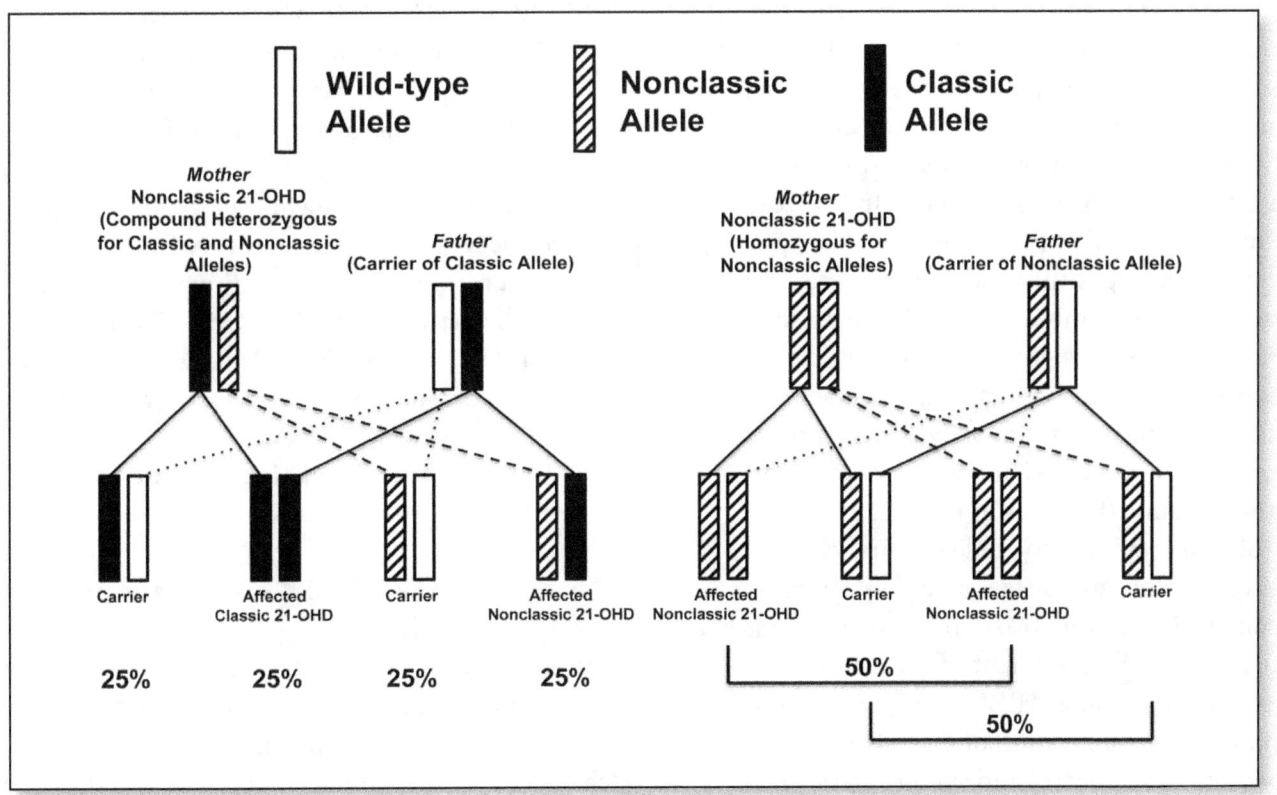

uptake in the colon. However, pheochromocytoma does not metastasize to the colon and the lesions seen in this patient are most likely related to his metformin therapy. Intestinal ^{18}F-fluorodeoxyglucose uptake is markedly increased in patients with type 2 diabetes mellitus who take metformin. Uptake occurs in all segments of the intestine and it is typically intense and diffuse in the small and large intestine above the bowel wall and lumen. The pattern can be variable, with some patients having focal or segmental uptake. Therefore, radiotherapy to the colon (Answer B) is not indicated. Discontinuation of metformin reverses intestinal ^{18}F-fluorodeoxyglucose uptake.

The clinical course of metastatic pheochromocytoma and paraganglioma is highly variable with a reported 5-year survival rate that ranges widely from 12% to 84%. Some patients may have stable disease for 10 to 20 years. The prognosis is influenced by tumor burden and location of metastases. Patients with brain, liver, and lung metastasis tend to have a worse prognosis than those with isolated bone lesions. Because this man has stable disease, no additional antitumor therapy is warranted now and follow-up biochemical studies and imaging in 6 to 12 months would be the most reasonable approach. Because he has bone involvement, antiresorptive therapy (Answer E) would generally be indicated.

Systemic treatment options for progressive metastatic pheochromocytoma include cytotoxic chemotherapy, with the best evidence supporting the use of cyclophosphamide, vincristine, and doxorubicin in combination with capecitabine and temozolomide (Answer C) as a reasonable first-line therapeutic alternative. This has been associated with a median survival of 3.3 years after initiating therapy. There are no comparator studies for any of the systemic therapies in malignant pheochromocytoma to guide the first choice of therapy in this circumstance. Iodine ^{131}I *meta-iodobenzylguanidine* (MIBG) (Answer A) has been approved for the treatment of metastatic pheochromocytoma. MIBG may cause partial responses or stabilization of disease with better blood pressure control and symptomatic and

performance status improvement. However, this therapy is considered only palliative. Cabozantinib (Answer D) is an oral tyrosine kinase inhibitor with some effect on pheochromocytoma, but it is not indicated in this patient with stable disease.

EDUCATIONAL OBJECTIVE
Recommend an appropriate management approach in a patient with metastatic pheochromocytoma/paraganglioma, bearing in mind the variable and often indolent course of this disease.

REFERENCE(S)

Plouin PF, Fitzgerald P, Rich T, et al. Metastatic pheochromocytoma and paraganglioma: focus on therapeutics. *Horm Metab Res.* 2012;44(5):390-399. PMID: 22314389

Hescot S, Leboulleux S, Amar L, et al; French group of Endocrine and Adrenal tumors (Groupe des Tumeurs Endocrines-REseau NAtional des Tumeurs ENdocrines and COrtico-Medullo Tumerus Endocrines networks). One-year progression-free survival of therapy-naïve patients with malignant pheochromocytoma and paraganglioma. *J Clin Endocrinol Metab.* 2013;98(10):4006-4012. PMID: 23884775

Oh JR, Song H, Chong A, et al. Impact of medication discontinuation on increased intestinal FDG accumulation in diabetic patients treated with metformin. *Am J Roentgenol.* 2010;195(6):1404-1410. PMID: 21098202

Joshua AM, Ezzat S, Asa SL, et al. Rationale and evidence for sunitinib in the treatment of malignant paraganglioma/pheochromocytoma. *J Clin Endocrinol Metab.* 2009;94(1):5-9. PMID: 19001511

Pryma DA, Chin BB, Noto RB, et al. Efficacy and safety of high-specific-activity ^{131}I-MIBG therapy in patients with advanced pheochromocytoma or paraganglioma. *J Nucl Med.* 2019;60(5):623-630. PMID: 30291194

21 ANSWER: C) CT of the adrenal glands

Determining the cause of endogenous Cushing syndrome is essential to recommending appropriate therapy. The differential diagnostic challenge in this woman is deciding whether she has ACTH-dependent or ACTH-independent hypercortisolism. Reliable ACTH assays are necessary to distinguish between elevated and, more importantly, subnormal ACTH levels. Plasma ACTH assays have certainly improved since the first radioimmunoassays; however, a recent critical evaluation of plasma ACTH assays demonstrates a high degree of variability. Most ACTH assays cannot correctly identify patients with suppressed ACTH concentrations. This patient poses a particular diagnostic difficulty because her plasma ACTH concentration is 17.0 pg/mL (3.7 pmol/L). This plasma ACTH level does not establish the diagnosis of ACTH-dependent Cushing syndrome. A repeated ACTH measurement (possibly in a different reference laboratory) should be obtained to see if a more definitive value is secured. Another reasonable approach is to perform an ovine corticotropin-releasing hormone–stimulation test (1 mcg/kg intravenously with ACTH and cortisol measurements at 15-minute intervals for 1 hour). Patients with ACTH-independent (adrenal-dependent) Cushing syndrome would be expected to have a blunted ACTH response, and those with pituitary ACTH-dependent hypercortisolism would be expected to exhibit a robust ACTH response.

The major clue in this woman is the very low DHEA-S level and the failure of any cortisol suppression even after an 8-mg overnight dexamethasone-suppression test. DHEA-S is usually low in patients with benign causes of adrenal-dependent (ACTH-independent) Cushing syndrome, while it is usually normal (sometimes elevated) in patients with ACTH-dependent hypercortisolism. In addition, most patients with mild-to-moderate hypercortisolism due to Cushing disease demonstrate some reduction in basal cortisol after even a 1-mg overnight dexamethasone-suppression test, and you would expect some suppression of cortisol after a high dose of dexamethasone in a young woman with mild pituitary Cushing syndrome. This patient is more likely to have adrenal-dependent hypercortisolism and, therefore, CT of the adrenal glands (Answer C) should be performed.

Because most plasma ACTH assays cannot reliably detect subnormal or suppressed levels, experts suggest proceeding with adrenal imaging in patients with endogenous hypercortisolism who have ACTH concentrations less than 25 pg/mL (<5.5 pmol/L).

The finding of a 2-mm pituitary lesion should be viewed with great caution. Endocrinologists should carefully review all pituitary imaging in patients with Cushing syndrome. In this case, no evidence of a pituitary tumor was seen by an experienced endocrinologist. Thus, under no circumstances should this woman undergo pituitary surgery (Answer E) without further evaluation. Inferior petrosal sinus sampling for ACTH (Answer B) is recommended in patients with ACTH-dependent hypercortisolism in whom there are normal or equivocal findings on pituitary imaging. However, the diagnosis of ACTH-dependent Cushing syndrome has not yet been confirmed in this young woman.

Although the patient had relatively rapid onset of Cushing syndrome, ectopic ACTH syndrome seems very unlikely. Most patients with ectopic ACTH secretion have elevated (or at least high-normal) plasma ACTH levels. Furthermore, CT of the chest (Answer D) and octreotide acetate scintigraphy (Answer A) should only be performed if inferior petrosal sinus sampling demonstrates the lack of a pituitary ACTH gradient. Without establishing a clear differential diagnosis, extensive imaging in patients with Cushing syndrome can lead to surgical misadventures.

Another measurement of this patient's basal ACTH concentration (performed at a more reliable laboratory) was less than 1.0 pg/mL (<0.22 pmol/L) and it did not stimulate after administration of ovine corticotropin-releasing hormone. CT of the adrenal glands showed a 3-cm right adrenal nodule with low attenuation values. Removal of the cortisol-secreting adrenal adenoma resulted in secondary adrenal insufficiency. She had complete resolution of her Cushing syndrome.

Calcium and Bone Board Review

Natalie E. Cusano, MD, MS

1 **ANSWER: D) Measure vitamin B₆ and order genetic testing for *ALPL* pathogenic variants**

Hypophosphatasia is a rare genetic disease caused by loss-of-function pathogenic variants in the *ALPL* gene, which encodes the tissue-nonspecific isoenzyme of alkaline phosphatase (TNSALP). TNSALP is particularly abundant in the bone, liver, and kidneys but is also expressed in other tissues, including cartilage and teeth. The main physiologic substrates of TNSALP are inorganic pyrophosphate and pyridoxal-5′-phosphate (the active metabolite of vitamin B₆). The loss of function of TNSALP in patients with hypophosphatasia results in a generalized reduction in alkaline phosphatase activity and accumulation of TNSALP substrates, including inorganic pyrophosphate and vitamin B₆. The prevalence of severe hypophosphatasia is approximately 1 in 100,000 among Anglo-Saxon populations and is more prevalent among the Mennonites in Manitoba, Canada, where 1 in every 25 persons is a carrier. Inheritance is autosomal recessive for the infantile forms but either autosomal recessive or autosomal dominant for the milder adult forms, with variable penetrance. The clinical presentation and severity of hypophosphatasia are variable due to the large number of described variants in the *ALPL* gene. This patient has a history of short stature, chronic dental issues, and multiple symptoms dating from childhood associated with a low alkaline phosphatase level. Hypophosphatasia was of concern in this patient, and measurement of vitamin B₆ and genetic testing for *ALPL* pathogenic variants were pursued (Answer D). A diagnosis of hypophosphatasia was confirmed, and enzyme replacement therapy with asfotase alfa improved his bone mineral density.

Pathogenic variants in the *PHEX* gene (Answer C) cause X-linked hypophosphatemic rickets, which presents with low phosphate, not low alkaline phosphatase. While this patient has osteoporosis and pharmacologic therapy should be considered (Answer B), the best next step is evaluation for hypophosphatasia. He has no symptoms of testosterone deficiency, and testosterone measurement (Answer A) is not indicated, especially given previous normal results. While small bone size (Answer E) can contribute to low bone density as it is a 2-dimensional measurement, therapy is still indicated if osteoporosis is present.

EDUCATIONAL OBJECTIVE
Diagnose hypophosphatasia.

REFERENCE(S)
Bianchi ML, Bishop NJ, Guañabens N, et al; Rare Bone Disease Action Group of the European Calcified Tissue Society. Hypophosphatasia in adolescents and adults: overview of diagnosis and treatment. *Osteoporos Int.* 2020;31(8):1445-1460. PMID: 32162014

Lewiecki EM. New and emerging concepts in the use of denosumab for the treatment of osteoporosis. *Ther Adv Musculoskelet Dis.* 2018;10(11):209-223. PMID: 30386439

2 **ANSWER: A) Refer to a parathyroid surgeon for bilateral neck exploration**

This patient has met criteria for a diagnosis of normocalcemic primary hyperparathyroidism and meets criteria for parathyroid surgery due to nephrolithiasis and osteoporosis. Patients with hypercalcemic or normocalcemic primary hyperparathyroidism who meet criteria for surgery should be considered for parathyroidectomy even if preoperative imaging studies are negative. Patients with normocalcemic primary hyperparathyroidism may be less likely to have a positive localization study due to a higher risk for multiglandular disease, as well as smaller adenoma size. This patient should be referred for bilateral neck exploration (Answer A) to address osteoporosis and risk for nephrolithiasis.

Selective venous sampling (Answer C) is an invasive test with limited expertise and it has not been studied in normocalcemic patients. Repeating ultrasonography and sestamibi imaging in 1 year (Answer B) is not appropriate since he has symptomatic disease and these studies may remain nonlocalizing. Parathyroid surgery in normocalcemic patients has been demonstrated in small cohort studies to improve biochemical parameters and bone density similar to that observed in hypercalcemic patients. This patient's urinary calcium excretion is not elevated, and hydrochlorothiazide (Answer D) is not indicated after a single episode of nephrolithiasis. In addition, hydrochlorothiazide would not address his osteoporosis. In a small study in postmenopausal women, alendronate (Answer E) improved bone density in normocalcemic patients similar to what was observed in hypercalcemic patients. However, alendronate would not reduce this patient's risk of future nephrolithiasis.

EDUCATIONAL OBJECTIVE
Identify patients with normocalcemic primary hyperparathyroidism who are surgical candidates and provide preoperative counseling.

REFERENCE(S)
Cusano NE, Cipriani C, Bilezikian JP. Management of normocalcemic primary hyperparathyroidism. *Best Pract Res Clin Endocrinol Metab.* 2018;32(6):837-845. PMID: 30665550

Cesareo R, Di Stasio E, Vescini F, et al. Effects of alendronate and vitamin D in patients with normocalcemic primary hyperparathyroidism. *Osteoporos Int.* 2015;26(4):1295-1302. PMID: 25524023

Pandian TK, Lubitz CC, Bird SH, Kuo LE, Stephen AE. Normocalcemic hyperparathyroidism: a Collaborative Endocrine Surgery Quality Improvement Program analysis. *Surgery.* 2020;167(1):168-172. PMID: 31543325

3 **ANSWER: C) Hypomagnesemia**
Hypomagnesemia (Answer C) impairs PTH release in response to low calcium and causes skeletal resistance to PTH. PTH resistance can occur with magnesium levels below 0.8 mEq/L (<0.3 mmol/L), with a decrease in PTH secretion occurring with more profound hypomagnesemia. Hypomagnesemia is most commonly due to malabsorption; chronic alcoholism; and medications such as proton-pump inhibitors, diuretics, and cisplatin. Despite relative hypoparathyroidism and PTH resistance, phosphate levels in these patients are usually normal or low, most likely due to poor intake. Magnesium disorders are the only reversible cause of hypoparathyroidism, and parenteral magnesium repletion resulted in a significant rise in this patient's PTH concentration. Calcium supplementation alone cannot correct hypocalcemia in the setting of magnesium deficiency.

While profound vitamin D deficiency (Answer D) can result in hypocalcemia and most likely contributed to this patient's low serum calcium, hypomagnesemia is the primary etiology in this case as evidenced by the low, not elevated, PTH concentration. Chronic hypoparathyroidism (Answer B) is a rare disorder usually occurring after parathyroid surgery or associated with autoimmune disease. This patient has no evidence of neck surgery or other autoimmune conditions on physical examination. Acute alcohol intoxication can cause transient hypoparathyroidism associated with hypocalcemia, hypercalciuria, and hypermagnesuria; however, alcohol withdrawal (Answer A) has not been associated with low calcium. Pancreatitis (Answer E) can result in hypocalcemia associated with precipitation of calcium soaps in the abdominal cavity. However, her amylase and lipase levels are only borderline elevated, which can occur with chronic alcohol abuse.

EDUCATIONAL OBJECTIVE
Identify hypomagnesemia as a cause of hypocalcemia.

REFERENCE(S)
Chase LR, Slatopolsky E. Secretion and metabolic efficacy of parathyroid hormone in patients with severe hypomagnesemia. *J Clin Endocrinol Metab.* 1974;38(3):363-371. PMID: 4360918

Fatemi S, Ryzen E, Flores J, Endres DB, Rude RK. Effect of experimental human magnesium depletion on parathyroid hormone secretion and 1,25-dihydroxyvitamin D metabolism. *J Clin Endocrinol Metab.* 1991;73(5):1067-1072. PMID: 1939521

4 ANSWER: E) Refer for parathyroid surgery for primary hyperparathyroidism

Lithium alters feedback mechanisms within the parathyroid gland, increasing the set point at which calcium suppresses PTH secretion. It also increases calcium reabsorption within the loop of Henle, decreasing urinary calcium excretion. Serum calcium remains within the normal range for most patients. While estimates vary, up to 20% of patients on lithium develop hypercalcemia. If lithium can be discontinued safely, serum calcium may normalize after 1 to 4 weeks in patients taking lithium for up to a few years. Normalization of serum calcium is less likely in patients who have been taking lithium for more than 10 years. Thus, discontinuing lithium to resolve her hypercalcemia (Answer C) is incorrect. This patient meets criteria for parathyroid surgery due to osteoporosis, and patients on lithium who develop primary hyperparathyroidism should receive surgical or medical therapy as indicated (thus, Answer E is correct and Answer B is incorrect). Of note, patients with a history of long-term lithium therapy have a higher risk of multiglandular disease, and bilateral neck exploration should be considered. There is no indication to restrict calcium intake (Answer D) in patients with primary hyperparathyroidism from any etiology.

Familial hypocalciuric hypercalcemia (Answer A) is a rare, benign disorder caused by loss-of-function pathogenic variants in the gene encoding the calcium-sensing receptor. The extremely high penetrance of familial hypocalciuric hypercalcemia ensures that virtually all affected individuals develop hypercalcemia by their third decade. In familial hypocalciuric hypercalcemia, 24-hour urinary calcium excretion is typically less than 100 mg with a calcium-to-creatinine clearance ratio less than 0.01, while the ratio is typically greater than 0.02 in patients with primary hyperparathyroidism. Manifesting familial hypocalciuric hypercalcemia later in life is unlikely, and her relatively low urinary calcium excretion can be explained by the increased urinary calcium reabsorption occurring with lithium therapy.

EDUCATIONAL OBJECTIVE
Diagnose primary hyperparathyroidism in a patient on lithium therapy.

REFERENCE(S)
Bilezikian JP, Brandi ML, Eastell R, et al. Guidelines for the management of asymptomatic primary hyperparathyroidism: summary statement from the Fourth International Workshop. *J Clin Endocrinol Metab.* 2014;99(10):3561-3569. PMID: 25162665

Haden ST, Stoll AL, McCormick S, Scott J, Fuleihan G el-H. Alterations in parathyroid dynamics in lithium-treated subjects. *J Clin Endocrinol Metab.* 1997;82(9):2844-2848. PMID: 9284708

5 ANSWER: B) Adjust FRAX score for trabecular bone score

Patients with type 1 and type 2 diabetes are at increased risk for fracture, above that predicted based on bone mineral density. The pathophysiology is most likely multifactorial and may be related to the accumulation of advanced glycosylation endpoints in the bone matrix resulting in more brittle bone and decreased bone formation due to interference with osteoblasts. No studies have directly assessed the performance of

FRAX for predicting fractures in patients with type 1 diabetes. However, several have studied patients with type 2 diabetes. To account for the increased fracture risk in patients with type 2 diabetes, proposed adjustments include: (1) using trabecular bone score; (2) using rheumatoid arthritis in the FRAX calculator as a proxy; and (3) decreasing bone density downwards by 0.5 SD.

The trabecular bone score is a gray-level textural analysis that can be used to estimate trabecular microarchitecture, and it has been associated with fragility fractures in postmenopausal women and men, independent of bone density measurements. Trabecular bone score analysis is readily available from the lumbar spine DXA image without further imaging. The FRAX score can be adjusted for trabecular bone score on the website by clicking the box that appears after the fracture risk probabilities have been generated. By adjusting this patient's bone density for trabecular bone score (Answer B), her risk for hip fracture increases to 3.0%, above the treatment threshold, and pharmacologic osteoporosis therapy should be initiated.

While many experts would advocate that she should maintain a 25-hydroxyvitamin D concentration above 30 ng/mL (>74.9 nmol/L), further assessment of her fracture risk and initiation of pharmacologic osteoporosis therapy is the best next step, rather than increasing her vitamin D supplementation (Answer C). Pioglitazone and canagliflozin have both been associated with increased fracture risk, and substitution of one for the other (Answer A) would not be of substantial benefit. While adding dulaglutide (Answer D) should improve her hemoglobin A_{1c} and most likely decrease her fracture risk over time, it is not the best next step for her skeletal health. This patient should receive pharmacologic therapy now for her bone health; waiting 2 years for interval bone density testing (Answer E) is not appropriate.

EDUCATIONAL OBJECTIVE
Manage bone health in patients with type 2 diabetes mellitus at increased fracture risk.

REFERENCE(S)
Camacho PM, Petak SM, Binkley N, et al. American Association of Clinical Endocrinologists/American College of Endocrinology clinical practice guidelines for the diagnosis and treatment of postmenopausal osteoporosis-2020 update. *Endocr Pract.* 2020;26(5):564-570. PMID: 32427503

Schacter GI, Leslie WD. DXA-dased measurements in diabetes: can they predict fracture risk? *Calcif Tissue Int.* 2017;100(2):150-164. PMID: 27591864

World Health Organization Collaborating Centre for Metabolic Bone Diseases, University of Sheffield, UK. FRAX. Who Fracture Risk Assessment Tool. Available at: http://www.shef.ac.uk/FRAX. Accessed for verification January 2021.

6 ANSWER: D) Low calcium, high PTH, high phosphate

This patient has Albright hereditary osteodystrophy with pseudohypoparathyroidism. Albright hereditary osteodystrophy is characterized by brachydactyly (classically described as shortening of the third, fourth, and fifth metacarpals), round facies, short stature, obesity, developmental delay, and subcutaneous calcifications. Albright hereditary osteodystrophy was described by Albright and colleagues in 1942 together with pseudohypoparathyroidism, historically the first reported hormone resistance syndrome. It is characterized by end-organ resistance to PTH associated with hypocalcemia, elevated PTH, and hyperphosphatemia (Answer D). Pseudohypoparathyroidism type 1A is the most common form of the disorder due to pathogenic variants in the *GNAS* gene, which encodes the α-subunit of G-protein coupled to the PTH receptor. Pathogenic variants prevent generation of adenyl cyclase when PTH binds to its receptor and, therefore, failure of signal transduction by PTH.

Interestingly, *GNAS* is imprinted in humans, so that expression of the allele for a specific tissue is dependent on whether the allele is inherited from the mother or father. Renal expression of *GNAS* is determined only by the maternal allele; a defect in the maternal allele results in pseudohypoparathyroidism. Patients with pseudohypoparathyroidism type 1A may have resistance to various other G-protein–coupled hormones, including TSH, LH, FSH, and GnRH. Paternally transmitted pathogenic variants in *GNAS* result in pseudopseudohypoparathyroidism, in which patients demonstrate the physical features of Albright hereditary osteodystrophy with no evidence of PTH resistance. As there is no renal tubular resistance to PTH, affected patients present with normal concentrations of calcium, phosphate, and PTH (Answer E); this answer is incorrect as this patient has symptoms of hypocalcemia (perioral and extremity numbness/tingling) and apparently inherited a *GNAS* pathogenic variant from his mother.

Low calcium, low PTH, and low phosphate (Answer A) can be seen with severe hypomagnesemia and nutritional deficiency. Low calcium, low PTH, and high phosphate (Answer B) can be seen with hypoparathyroidism. Low calcium, high PTH, and low phosphate (Answer C) can be seen with significant vitamin D deficiency or malabsorption. None of these disorders would present with evidence of Albright hereditary osteodystrophy.

EDUCATIONAL OBJECTIVE
Identify the physical and biochemical features of pseudohypoparathyroidism type 1A.

REFERENCE(S)

Linglart A, Levine MA, Jüppner H. Pseudohypoparathyroidism. *Endocrinol Metab Clin North Am.* 2018;47(4):865-888. PMID: 30390819

Mantovani G. Clinical review: pseudohypoparathyroidism: diagnosis and treatment. *J Clin Endocrinol Metab.* 2011;96(10):3020-3030. PMID: 21816789

7   ANSWER: E) Reduced calcium and calcitriol requirements during pregnancy

Alterations in calcium metabolism and requirements during pregnancy provide for adequate mineralization of the fetal skeleton. Calcitriol levels increase 2- to 5-fold in euparathyroid women in the first trimester of pregnancy to increase intestinal absorption of calcium. PTHrP levels increase by up to 3-fold by the third trimester, due to both placental and breast production. In women with hypoparathyroidism, these increased serum levels of calcitriol and PTHrP lead to a marked reduction in calcitriol and calcium requirements during pregnancy and nursing (Answer E). Serum calcium should be monitored closely, with a decrease in supplementation as needed.

The patient's increased 1,25-dihydroxyvitamin D level is due to increased production during pregnancy, as well as ingestion of calcitriol, and not due to granulomatous disease (Answer C). The patient's increased PTHrP is due to production during pregnancy and not due to humoral hypercalcemia of malignancy (Answer D). Recurrence of primary hyperparathyroidism (Answer A) has not been reported in a patient with chronic postoperative hypoparathyroidism. A diagnosis of milk-alkali syndrome (Answer B) can be made in a patient with a history of hypercalcemia, alkalosis, and renal impairment in the setting of a history of ingestion of calcium-rich products and exclusion of other causes of hypercalcemia. This patient has normal serum bicarbonate and kidney function, excluding this diagnosis.

EDUCATIONAL OBJECTIVE
Identify the reduction in calcitriol and calcium requirements during pregnancy and nursing in patients with hypoparathyroidism.

REFERENCE(S)

Khan AA, Clarke B, Rejnmark L, Brandi ML. Management of endocrine disease: hypoparathyroidism in pregnancy: review and evidence-based recommendations for management. *Eur J Endocrinol.* 2019;180(2):R37-R44. PMID: 30444723

Dobnig H, Kainer F, Stepan V, et al. Elevated parathyroid hormone related peptide levels after human gestation: relationship to changes in bone and mineral metabolism. *J Clin Endocrinol Metab.* 1995;80(12):3699-3707. PMID: 8530622

8 ANSWER: C) Fracture risk reduction = 50%, atypical femoral fracture risk = 5/10,000, osteonecrosis of the jaw risk = 1/100,000

This patient's calculated major osteoporotic fracture risk is 25% if untreated. Alendronate, risedronate, zoledronic acid, and denosumab have all been demonstrated to reduce the risk of vertebral and nonvertebral fractures, including hip fractures. While patients should be adequately counseled regarding risks of treatment, for patients with osteoporosis, the benefits of pharmacologic osteoporosis therapy far outweigh the risks. Her estimated fracture risk reduction with treatment is 50%, while her risk of atypical femoral fracture is approximately 5/10,000 person-years and her risk of osteonecrosis of the jaw is approximately 1/100,000 person-years (Answer C). The risks of atypical femoral fracture and osteonecrosis of the jaw increase with increasing duration of antiresorptive use, with higher risk generally beyond 5 years of use. The other answers overestimate or underestimate the benefits and risks.

EDUCATIONAL OBJECTIVE
Counsel a patient with osteoporosis regarding benefits and risks of antiresorptive therapy.

REFERENCE(S)

Camacho PM, Petak SM, Binkley N, et al. American Association of Clinical Endocrinologists/American College of Endocrinology clinical practice guidelines for the diagnosis and treatment of postmenopausal osteoporosis-2020 update. *Endocr Pract.* 2020;26(5):564-570. PMID: 32427503

Khosla S, Burr D, Cauley J, et al; American Society for Bone and Mineral Research. Bisphosphonate-associated osteonecrosis of the jaw: report of a task force of the American Society for Bone and Mineral Research. *J Bone Miner Res.* 2007;22(10):1479-1491. PMID: 17663640

Shane E, Burr D, Ebeling PR, et al. Atypical subtrochanteric and diaphyseal femoral fractures: report of a task force of the American Society for Bone and Mineral Research. *J Bone Miner Res.* 2010;25(11):2267-2294. PMID: 20842676

Schilcher J, Koeppen V, Aspenberg P, Michaëlsson K. Risk of atypical femoral fracture during and after bisphosphonate use. *N Engl J Med.* 2014;371(10):974-976. PMID: 25184886

Black DM, Geiger EJ, Eastell R, et al. Atypical femur fracture risk versus fragility fracture prevention with bisphosphonates. *N Engl J Med.* 2020;383(8):743-753. PMID: 32813950

9 ANSWER: E) No treatment necessary

Fifty percent of circulating calcium is bound to serum proteins, primarily to albumin. In this patient with multiple myeloma, the serum albumin is normal. However, in some patients with multiple myeloma, high circulating levels of serum immunoglobulins can also bind calcium, leading to "pseudohypercalcemia." The key to recognizing this condition is to note the marked discordance between the serum calcium (very high) and the patient's symptoms (almost none). No therapy is needed (Answer E).

Normal saline intravenously (Answer A), cinacalcet therapy (Answer B), pamidronate therapy (Answer C), and emergency plasmapheresis (Answer D) are reasonable steps in the treatment of true, severe hypercalcemia, but they are not needed in this case.

EDUCATIONAL OBJECTIVE
Diagnose "pseudohypercalcemia" and guide management.

REFERENCE(S)

Jacobs TP, Bilezikian JP. Clinical review: rare causes of hypercalcemia. *J Clin Endocrinol Metab.* 2005;90(11):6316-6322. PMID: 16131579

Schwab JD, Strack MA, Hughes LD, Shaker JL. Pseudohypercalcemia in an elderly patient with multiple myeloma: report of a case and review of literature. *Endocr Pract.* 1995;1(6):390-392. PMID: 15251564

10 ANSWER: C) Adynamic bone disease

The bone biopsy in this patient is most likely to show adynamic bone disease (Answer C), a variety of chronic kidney disease–mineral bone disorder (previously referred to as renal osteodystrophy). Adynamic bone disease is characterized by reduced osteoblasts and osteoclasts, markedly low bone turnover, and no accumulation of osteoid. It occurs in a high percentage of patients on dialysis (either peritoneal or hemodialysis), but also in patients with chronic kidney disease on conservative treatment. Serum PTH levels in patients with adynamic bone disease are relatively low; however, serum PTH levels in patients with chronic kidney disease without adynamic bone disease are generally higher than normal, so the PTH level in this patient is much lower than expected. In patients with end-stage kidney disease, there is resistance to PTH, due at least in part to increased N-terminal truncated PTH (7-84), which counteracts the effect of the 1-84 whole molecule on bone. This can be exacerbated by the use of cinacalcet, as well as overly aggressive treatment with calcitriol, both of which reduce PTH secretion. The low alkaline phosphatase is consistent with a low bone turnover state.

Osteomalacia (Answer B) would be characterized by a much lower 25-hydroxyvitamin D level and a higher alkaline phosphatase level. Osteitis fibrosa cystica (Answer A) would be associated with very high PTH levels and secondary or tertiary hyperparathyroidism. Mixed renal osteodystrophy (Answer D) would be associated with elements of both hyperparathyroidism and osteomalacia. Osteoporosis (Answer E) may be present to some degree in patients with end-stage kidney disease, especially in those who have osteoporosis that predates the kidney disease. However, after 8 years of hemodialysis and suppression of PTH, the most likely cause of the bone fragility in this patient is adynamic bone disease, not osteoporosis.

EDUCATIONAL OBJECTIVE
Diagnose adynamic bone disease in a patient undergoing dialysis.

REFERENCE(S)

Kidney Disease: Improving Global Outcomes (KDIGO) CKD-MBD Update Work Group. KDIGO 2017 clinical practice guideline update for the diagnosis, evaluation, prevention, and treatment of chronic kidney disease-mineral and bone disorder (CKD-MBD). *Kidney Int Suppl (2011)*. 2017;7(1):1-59. PMID: 30675420

Damasiewicz MJ, Nickolas TL. Rethinking bone disease in kidney disease. *JBMR Plus.* 2018;2(6):309-322. PMID: 30460334

11 ANSWER: A) Foreign-body granulomas

This patient has non–PTH-mediated hypercalcemia. In the setting of hypercalcemia and low PTH, 1,25-dihydroxyvitamin D should be suppressed, not elevated. Calciphylaxis (Answer D) is an incorrect diagnosis because it occurs in cases where calcium, phosphate, and PTH are all high and it is associated with necrosis of the skin. Calciphylaxis typically occurs in patients with end-stage kidney disease. Fibrodysplasia ossificans progressiva (Answer E) is an inherited disorder that does not present with hypercalcemia. Sarcoidosis (Answer C) and T-cell lymphoma (Answer B) can result in 1,25-dihydroxyvitamin D–mediated hypercalcemia, but this patient's history, physical examination findings, and imaging all point to foreign-body granulomas (Answer A) due to silicone injections as the cause of her hypercalcemia. This suspicion was confirmed by biopsy of one of the nodular masses. Certain lymphomas and granulomas with activated macrophages contain the 1a-hydroxylase enzyme that converts 25-hydroxyvitamin D to 1,25-dihydroxyvitamin D. This activated vitamin D causes hypercalcemia primarily by increasing the gut absorption of calcium (and phosphate), but also by directly causing bone resorption.

Image in vignette from Leyva A, Tran T, Cibulas AT, et al. Filler migration and granuloma formation after gluteal augmentation with free-silicone injections. *Cureus*. 2018;10(9):e3294. © The Authors.

EDUCATIONAL OBJECTIVE
Diagnose 1,25-dihydroxyvitamin D–mediated hypercalcemia due to foreign-body granulomas.

REFERENCE(S)

Agrawal N, Altiner S, Mezitis NH, Helbig S. Silicone-induced granuloma after injection for cosmetic purposes: a rare entity of calcitriol-mediated hypercalcemia. *Case Rep Med.* 2013;2013:807292. PMID: 24363673

Visnyei K, Samuel M, Heacock L, Cortes JA. Hypercalcemia in a male-to-female transgender patient after body contouring injections: a case report. *J Med Case Rep.* 2014;8:71. PMID: 24572248

Camuzard O, Dumas P, Foissac R, et al. Severe granulomatous reaction associated with hypercalcemia occurring after silicone soft tissue augmentation of the buttocks: a case report. *Aesthetic Plast Surg.* 2014;38(1):95-99. PMID: 24281899

Loke SC, Leow MK-S. Calcinosis cutis with siliconomas complicated by hypercalcemia. *Endocr Pract.* 2005;11(5):341-345. PMID: 16191496

12 ANSWER: C) 21-Hydroxylase antibodies

This patient has autoimmune polyendocrine syndrome type 1 (APS type 1) due to a pathogenic variant in the autoimmune regulator gene (*AIRE*). APS type 1 is also known by the acronym APECED (autoimmune polyendocrinopathy-candidiasis-ectodermal dystrophy). The classic presentation includes at least 2 of the following 3 major clinical components: chronic mucocutaneous candidiasis, primary hypoparathyroidism, and autoimmune adrenal insufficiency. Premature ovarian insufficiency occurs in about 60% of patients. Malabsorption and other gastrointestinal issues occur in 25% of patients with APS type 1. Studies have shown that primary adrenal insufficiency may be diagnosed before clinical symptoms by checking for antibodies against the 21-hydroxylase enzyme (Answer C). Note that screening with an 8-AM serum cortisol level is not sensitive enough to detect preclinical disease, although inclusion of an ACTH measurement with the morning cortisol might show early adrenal insufficiency.

Antiphospholipid antibodies (Answer A) are found in the setting of antiphospholipid antibody syndrome, an autoimmune disorder occurring mainly in young women. Clinical presentations include deep vein thrombosis, stroke, pregnancy complications, and recurrent miscarriage. Glutamic acid decarboxylase (GAD-65) antibodies (Answer B) are often present in individuals with APS type 1, but they have not been shown to predict the development of type 1 diabetes, which occurs in about 18% of those with the syndrome.

Islet-cell antibodies are a better predictor. Tissue transglutaminase antibodies (Answer D) are used to diagnose celiac disease, which is not a feature of APS type 1. TPO antibodies (Answer E) as a predictor of autoimmune thyroid disease is not the best answer. About 12% of patients with APS type 1 develop hypothyroidism in contrast to 60% who develop Addison disease. Screening for adrenal insufficiency is much more critical.

EDUCATIONAL OBJECTIVE
Diagnose autoimmune polyendocrine syndrome type 1 as a cause of hypoparathyroidism and recommend appropriate adrenal screening.

REFERENCE(S)
Weiler FG, Dias-da-Silva MR, Lazaretti-Castro M. Autoimmune polyendocrine syndrome type 1: case report and review of literature. *Arq Bras Endocrinol Metabol.* 2012;56(1):54-66. PMID: 22460196

Akirav EM, Ruddle NH, Herold KC. The role of AIRE in human autoimmune disease. *Nat Rev Endocrinol.* 2011;7(1):25-33. PMID: 21102544

Eisenbarth GS, Gottlieb PA. Autoimmune polyendocrine syndromes. *N Engl J Med.* 2004;350(20):2068-2079. PMID: 15141045

13 ANSWER: D) Tissue transglutaminase antibody assessment

When a patient on potent antiosteoporosis therapy shows a poor response, such as a significant decline in bone mineral density, it is important to review the history, physical examination findings, medications, and laboratory results to look for any secondary causes that may have been missed or developed in the interim. The most common cause for a poor outcome, particularly with self-administered medications, is nonadherence. It is estimated that 50% of patients starting on oral bisphosphonates stop the drugs within 3 to 6 months. Many others take the drugs intermittently or improperly. Consequences of nonadherence include loss of bone mineral density, increased fracture risk, and higher health care costs. Other etiologies of nonresponse include calcium and/or vitamin D deficiencies, poor absorption of oral bisphosphonates, errors in DXA measurements, or underlying diseases that remain undiagnosed or untreated.

This patient has laboratory evidence of inadequate calcium and vitamin D with a low 25-hydroxyvitamin level and secondary hyperparathyroidism. Additionally, she notes unexplained weight loss, fatigue, and gastrointestinal upset. The single best explanation for this clinical scenario would be celiac disease with positive tissue transglutaminase antibodies (Answer D). While some patients with celiac disease present with severe symptoms such as diarrhea, abdominal gas, and cramping, others have more subtle presentations as in this case. Multiple myeloma should always be ruled out in cases of unexplained bone loss, osteoporosis, or fractures, but the clinical presentation and laboratory findings would be different, so serum protein electrophoresis (Answer A) is incorrect. While it is not wrong to measure 24-hour urinary calcium excretion (Answer B), this would not provide a definitive diagnosis. In celiac disease, the urinary calcium excretion would be low as a result of calcium malabsorption and secondary hyperparathyroidism. A cosyntropin-stimulation test (Answer C) to diagnose adrenal insufficiency could explain weight loss and gastrointestinal upset, but it would not explain findings consistent with malabsorption or bone loss; serum calcium would usually be normal or elevated in Addison disease, not low. Finally, a marker of bone resorption (Answer E) could be elevated in a case of oral bisphosphonate nonadherence/malabsorption, but again, this would not point to a specific diagnosis.

EDUCATIONAL OBJECTIVE
Identify a secondary cause for nonresponse to osteoporosis therapy (celiac disease).

REFERENCE(S)

Modi A, Siris ES, Tang J, Sen S. Cost and consequences of noncompliance with osteoporosis treatment among women initiating therapy. *Curr Med Res Opin.* 2015;31(4):757-765. PMID: 25661017

Mirza F, Canalis E. Management of endocrine disease: secondary osteoporosis: pathophysiology and management. *Eur J Endocrinol.* 2015;173(3): R131-R151. PMID: 25971649

Heikkilä K, Pearce J, Mäki M, Kaukinen K. Celiac disease and bone fractures: a systematic review and meta-analysis. *J Clin Endocrinol Metab.* 2015;100(1): 25-34. PMID: 25279497

Painter SE, Kleerekoper M, Camacho PM. Secondary osteoporosis: a review of the recent evidence. *Endocr Pract.* 2006;12(4):436-445. PMID: 16901802

Lewiecki EM, Watts NB. Assessing response to osteoporosis therapy. *Osteoporos Int.* 2008;19(10): 1363-1368. PMID: 18546030

14 ANSWER: B) Stop calcitonin and continue current hydration and monitoring

This is a classic case of humoral hypercalcemia of malignancy leading to a hypercalcemic crisis. The underlying etiology is secretion of PTHrP from a squamous cell carcinoma of the lung. Hypercalcemic crisis is defined as a corrected serum calcium value of 14 mg/dL (3.5 mmol/L) or higher with rapid deterioration of multiple organs (eg, central nervous system, cardiac, gastrointestinal, and kidney). Acute management of hypercalcemic crisis involves saline hydration, subcutaneous calcitonin for 24 to 48 hours, intravenous bisphosphonate (or subcutaneous denosumab in selected cases), and treatment of the underlying disease. Furosemide (Answer A) should be added only when there is clinical evidence of volume overload or congestive heart failure. In cases of vitamin D–mediated hypercalcemia, prednisone 40 to 60 mg daily, or another glucocorticoid equivalent (Answer E) may be useful, but it should not be given without biochemical evidence of inappropriate vitamin D levels. Finally, in patients with hypercalcemic crisis due to primary hyperparathyroidism, cinacalcet can be a "bridge" to parathyroidectomy.

The peak hypocalcemic action of intravenous bisphosphonate starts around 48 hours after administration and peaks around day 6. Because this patient is clinically improving after only 48 hours, the best next step is to stop calcitonin and continue current hydration and monitoring (Answer B). To give another dose of zoledronic acid (Answer C) so quickly would be unnecessary and could potentially lead to prolonged hypocalcemia. Denosumab (Answer D) is also approved for treatment of hypercalcemia from solid tumors, but it would not be needed now for the same reason. Ultimately, the key to treating malignant hypercalcemia is to treat the underlying cancer with surgery, chemotherapy, and other modalities.

EDUCATIONAL OBJECTIVE
Manage hypercalcemic crisis in a patient with humoral hypercalcemia of malignancy.

REFERENCE(S)

Hu MI, Glezerman IG, Leboulleux S, et al. Denosumab for treatment of hypercalcemia of malignancy. *J Clin Endocrinol Metab.* 2014;99(9):3144-3152. PMID: 24915117

Stewart AF. Clinical practice. Hypercalcemia associated with cancer. *N Engl J Med.* 2005;352(4):373-379. PMID: 15673803

Ahmad S, Kuraganti G, Steenkamp D. Hypercalcemic crisis: a clinical review. *Am J Med.* 2015;128(3):239-245. PMID: 25447624

15 ANSWER: D) Revise the region of interest for the total hip measurement

Reviewing the images and numbers from a DXA study is always important, particularly when the results do not make sense. It is common for bone mineral density at one site to go down and bone density at another site to stay the same, and sometimes there are "gains" in the spine and losses in the hip (the "gains" being either a vertebral fracture or worsening degenerative change in the spine that drives the measured bone density up). It would be most unusual to see a true gain in the spine and simultaneous loss in the hip unless the patient had become immobilized or disabled in some way and unable to walk. Teriparatide therapy can also lead to this pattern (gain of bone mineral density at the spine, but loss at the hip), particularly after the first year of treatment.

A mistake in DXA measurement can be incorrect placement of the region of interest of the total hip. In this case, the area included in the total hip region is too small. The lower edge of the hip region of interest should be approximately 2.5 cm below the lesser trochanter. When reanalyzed, this patient's total hip bone mineral density was not significantly different between the 2 studies. The increase in the bone mineral density at the lumbar spine is most likely real and indicates a good treatment response to alendronate.

The corrected image is shown (*see image*) and it reveals stable bone mineral density at the total hip compared with the previous scan (thus, Answer D is correct).

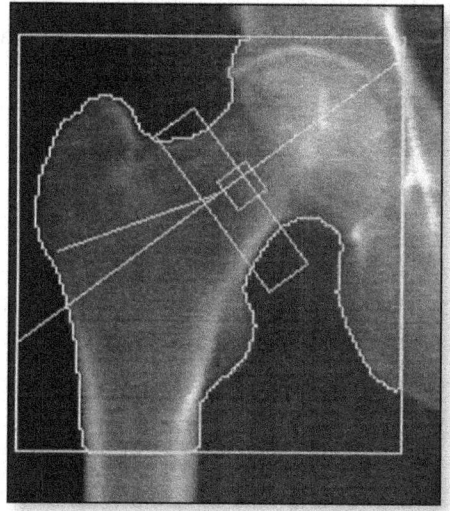

DXA Results Summary:

Region	Area (cm²)	BMC (g)	BMD (g/cm²)	T-Score	PR (%)	Z-Score	AM (%)
Neck	5.53	3.68	0.665	-1.9	72	-0.5	91
Troch	14.12	9.65	0.684	-0.7	88	-0.1	98
Inter	29.19	27.54	0.944	-1.4	79	-0.5	91
Total	**48.84**	**40.87**	**0.837**	**-1.3**	**81**	**-0.4**	**94**
Ward's	1.15	0.68	0.594	-1.4	76	0.9	126

Total BMD CV 1.0%, ACF = 1.019, BCF = 1.001, TH = 5.779

BMC = bone mineral content; BMD = bone mineral density.

Continuation of the current regimen (Answer A) is reasonable, but this approach should not be considered until the DXA image is reanalyzed. Performing an extensive workup for secondary causes of bone loss (Answer B) is reasonable if the original DXA image were not technically flawed. An intensive weight-bearing exercise program (Answer C) is usually not adequate to reverse significant bone loss at the hip and is not necessary in this case. Finally, switching from alendronate to intravenous zoledronic acid (Answer E) would make sense if the patient were a true "nonresponder" and had poor absorption or poor adherence to the oral bisphosphonate regimen.

EDUCATIONAL OBJECTIVE
Carefully review DXA images and identify common technical errors.

REFERENCE(S)
Watts NB. Fundamentals and pitfalls of bone densitometry using dual-energy X-ray absorptiometry (DXA). *Osteoporos Int.* 2004;15(11):847-854. PMID: 15322740

Schousboe JT, Shepherd JA, Bilezikian JP, Baim S. Executive summary of the 2013 international society for clinical densitometry position development conference on bone densitometry. *J Clin Densitom.* 2013;16(4):455-466. PMID: 24183638

16 ANSWER: B) Continue calcium and vitamin D and repeat DXA in 2 years

According to the National Osteoporosis Foundation, osteoporosis can be diagnosed by a T-score in the hip or spine of less than –2.5 or by a low-trauma fracture of the hip or spine. Fractures of ribs do not meet the diagnostic criteria for osteoporosis. Therefore, this patient has low bone mass (osteopenia), and the best tool to determine whether she should be treated pharmacologically is the FRAX calculator. Relying on FRAX results, patients who have an absolute 10-year fracture risk of 20% or higher for any major fracture or 3% or higher for hip fracture should be treated pharmacologically. This patient's fracture risk is well below the treatment threshold, and she should therefore continue with her dietary calcium and vitamin D for now and undergo DXA again in 2 years (Answer B). Treating her with a bisphosphonate (Answer A), the selective estrogen receptor modulator raloxifene (Answer C), or nasal calcitonin (Answer E) is incorrect. Estrogen replacement therapy (Answer D) is not approved by the US FDA for treatment of osteoporosis and is only given to postmenopausal women with significant menopausal symptoms.

EDUCATIONAL OBJECTIVE
Use the FRAX tool to determine treatment of patients with low bone mass.

REFERENCE(S)
Eastell R, Rosen CJ, Black DM, Cheung AM, Murad MH, Shoback D. Pharmacologic management of osteoporosis in postmenopausal women: an Endocrine Society clinical practice guideline. *J Clin Endocrinol Metab.* 2019;104(5):1595-1622. PMID: 30907953

Camacho PM, Petak SM, Binkley N, et al. American Association of Clinical Endocrinologists/American College of Endocrinology clinical practice guidelines for the diagnosis and treatment of postmenopausal osteoporosis-2020 update. *Endocr Pract.* 2020;26(5):564-570. PMID: 32427503

National Osteoporosis Foundation. *Clinician's Guide to Prevention and Treatment of Osteoporosis.* National Osteoporosis Foundation; 2014.

17 ANSWER: A) Nuclear medicine bone scan

This patient cannot recall any circumstances that might account for the fracture. In this case, it would be useful to know whether the fracture occurred within the past 2 years. A nuclear medicine bone scan (Answer A) will show uptake for 1 to 2 years after a fracture.

Although it is common to detect vertebral fractures on radiographs and radiographs may be more sensitive than vertebral fracture assessment for finding subtle fractures (grade 1), the age of the fracture cannot be determined from a radiograph (Answer B). Bone turnover markers, such as bone-specific alkaline phosphatase (Answer E), increase as part of fracture repair and may remain high for 6 to 12 months, but the magnitude and duration of the rise are not well characterized. MRI (Answer C) shows marrow edema soon after a fracture, but this usually resolves within 2 to 3 months. MRI (Answer C) or CT (Answer D) may be useful to rule out malignancy as a cause of the fracture. CT is fine for morphometry (determining whether there is a fracture), but it is not as good as MRI for dating acute fractures.

A fracture is not an indication of treatment failure; however, it is certainly not the desired outcome and changing medications would be reasonable.

EDUCATIONAL OBJECTIVE
Choose a nuclear medicine bone scan over MRI to determine the age of a vertebral fracture.

REFERENCE(S)
Kim JH, Kim JI, Jang BH, Seo JG, Kim JH. The comparison of bone scan and MRI in osteoporotic compression fractures. *Asian Spine J.* 2010;4(2):89-95. PMID: 21165311

Ishiyama M, Numaguchi Y, Makidono A, et al. Contrast-enhanced MRI for detecting intravertebral cleft formation: relation to the time since onset of vertebral fracture. *AJR Am J Roentgenol.* 2013;201(1):W117-W123. PMID: 23789683

Warwick R, Willatt JM, Singhal B, Borremans J, Meagher T. Comparison of computed tomographic and magnetic resonance imaging in fracture healing after spinal injury. *Spinal Cord.* 2009;47(12):874-877. PMID: 19528996

18 ANSWER: D) Multiple endocrine neoplasia type 1

Multiple endocrine neoplasia type 1 (Answer D) due to pathogenic variants in the *MEN1* gene is inherited as an autosomal dominant disorder, although occasionally de novo variants occur. It is critical to think about and recommend genetic testing for multiple endocrine neoplasia type 1 in all patients younger than 30 years who present with primary hyperparathyroidism. Up to 10% of all patients with primary hyperparathyroidism have a familial (germline) pathogenic variant. Hereditary syndromes should be suspected in patients with a personal history of other endocrine tumors (especially pancreatic-duodenal or pituitary) or a history of parathyroid disease, kidney stones, or pancreatic-duodenal/pituitary tumors in first-degree relatives. These syndromes should also be suspected and screened for in patients presenting with atypical or multigland parathyroid adenomas at any age. Only 2% to 4% of all patients with primary hyperparathyroidism present with multigland adenomas.

In addition to multiple endocrine neoplasia type 1, other more rare causes of multiorgan syndromic primary hyperparathyroidism include multiple endocrine neoplasia type 2, multiple endocrine neoplasia type 4, and hyperparathyroidism–jaw tumor syndrome (Answer E). The latter is caused by pathogenic variants in the *CDC73* gene, and inheritance is autosomal dominant with variable penetrance. It should be considered in the following clinical situations:

- Familial hyperparathyroidism (at least 2 first- or second-degree relatives have primary hyperparathyroidism)
- Primary hyperparathyroidism in a young person (<35 years)
- Ossifying fibromas of the maxilla or mandible in a patient or family member (found in 25%-50%)
- Kidney abnormalities such as Wilms tumor, renal cell carcinoma, hamartomas, polycystic kidneys (found in 15%)
- Uterine tumors (benign or malignant) (75% of females with the syndrome)
- Parathyroid carcinoma (found in 15%)

Familial "idiopathic" hyperparathyroidism (Answer A) may be a subtype of hyperparathyroidism–jaw tumor syndrome. It is less likely to be the correct diagnosis in this patient because of the father's history of diarrhea and the sibling's history of peptic ulcers (gastrinomas) suggesting a multiple endocrine neoplasia. Multiple endocrine neoplasia type 2 is associated with primary hyperparathyroidism in about 30% of cases, but it is ruled out in this case by the absence of hypertension, spells, or medullary thyroid carcinoma in any of the affected individuals.

Hereditary "renal leak" hypercalciuria (Answer B) can cause kidney stones and secondary hyperparathyroidism but not primary hyperparathyroidism, and it would not explain the additional family history. Hereditary activation of the calcium-sensing receptor

(Answer C) would result in hypocalcemia, not hypercalcemia.

EDUCATIONAL OBJECTIVE
Pursue the diagnosis of multiple endocrine neoplasia type 1 in young patients presenting with primary hyperparathyroidism.

REFERENCE(S)
Thakker RV, Newey PJ, Walls GV, et al; Endocrine Society. Clinical practice guidelines for multiple endocrine neoplasia 1 (MEN1). *J Clin Endocrinol Metab.* 2012;97(9):2990-3011. PMID: 22723327

Eastell R, Brandi ML, Costa AG, D'Amour P, Shoback DM, Thakker RV. Diagnosis of asymptomatic primary hyperparathyroidism: proceedings of the Fourth International Workshop. *J Clin Endocrinol Metab.* 2014;99(10):3570-3579. PMID: 25162666

Lassen T, Friis-Hansen L, Rasmussen AK, Knigge U, Feldt-Rasmussen U. Primary hyperparathyroidism in young people. When should we perform genetic testing for multiple endocrine neoplasia 1 (MEN-1)? *J Clin Endocrinol Metab.* 2014;99(11):3983-3987. PMID: 24731012

19 ANSWER: A) X-linked hypophosphatemic rickets

X-linked hypophosphatemic rickets (Answer A) is an X-linked dominant form of rickets that is relatively unresponsive to vitamin D. The hypophosphatemia arises as a consequence of a defective *PHEX* gene product (phosphate-regulating gene with homology to endopeptidases on the X chromosome), which ultimately results in elevated FGF-23 levels and impaired renal proximal tubule phosphate reabsorption. In addition, despite severe hypophosphatemia, 1,25-dihydroxyvitamin D_3 production is not appropriately enhanced due to FGF-23–mediated suppression of 1α-hydroxylase activity. Thus, the "normal" level of 1,25-dihydroxyvitamin D_3 is inappropriate in the setting of elevated PTH and low serum phosphate.

Vitamin D–resistant rickets (Answer D) is characterized by low serum calcium, low serum phosphate, high PTH, and normal 25-hydroxyvitamin D levels. The key to distinguishing vitamin D–resistant rickets from other forms of rickets is to measure the 1,25-dihydroxyvitamin D level. There are 2 different types of "vitamin D–resistant rickets." Persons with the first type have inactivating pathogenic variants in the gene encoding the 1α-hydroxylase enzyme. They are unable to synthesize 1,25-dihydroxyvitamin D, and they present with very low or undetectable 1,25-dihydroxyvitamin D levels. These patients respond quite well to treatment with exogenous activated vitamin D metabolites but not as well to the usual vitamin D supplementation (hence, they were considered "resistant" to vitamin D in the era before activated vitamin D supplements were available). In contrast, patients with true vitamin D–resistant rickets have inactivating pathogenic variants in the gene encoding the vitamin D receptor, resulting in high 1,25-dihydroxyvitamin D levels and generally poor response to exogenous activated vitamin D metabolites. This patient does not have vitamin D–resistant rickets in view of her normal serum calcium level and lack of an elevated 1,25-dihydroxyvitamin D level.

Oncogenic osteomalacia (Answer B) is highly unlikely given the childhood presentation in this case. In the setting of oncogenic osteomalacia, 1,25-dihydroxyvitamin D levels are severely reduced due to suppression by high FGF-23 levels from these often small mesenchymal tumors. McCune-Albright syndrome (Answer C) can be associated with rickets and osteomalacia due to hyperphosphaturic hypophosphatemia, but one would expect polyostotic fibrous dysplasia, café-au-lait macules, and other endocrine disorders. Finally, this patient's 25-hydroxyvitamin D concentration of 24 ng/mL (59.9 nmol/L) is not low enough to result in such severe rickets/osteomalacia. In true vitamin D–deficient rickets (Answer E), 25-hydroxyvitamin D levels are often too low to be measured.

EDUCATIONAL OBJECTIVE
Diagnose X-linked hypophosphatemic rickets.

REFERENCE(S)

Connor J, Olear EA, Insogna KL, et al. Conventional therapy in adults with X-linked hypophosphatemia: effects on enthesopathy and dental disease. *J Clin Endocrinol Metab.* 2015;100(10):3625-3632. PMID: 26176801

Dahir K, Roberts MS, Krolczyk S, Simmons JH. X-linked hypophosphatemia: a new era in management. *J Endocr Soc.* 2020;4(12):bvaa151. PMID: 33204932

20 ANSWER: B) 1000 IU daily

Vitamin D deficiency is not uncommon among patients with primary hyperparathyroidism. In asymptomatic primary hyperparathyroidism, low levels of 25-hydroxyvitamin D are associated with higher bone turnover, lower bone density, and greater cardiovascular risk factors in some, but not all, studies. A number of trials have shown that correction of 25-hydroxyvitamin D levels from less than 20 ng/mL (<49.9 nmol/L) to approximately 30 ng/mL (74.9 nmol/L) reduces serum PTH levels without significant increases in serum calcium or hypercalciuria. Given the possibility that some patients may be at risk for symptomatic worsening of hypercalcemia or hypercalciuria with vitamin D supplementation, it is recommended to start with cholecalciferol dosages of 600 to 1000 IU daily (Answer B) rather than much higher dosages, such as 4000 IU daily or 50,000 IU weekly (Answers C and D). A randomized controlled trial demonstrated that vitamin D supplementation up to 2800 IU daily was safe in patients with primary hyperparathyroidism. In this older man with low bone mineral density, providing no supplementation (Answer E) would potentially worsen his bone loss over time and is therefore is not recommended. A regimen of 400 IU daily (Answer A) is too modest to correct the vitamin D deficiency and help prevent bone loss.

The average serum 25-hydroxyvitamin D response to 1000 IU of vitamin D daily would be an increase of about 10 ng/mL (25.0 nmol/L) (in this vignette, the patient's level would be expected to increase from 18 ng/mL to 28 ng/mL [44.9 nmol/L to 69.9 nmol/L]). It takes 2 to 3 months of daily dosing to reach a steady state. The magnitude of increase varies widely, so it would be important to test him again.

EDUCATIONAL OBJECTIVE

Recommend appropriate vitamin D supplementation in patients with primary hyperparathyroidism.

REFERENCE(S)

Marcocci C, Bollerslev J, Khan AA, Shoback DM. Medical management of primary hyperparathyroidism: proceedings of the fourth International Workshop on the Management of Asymptomatic Primary Hyperparathyroidism. *J Clin Endocrinol Metab.* 2014;99(10):3607-3618. PMID: 25162668

Rolighed L, Rejnmark L, Sikjaer T, et al. Vitamin D treatment in primary hyperparathyroidism: a randomized placebo controlled trial. *J Clin Endocrinol Metab.* 2014;99(3):1072-1080. PMID: 24423366

Shah VN, Shah CS, Bhadada SK, Rao DS. Effect of 25 (OH) D replacements in patients with primary hyperparathyroidism (PHPT) and coexistent vitamin D deficiency on serum 25(OH) D, calcium and PTH levels: a meta-analysis and review of literature. *Clin Endocrinol (Oxf).* 2014;80(6):797-803. PMID: 24382124

21 ANSWER: E) Strongly recommended because of her hip fracture

Osteoporosis is a skeletal disorder classified by increased fracture risk. According to the National Osteoporosis Foundation guidelines, as well as others, the diagnosis of osteoporosis can be made after a fracture of the hip or spine, regardless of T-score, or by a T-score less than −2.5 in the hip or spine. This patient has osteoporosis, diagnosed by her hip fracture (thus, Answer A is incorrect), and treatment is strongly recommended (Answer E). Only half of patients who have a hip fracture also have a T-score in the osteoporosis range. Use of the FRAX tool to decide on this patient's treatment (Answer B) is inappropriate. Age alone (Answer C) is not a reason to recommend treatment. While current tobacco use is a risk factor for fracture as per FRAX, prior tobacco use (Answer D) is not considered a risk.

EDUCATIONAL OBJECTIVE
Diagnose osteoporosis on the basis of a hip fracture.

REFERENCE(S)
World Health Organization Collaborating Centre for Metabolic Bone Diseases, University of Sheffield, UK. FRAX. Who Fracture Risk Assessment Tool. Available at: http://www.shef.ac.uk/FRAX. Accessed for verification January 2021.

Dawson-Hughes B, Looker AC, Tosteson ANA, Johansson H, Kanis JA, Melton LF 3rd. The potential impact of new National Osteoporosis Foundation guidance on treatment patterns. *Osteoporos Int.* 2009;21(1):41-52. PMID: 19705046

National Osteoporosis Foundation. Clinician's Guide to Prevention and Treatment of Osteoporosis. National Osteoporosis Foundation; 2014.

22 ANSWER: B) History of radiation treatment

Teriparatide increases the risk of osteosarcoma in rats. Although there is no evidence of an increased risk in humans, use of teriparatide in patients whose risk of osteosarcoma is higher than baseline is not recommended. This includes children and adolescents with unfused epiphyses, patients with Paget disease, and those with a history of skeletal irradiation (thus, Answer B is correct and Answer E is incorrect).

Age (Answer A) is not a contraindication to the use of teriparatide. Pharmacovigilance surveys have not confirmed any increased signal of osteosarcoma in users of teriparatide. Teriparatide should not be used by any patient with a malignant bone tumor, skeletal metastasis, or high risk for skeletal metastasis. However, breast cancer (Answer D) and other malignancies, in the absence of high risk of skeletal metastases, are not a contraindication. Teriparatide probably should not be used in patients with elevated PTH levels, although the evidence for this is not conclusive. Previous bisphosphonate therapy (Answer C) may blunt the anabolic effect of teriparatide, but it is not a contraindication.

EDUCATIONAL OBJECTIVE
Identify radiation as a contraindication to the use of teriparatide.

REFERENCE(S)
Silverman SL, Nasser K. Teriparitide update. *Rheum Dis Clin North Am.* 2011;37(3):471-477. PMID: 22023903

Cosman F. Parathyroid hormone treatment for osteoporosis. *Curr Opin Endocrinol Diabetes Obes.* 2008;15(6):495-501. PMID: 18971677

Andrews EB, Gilsenan AW, Midkiff K, et al. The US postmarketing surveillance study of adult osteosarcoma and teriparatide: study design and findings from the first 7 years. *J Bone Miner Res.* 2012;27(12):2429-2437. PMID: 22991313

23 ANSWER: C) 3 months

The average serum 25-hydroxyvitamin D response to 2000 IU of vitamin D daily would be an increase of about 20 ng/mL (in this vignette, the patient's level would be expected to increase from 18 to 38 ng/mL [44.9 to 94.8 nmol/L]), and it takes 2 to 3 months of daily dosing to reach a steady state. The magnitude of increase varies widely, so it would be important to test her again, and waiting 3 months (Answer C) would make sense. Checking her level again in 2 weeks or 1 month (Answers A and B) would be too soon and there is no need to wait 6 to 12 months (Answers D and E) to retest.

In this patient, it would probably be safe to start treatment with alendronate now. In the 1980s and 1990s, the days of the early osteoporosis trials with alendronate and risedronate, the lower bound of the "normal" range for 25-hydroxyvitamin D was as low as 12 ng/mL (30.0 nmol/L) in some labs, and a minimum level of 17 ng/mL (42.4 nmol/L) was sufficient for entry into those trials. Hypocalcemia was not a problem.

EDUCATIONAL OBJECTIVE
Determine when to assess the effectiveness of vitamin D supplementation and anticipate the effect on 25-hydroxyvitamin D levels depending on dosage.

REFERENCE(S)

Heaney RP, Davies KM, Chen TC, Holick MF, Barger-Lux MJ. Human serum 25-hydroxychole-calciferol response to extended oral dosing with cholecalciferol [published correction appears in *Am J Clin Nutr.* 2003;78(5):1047]. *Am J Clin Nutr.* 2003;77(1):204-210. PMID: 12499343

Harris ST, Watts NB, Genant HK, et al. The effects of risedronate treatment on vertebral and nonverte-bral fractures in women with postmenopausal osteoporosis. *JAMA.* 1999;282(14):1344-1352. PMID: 10527181

24 ANSWER: D) MRI of the right tibia

This patient has developed an osteosarcoma in her tibia, a rare complication of Paget disease (0.5%-1%), but an important one to consider when a patient presents with severe pain in a pagetic bone and an increase in alkaline phosphatase from baseline. In this case, MRI (Answer D) or CT of her tibia is the next step to assess for tumor. A whole-body bone scan (Answer C) is most likely to show increased uptake in the tibia, but it will not result in a diagnosis of tumor. Bone biopsies (Answer B) in Paget disease generally need to be done open, rather than percutaneously, to be diagnostic and this would not be done in her case before further imaging, which is less invasive. C-telopeptide (Answer A) is expected to be elevated in Paget disease, but its measurement will not help to distinguish between active Paget disease and osteosarcoma. Zoledronic acid (Answer E) is an appropriate therapy for Paget disease, but not osteosarcoma.

EDUCATIONAL OBJECTIVE

Recognize the clinical presentation of osteosarcoma and recommend appropriate evaluation.

REFERENCE(S)

Deyrup AT, Montag AG, Inwards CY, Xu Z, Swee RG, Krishnan Unni K. Sarcomas arising in Paget disease of bone: a clinicopathologic analysis of 70 cases. *Arch Pathol Lab Med.* 2007;131(6):942-946. PMID: 17550323

Reid IR. Pharmacotherapy of Paget's disease of bone. *Expert Opin Pharmacother.* 2012;13(5):637-646. PMID: 22339140

Ralston SH. Clinical practice. Paget's disease of bone. *N Engl J Med.* 2013;368(7):644-650. PMID: 23406029

25 ANSWER: C) Hydrochlorothiazide, 25 mg once daily

According to the 2013 American College of Physicians guidelines, in patients who had a single kidney stone, increased fluid intake was the one intervention that was clearly shown to reduce recurrent stone disease. This patient's urine volume is already at goal (>2.5 L/24 h) and increasing his fluids is unlikely to further reduce stone risk. In patients with multiple stone episodes and hypercalciuria, thiazide diuretics (Answer B) are effective in reducing urinary calcium and the incidence of future stones. The hydrochlorothiazide dosage shown to reduce stone frequency is 50 mg daily. However, starting with 25 mg daily is reasonable until documenting that serum potassium remains normal on this dosage. Hydrochlorothiazide dosages lower than 25 mg have not been studied.

Although potassium citrate supplementation may also be effective in reducing stones in this patient, sodium increases urinary calcium excretion, so sodium citrate (Answer A) would not be a good choice for him. Hydrochlorothiazide acts to enhance renal calcium reabsorption to reduce urinary calcium excretion. As noted above, increased sodium intake leads to increased sodium excretion and an obligatory loss of calcium in the urine; however, this patient's normal urinary sodium excretion indicates that is not the case here. Thus, reducing his dietary sodium (Answer D) is incorrect. His urinary oxalate level is not elevated, so there would be no benefit in reducing his dietary intake of oxalate (Answer E). Allopurinol (Answer B) can be used for patients with hyperuricosuria who continue to have active disease despite attempted dietary modification. However, this patient's urinary uric acid is not elevated.

EDUCATIONAL OBJECTIVE

Recommend hydrochlorothiazide to reduce hypercalciuria as a means to reduce the risk of additional kidney stones.

REFERENCE(S)

Voskaki I, al Qadreh A, Mengreli C, Sbyrakis S. Effect of hydrochlorothiazide on renal hypercalciuria. *Child Nephrol Urol.* 1992;12(1):6-9. PMID: 1606587

Yendt ER, Cohanim M. Prevention of calcium stones with thiazides. *Kidney Int.* 1978;13(5):397-409. PMID: 351268

Fink HA, Wilt TJ, Eidman KE, et al. Medical management to prevent recurrent nephrolithiasis in adults: a systematic review for an American College of Physicians Clinical Guideline [published correction appears in *Ann Intern Med.* 2013;159(3): 230-232]. *Ann Intern Med.* 2013;158(7):535-543. PMID: 23546565

Reilly RF, Peixoto AJ, Desir GV. The evidence-based use of thiazide diuretics in hypertension and nephrolithiasis. *Clin J Am Soc Nephrol.* 2010;5(10):1893-1903. PMID: 20798254

26 ANSWER: A) Potassium phosphate and calcitriol

This patient has tumor-induced osteomalacia caused by a benign mesenchymal tumor that is secreting FGF-23, which causes renal tubular loss of phosphorus and inhibits 1α-hydroxylase, resulting in low 1,25-dihydroxyvitamin D levels. Treatment should include both potassium phosphate and calcitriol (Answer A). Potassium phosphate alone (Answer C) can result in secondary hyperparathyroidism since phosphate loading reduces serum calcium, thereby stimulating PTH release. Treating with only cholecalciferol and calcitriol (Answer B) will not correct the hypophosphatemia. These tumors are typically located in the skin, bones, or connective tissue (eg, sinuses) and may be difficult to localize. Imaging to localize the tumor includes nuclear medicine imaging techniques such as bone scan, octreotide scan, or PET. In difficult cases, serum FGF-23 on selective venous sampling may be used to localize the extremity from which FGF-23 is being secreted. Tumor removal (if it can be located and removed) normalizes renal phosphate handling within hours to days. Burosumab has been approved for FGF-23–related hypophosphatemia in tumor-induced osteomalacia associated with mesenchymal tumors that cannot be localized or curatively resected in adults and children 2 years and older. Neither alendronate (Answer D) nor zoledronic acid (Answer E) would improve his serum phosphate or osteomalacia.

EDUCATIONAL OBJECTIVE

Recommend appropriate treatment of hypophosphatemia due to tumor-induced osteomalacia.

REFERENCE(S)

Chong WH, Molinolo AA, Chen CC, Collins MT. Tumor-induced osteomalacia. *Endocr Relat Cancer.* 2011;18(3):R53-R77. PMID: 21490240

Hodgson SF, Clarke BL, Tebben PJ, Mullan BP, Cooney WP 3rd, Shives TC. Oncogenic osteomalacia: localization of underlying peripheral mesenchymal tumors with use of Tc 99m sestamibi scintigraphy. *Endocr Pract.* 2006;12(1):35-42. PMID: 16524861

Chong WH, Yavuz S, Patel SM, Chen CC, Collins MT. The importance of whole body imaging in tumor-induced osteomalacia. *J Clin Endocrinol Metab.* 2011;96(12):3599-3600. PMID: 22143830

Jan de Beur SM, Miller PD, Weber TJ, et al. Burosumab for the treatment of tumor-induced osteomalacia. *J Bone Miner Res.* 2021;36(4):627-635. PMID: 33338281

27 ANSWER: A) Nonadherence to treatment

When a patient on potent antiosteoporosis therapy has a poor response, such as a significant decline in bone mineral density, it is important to review the history, physical examination findings, medications, and laboratory results to look for secondary causes that may have been missed or developed in the interim. However, the most common cause for a poor outcome, particularly with self-administered medications, is treatment nonadherence (Answer A). Fifty percent of patients who start oral bisphosphonates are estimated to stop the drugs within 3 to 6 months. Many others take the drugs intermittently or improperly. Consequences of nonadherence include loss of bone mineral density, increased fracture risk, and higher health care costs. Other etiologies of nonresponse include calcium and/or vitamin D deficiencies, poor absorption of oral bisphosphonates, errors in DXA measurements, or underlying diseases that remain undiagnosed or untreated.

Malabsorption (Answer B) is unlikely given the adequate levels of calcium and vitamin D and the normal 24-hour urinary calcium excretion. Although patients who adhere to their treatment regimen may occasionally have inadequate absorption of bisphosphonates, this is much less common than nonadherence. There is nothing in her laboratory findings to suggest an eating disorder (Answer C), and patients with an eating disorder should respond to oral bisphosphonate therapy if taken appropriately. Positioning error by the DXA technician (Answer D) is unlikely to result in "bone loss" at both the spine and hip. Finally, all oral bisphosphonates, when taken properly, have been shown to greatly reduce postmenopausal bone loss, although risedronate may be slightly less potent than alendronate (thus, Answer E is incorrect).

EDUCATIONAL OBJECTIVE
Identify treatment nonadherence as the reason for poor response to osteoporosis therapy.

REFERENCE(S)
Modi A, Siris ES, Tang J, Sen S. Cost and consequences of noncompliance with osteoporosis treatment among women initiating therapy. *Curr Med Res Opin.* 2015;31(4):757-765. PMID: 25661017

Lewiecki EM, Watts NB. Assessing response to osteoporosis therapy. *Osteoporos Int.* 2008;19(10):1363-1368. PMID: 18546030

28 ANSWER: E) Begin hydrochlorothiazide

Patients with hypoparathyroidism cannot stimulate renal tubular reabsorption of filtered calcium due to lack of PTH effect on the kidneys. Therefore, calcium and calcitriol supplementation in the management of chronic hypoparathyroidism can lead to hypercalciuria, nephrolithiasis, nephrocalcinosis, and renal insufficiency. Epidemiologic studies have shown markedly increased relative risks (3- to 6-fold) of kidney dysfunction among those with both surgical and nonsurgical hypoparathyroidism. Because of this, it is important to encourage patients to minimize excessive calcium intake, to take the lowest possible calcitriol dosage, and to try to maintain serum calcium in the low-normal or even slightly low range. It is also important to monitor urinary calcium excretion and avoid hypercalciuria. Because this patient has hypercalciuria, continuing the current regimen (Answer A) is not optimal. Increasing the calcium dosage (Answer B) is not needed since her serum calcium is at goal (8-9 mg/dL [2.0-2.3 mmol/L]) and will worsen her hypercalcuria. Increasing the calcitriol dosage (Answer C) may allow her to cut down on extra doses of calcium, but it will also increase serum phosphate and hypercalciuria. Sevelamer (Answer D), a phosphate binder, is not indicated for this mild hyperphosphatemia and would not address her hypercalciuria.

Thiazide diuretics (Answer E) may be useful adjunctive therapy for some patients with persistent hypercalciuria who are unable to lower calcium intake due to hypocalcemic symptoms. It is reasonable to try a thiazide diuretic in this patient. Often, high dosages (such as 50 mg daily of hydrochlorothiazide or higher) are needed to normalize urinary calcium excretion, but some patients respond well to lower dosages. Concomitant potassium-sparing diuretics such as amiloride and low-salt diets may be useful adjunctive therapies. When starting thiazides, serum calcium may rise, allowing reduction in the calcitriol dosage.

Other risks for patients with permanent surgical hypoparathyroidism include neuropsychiatric disease, infections, and seizures. Among those with nonsurgical hypoparathyroidism, there is a higher occurrence of ischemic cardiovascular disease, cataracts, and fractures. The risk of malignancy in patients with nonsurgical hypoparathyroidism is actually decreased (hazard ratio = 0.44) compared with that in the general population.

EDUCATIONAL OBJECTIVE
Manage chronic surgical hypoparathyroidism.

REFERENCE(S)

Bilezikian JP, Khan A, Potts JT Jr, et al. Hypoparathyroidism in the adult: epidemiology, diagnosis, pathophysiology, target-organ involvement, treatment, and challenges for future research. *J Bone Miner Res.* 2011;26(10):2317-2337. PMID: 21812031

Clarke BL, Brown EM, Collins MT, et al. Epidemiology and diagnosis of hypoparathyroidism. *J Clin Endocrinol Metab.* 2016;101(6):2284-2299. PMID: 26943720

Bilezikian JP, Brandi ML, Cusano NE, et al. Management of hypoparathyroidism: present and future. *J Clin Endocrinol Metab.* 2016;101(6):2313-2324. PMID: 26938200

Diabetes Mellitus, Section 1 Board Review

Serge A. Jabbour, MD

1 ANSWER: B

In February 2019, the Advanced Technologies and Treatments for Diabetes Congress convened an international panel of physicians, researchers, and individuals with diabetes who are experts in CGM technologies and published consensus recommendations for relevant aspects of CGM data use and reporting among various diabetes populations.

Hemoglobin A_{1c} reflects blood glucose concentrations over 3 to 4 months and is the only parameter of glycemic control that has been strongly associated with chronic diabetes vascular complications. However, hemoglobin A_{1c} may be influenced by several conditions that affect the survival of red blood cells independent of glycemia. In addition, hemoglobin A_{1c} does not distinguish between individuals with similar average glycemia but with pronounced differences in hypoglycemic events and/or hyperglycemic excursions. CGM provides a continuous measurement of the interstitial glucose over time and offers the opportunity to detect glucose variations, hypoglycemic events, and time in range.

The following tables and figure summarize the CGM consensus recommendations (*see Tables 1, 2, and 3 and Figure*).

Table 1. Standardized CGM Metrics for Clinical Care: 2019

1. Number of days CGM worn (recommend 14 days) (42,43)	
2. Percentage of time CGM is active (recommend 70% of data from 14 days) (41,42)	
3. Mean glucose	
4. Glucose management indicator (GMI) (75)	
5. Glycemic variability (%CV) target ≤36% (90)*	
6. Time above range (TAR): % of readings and time >250 mg/dL (>13.9 mmol/L)	Level 2
7. Time above range (TAR): % of readings and time 181–250 mg/dL (10.1–13.9 mmol/L)	Level 1
8. Time in range (TIR): % of readings and time 70–180 mg/dL (3.9–10.0 mmol/L)	In range
9. Time below range (TBR): % of readings and time 54–69 mg/dL (3.0–3.8 mmol/L)	Level 1
10. Time below range (TBR): % of readings and time <54 mg/dL (<3.0 mmol/L)	Level 2
Use of Ambulatory Glucose Profile (AGP) for CGM report	

CV, coefficient of variation. *Some studies suggest that lower %CV targets (<33%) provide additional protection against hypoglycemia for those receiving insulin or sulfonylureas (45,90,91).

Table 2. Guidance on Targets for Assessment of Glycemic Control in Adults With Type 1 or Type 2 Diabetes and Older/High-Risk Individuals

Diabetes group	TIR		TBR		TAR	
	% of readings; time per day	Target range	% of readings; time per day	Below target level	% of readings; time per day	Above target level
Type 1*/type 2	>70%; >16 h, 48 min	70–180 mg/dL (3.9–10.0 mmol/L)	<4%; <1 h <1%; <15 min	<70 mg/dL (<3.9 mmol/L) <54 mg/dL (<3.0 mmol/L)	<25%; <6 h <5%; <1 h, 12 min	>180 mg/dL (>10.0 mmol/L) >250 mg/dL (>13.9 mmol/L)
Older/high-risk# type 1/type 2	>50%; >12 h	70–180 mg/dL (3.9–10 mmol/L)	<1%; <15 min	<70 mg/dL (<3.9 mmol/L)	<10%; <2 h, 24 min	>250 mg/dL (>13.9 mmol/L)

Each incremental 5% increase in TIR is associated with clinically significant benefits for individuals with type 1 or type 2 diabetes (26,27). *For age <25 years, if the A1C goal is 7.5%, set TIR target to approximately 60%. See the section CLINICAL APPLICATION OF TIME IN RANGES for additional information regarding target goal setting in pediatric management. #See the section OLDER AND/OR HIGH-RISK INDIVIDUALS WITH DIABETES for additional information regarding target goal setting.

Table 3. Guidance on Targets for Assessment of Glycemic Control During Pregnancy

Diabetes group	TIR		TBR		TAR	
	% of readings; time per day	Target range	% of readings; time per day	Below target level	% of readings; time per day	Above target level
Pregnancy, type 1§	>70%; >16 h, 48 min	63–140 mg/dL† (3.5–7.8 mmol/L†)	<4%; <1 h <1%; <15 min	<63 mg/dL† (<3.5 mmol/L†) <54 mg/dL (<3.0 mmol/L)	<25%; <6 h	>140 mg/dL (>7.8 mmol/L)
Pregnancy, type 2/GDM§	See PREGNANCY section	63–140 mg/dL† (3.5–7.8 mmol/L†)	See PREGNANCY section	<63 mg/dL† (<3.5 mmol/L†) <54 mg/dL (<3.0 mmol/L)	See PREGNANCY section	>140 mg/dL (>7.8 mmol/L)

Each incremental 5% increase in TIR is associated with clinically significant benefits for pregnancy in women with type 1 diabetes (59,60). †Glucose levels are physiologically lower during pregnancy. §Percentages of TIR are based on limited evidence. More research is needed.

Figure. Targets for Assessment of Glycemic Control

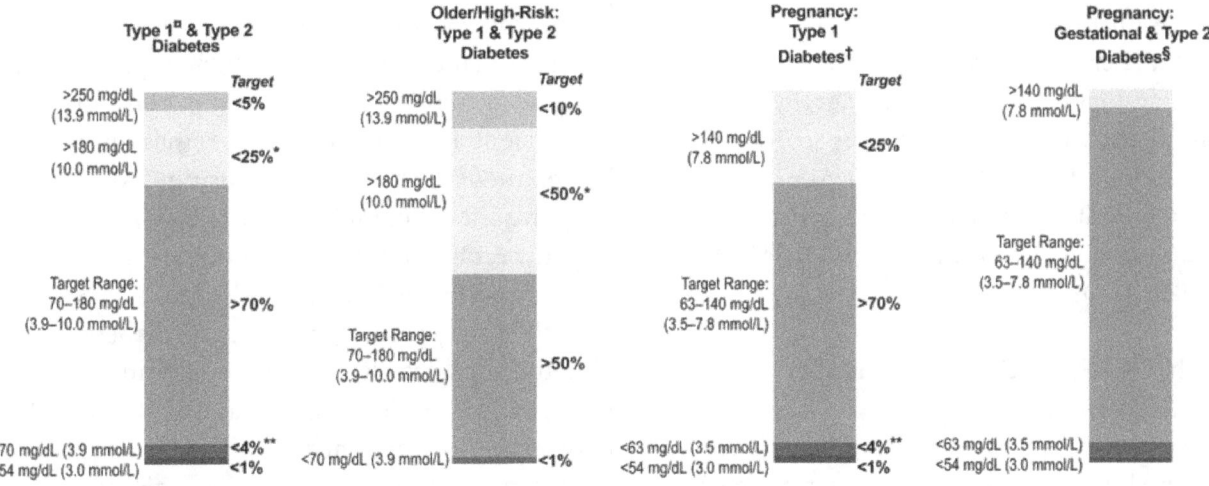

¤ For age <25 yr., if the A1C goal is 7.5%, then set TIR target to approximately 60%. (See Clinical Applications of Time in Ranges section in the text for additional information regarding target goal setting in pediatric management.)
† Percentages of time in ranges are based on limited evidence. More research is needed.

§ Percentages of time in ranges have not been included because there is very limited evidence in this area. More research is needed. Please see Pregnancy section in text for more considerations on targets for these groups.

* Includes percentage of values >250 mg/dL (13.9 mmol/L).
** Includes percentage of values <54 mg/dL (3.0 mmol/L).

Based on the above recommendations, this patient's CGM-based targets are best characterized by Answer B. Answers A and C do not have the correct percentage for each category of time-in-range, time-above-range, and time-below-range. Answer D has a time-in-range of 63 to 140 mg/dL used for pregnant women. Answer E has a time-in-range of 80 to 130 mg/dL, which is incorrect because this range is the American Diabetes Association goal for premeal blood glucose, not time-in-range used in CGM.

EDUCATIONAL OBJECTIVE
Interpret continuous glucose monitoring data and targets.

REFERENCE(S)

Battelino T, Danne T, Bergenstal RM, et al. Clinical targets for continuous glucose monitoring data interpretation: recommendations from the International Consensus on Time in Range. *Diabetes Care.* 2019;42(8):1593-1603. PMID: 31177185

Gabbay MAL, Rodacki M, Calliari LE, et al. Time in range: a new parameter to evaluate blood glucose control in patients with diabetes. *Diabetol Metab Syndr.* 2020;12:22. PMID: 32190124

Beck RW, Bergenstal RM, Cheng P, et al. The relationships between time in range, hyperglycemia metrics, and HbA1c. *J Diabetes Sci Technol.* 2019;13(4):614-626. PMID: 30636519

Advani A. Positioning time in range in diabetes management. *Diabetologia.* 2020;63(2):242-252. PMID: 31701199

2   ANSWER: D) Continue insulin indefinitely

This patient has immunotherapy-induced type 1 diabetes mellitus, consistent with the timing of initiating nivolumab and ipilimumab, the severity of diabetic ketoacidosis, and coexistent recent-onset primary hypothyroidism (induced by the checkpoint inhibitors).

Unleashing the power of the immune system with monoclonal antibodies targeting immune checkpoint receptors has been a major breakthrough, causing a paradigm shift in the treatment of many types of cancer. The deficient antitumor immune response can be restored by blocking inhibitory immune receptors of which cytotoxic T-lymphocyte antigen 4 (CTLA-4), programmed cell death 1 receptor (PD-1), and its ligand (PD-L1) have become part of standard-of-care options for many indications, including metastatic melanoma. Immune checkpoint blockade is associated with a unique risk for immune-related adverse effects, affecting the endocrine organs in 4% to 30% of patients. While hypophysitis and thyroid disorders (in this case primary hypothyroidism) are the most frequent endocrine immune-related adverse effects, autoimmune diabetes mellitus is a rare (1%) but potentially life-threatening effect.

The median duration until diabetes onset after the start of immune checkpoint inhibitors is 49 days. The shortest time to onset is 5 days and the longest time to onset is reported to be 448 days. Remarkably, of patients who develop new-onset type 1 diabetes, 71% do so within 3 months after the first exposure. Most affected patients (76%) present with diabetic ketoacidosis. Almost half of the cases are associated with traditional type 1 diabetes antibodies, most commonly glutamic acid decarboxylase 65 antibodies (as opposed to classic type 1 diabetes where 70%-90% of patients have those antibodies). All affected patients are insulin-deficient at presentation and require permanent treatment with exogenous insulin (Answer D) due to the almost complete destruction of the pancreatic β cells by immunotherapy.

Prednisone in this case had no effect on the patient's glycemic control or the diabetic ketoacidosis itself, as his hemoglobin A_{1c} level was at goal on a prednisone dosage of 10 mg daily. Stopping it would not significantly affect his glycemic control or his insulin regimen. Empagliflozin, along with all other SGLT-2 inhibitors, has been linked to euglycemic diabetic ketoacidosis in type 2 diabetes, often precipitated by an illness, infection, severe dehydration, etc. In this case, there was no precipitating factor and the diabetic ketoacidosis was not euglycemic.

Basal and mealtime insulins cannot be stopped or weaned (thus, Answers A, B, C, and E are incorrect).

EDUCATIONAL OBJECTIVE

Diagnose and manage immunotherapy-induced type 1 diabetes mellitus.

REFERENCE(S)

de Filette JMK, Pen JJ, Decoster L, et al. Immune checkpoint inhibitors and type 1 diabetes mellitus: a case report and systematic review. *Eur J Endocrinol.* 2019;181(3):363-374. PMID: 31330498

Akturk HK, Kahramangil D, Sarwal A, Hoffecker L, Murad MH, Michels AW. Systematic review or meta-analysis immune checkpoint inhibitor-induced type 1 diabetes: a systematic review and meta-analysis. *Diabet Med.* 2019;36(9):1075-1081. PMID: 31199005

Clotman K, Janssens K, Specenier P, Weets I. Programmed cell death-1 inhibitor-induced type 1 diabetes mellitus. *J Clin Endocrinol Metab.* 2018;103(9):3144-3154. PMID: 29955867

Barroso-Sousa R, Barry WT, Garrido-Castro AC, et al. Incidence of endocrine dysfunction following the use of different immune checkpoint inhibitor regimens: a systematic review and meta-analysis. *JAMA Oncol.* 2018;4(2):173-182. PMID: 28973656

3 ANSWER: D) Add dapagliflozin

This patient has well-controlled type 2 diabetes with a hemoglobin A_{1c} level less than 7.0% (<53 mmol/mol). However, he has HFrEF and stage 3 chronic kidney disease with a urinary albumin-to-creatinine ratio less than 300 mg/g creat (microalbuminuria). Typically, metformin is first-line therapy in type 2 diabetes, but this patient cannot take metformin because of unstable HFrEF and low estimated glomerular filtration rate (not recommended to start metformin when the glomerular filtration rate is <45 mL/min per 1.73 m²; in patients already on metformin, it must be stopped if it is <30 mL/min per 1.73 m²). Both conditions could predispose him to lactic acidosis.

DPP-4 inhibitors (except saxagliptin [Answer A]) are a safe choice in a patient with HFrEF and chronic kidney disease, but they do not offer any benefit when it comes to cardiovascular or renal outcomes. The Saxagliptin Assessment of Vascular Outcomes Recorded in Patients with Diabetes Mellitus (SAVOR) Thrombolysis in Myocardial Infarction (TIMI) 53 study showed that patients treated with saxagliptin were more likely to be hospitalized for heart failure than those given placebo (3.5% vs 2.8%, respectively; hazard ratio, 1.27; 95% CI, 1.07-1.51; *P* = .007), so saxagliptin is not recommended in patients with heart failure. In addition, this patient's hemoglobin A_{1c} level is already at goal; there is no need to add a glucose-lowering agent.

The current American Diabetes Association guidelines state the following: for patients with established atherosclerotic cardiovascular disease or indicators of high risk for atherosclerotic cardiovascular disease (ie, ≥55 years of age with coronary, carotid, or lower-extremity artery stenosis >50% or left ventricular hypertrophy), established kidney disease, or heart failure, an SGLT-2 inhibitor or GLP-1 receptor agonist with demonstrated cardiovascular disease benefit is recommended as part of the glucose-lowering regimen independent of hemoglobin A_{1c} and in consideration of patient-specific factors. When HFrEF and/or chronic kidney disease predominate, SGLT-2 inhibitors are the drugs of choice, specifically the one(s) with evidence-based outcomes based on randomized controlled trials.

Of the listed options, only dapagliflozin has the official indication to reduce the risk of cardiovascular death and hospitalization for heart failure in adults with heart failure with reduced ejection fraction based on the Dapagliflozin and Prevention of Adverse Outcomes in Heart Failure trial (DAPA-HF). DAPA-HF was an international, multicenter, randomized, double-blind, placebo-controlled study in patients with heart failure (New York Heart Association [NYHA] functional class II-IV) with reduced ejection fraction (left ventricular ejection fraction ≤40%) to determine whether dapagliflozin reduces the risk of cardiovascular death and hospitalization for heart failure. Of 4744 patients, 2373 were randomly assigned to dapagliflozin, 10 mg daily, and 2371 were assigned to placebo. Participants were followed for a median of 18 months. The mean age of the study population was 66 years, 77% were male, and 70% were White, 5% were Black or African American, and 24% were Asian. At baseline, 68% patients were classified as NYHA class II, 32% as class III, and 1% as class IV. Median left ventricular ejection fraction was 32%. History of type 2 diabetes mellitus was present in 45%. At baseline, 94% of patients were treated with ACE inhibitor, angiotensin receptor blocker, or angiotensin receptor–neprilysin inhibitor (including sacubitril/valsartan 11%); 96% were treated with a β-adrenergic blocker; 71% were treated with a mineralocorticoid receptor antagonist; 93% were treated with a diuretic; and 26% had an implantable device. Dapagliflozin reduced the incidence of the primary composite endpoint of cardiovascular death, hospitalization for heart failure, or urgent heart failure visit (hazard ratio, 0.74; 95% CI, 0.65-0.85; $P < .0001$). All 3 components of the primary composite endpoint individually contributed to the treatment effect. The results were similar between patients who had type 2 diabetes and those who did not for any estimated glomerular filtration rate above 30 mL/min per 1.73 m^2. Thus, adding dapagliflozin (Answer D) is correct based on the above data. Adding dapagliflozin would lower the risk of hospitalization for heart failure and cardiovascular death in this patient despite the estimated glomerular filtration rate being less than 45 mL/min per 1.73 m^2. No hemoglobin A_{1c} lowering would be expected (patient's hemoglobin A_{1c} is already at goal).

Liraglutide (Answer B) and dulaglutide (Answer C) are incorrect, as the GLP-1 receptor agonists listed have shown reduction in MACE (nonfatal myocardial infarction, nonfatal stroke, cardiovascular death), but not a statistically robust reduction in heart failure events (small reduction) or hard renal endpoints (in meta-analyses of GLP-1 receptor trials). Liraglutide and dulaglutide lower the urinary albumin-to-creatinine ratio, but they do not affect the progression of renal disease (low estimated glomerular filtration rate, dialysis, renal death). Recommending no treatment change (Answer E) is incorrect, because despite his

hemoglobin A_{1c} level being at goal, adding an SGLT-2 inhibitor would be beneficial as described.

EDUCATIONAL OBJECTIVE
Manage type 2 diabetes mellitus in a patient with heart failure with reduced ejection fraction and chronic kidney disease.

REFERENCE(S)

American Diabetes Association. Pharmacologic approaches to glycemic treatment: standards of medical care in diabetes-2021. *Diabetes Care.* 2021;44(Suppl 1):S111-S124. PMID: 33298420

McMurray JJV, Solomon SD, Inzucchi SE, et al; DAPA-HF Trial Committees and Investigators. Dapagliflozin in patients with heart failure and reduced ejection fraction. *N Engl J Med.* 2019;381(21):1995-2008. PMID: 31535829

Petrie MC, Verma S, Docherty KF, et al. Effect of dapagliflozin on worsening heart failure and cardiovascular death in patients with heart failure with and without diabetes. *JAMA.* 2020;323(14):1353-1368. PMID: 32219386

Rosenstock J, Kahn SE, Johansen OE, et al; CARMELINA Investigators. Effect of linagliptin vs placebo on major cardiovascular events in adults with type 2 diabetes and high cardiovascular and renal risk: the CARMELINA randomized clinical trial. *JAMA.* 2019;321(1):69-79. PMID: 30418475

Kristensen SL, Rorth R, Jhund PS, et al. Cardiovascular, mortality, and kidney outcomes with GLP-1 receptor agonists in patients with type 2 diabetes: a systematic review and meta-analysis of cardiovascular outcome trials. *Lancet Diabetes Endocrinol.* 2019;7(10):776-785. PMID: 31422062

Scirica BM, Bhatt DL, Braunwald E, et al; SAVOR-TIMI 53 Steering Committee and Investigators. Saxagliptin and cardiovascular outcomes in patients with type 2 diabetes mellitus. *N Engl J Med.* 2013;369(14):1317-1326. PMID: 23992601

4 ANSWER: C) Tacrolimus
An international consensus meeting in 2014 recommended changing the term "new-onset diabetes after transplantation (NODAT)" to posttransplant diabetes mellitus (PTDM) because pretransplant diabetes is not always accurately

identified. Hyperglycemia is very common (up to 90% of patients) in the immediate-to-early posttransplant period. This generally occurs as a result of postsurgical stress or with the administration of high-dosage glucocorticoids. In most cases, posttransplant hyperglycemia is transient and resolves within the first few weeks after transplant. Thus, to avoid labeling most kidney transplant recipients as having PTDM in the immediate-to-early posttransplant period, a formal diagnosis of PTDM should not be made within the first 6 weeks after transplant.

PTDM is associated with increased mortality and morbidity and, in particular, higher rates of cardiovascular disease and infection, which are the leading causes of death in kidney transplant recipients. Risk factors for PTDM are older age (≥45 years), obesity (BMI ≥30 kg/m²), African American race, Hispanic ethnicity, history of gestational diabetes or family history of diabetes, hepatitis C infection, as well as transplant-specific risk factors, including glucocorticoids and immunosuppressive agents. Both cyclosporine and tacrolimus increase the risk of PTDM. Tacrolimus (Answer C) is significantly more diabetogenic than cyclosporine (Answer B). Both calcineurin inhibitors cause reversible toxicity to islet cells and may directly affect transcriptional regulation of insulin expression.

The antimetabolite agents azathioprine (Answer A) and mycophenolate mofetil (Answer D) do not have independent diabetogenic effects. Costimulatory blockade agents such as belatacept (Answer E) do not have diabetogenic effects. mTOR (mammalian [mechanistic] target of rapamycin) inhibitors such as sirolimus and everolimus are both diabetogenic. Neither is listed as an answer option in this vignette.

EDUCATIONAL OBJECTIVE
Describe the diabetogenic potential of immunosuppressive agents in posttransplant diabetes mellitus.

REFERENCE(S)

Tomkins M, Tudor RM, Cronin K, et al. Risk factors and long-term consequences of new-onset diabetes after renal transplantation. *Ir J Med Sci.* 2020;189(2): 497-503. PMID: 31631244

Dai C, Walker JT, Ashostak A, et al. Tacrolimus- and sirolimus-induced human β-cell dysfunction is reversible and preventable. *JCI Insight.* 2020; 5(1):e130770. PMID: 31941840

Ahmed SH, Biddle K, Augustine T, Azmi S. Post-transplantation diabetes mellitus. *Diabetes Ther.* 2020;11(4):779-801. PMID: 32095994

Bhat M, Pasini E, Das A, et al. Diabetogenic effects of immunosuppression: an integrative analysis. *Transplantation.* 2020;104(1):211-221. PMID: 31283677

El Essawy B, Kandeel F. Pre, peri and posttransplant diabetes mellitus. *Curr Opin Nephrol Hypertens.* 2019;28(1):47-57. PMID: 30418189

Sharif A, Hecking M, de Vries APJ, et al. Proceedings from an international consensus meeting on posttransplantation diabetes mellitus: recommendations and future directions. *Am J Transplant.* 2014;14(9):1992-2000. PMID: 25307034

5 ANSWER: D) Panretinal laser photocoagulation

This photograph reveals proliferative retinopathy with florid neovascularization (*blue arrow*) arising from the disc and retinal vessels (*red arrow*), as well as intraretinal hemorrhages (*see image*).

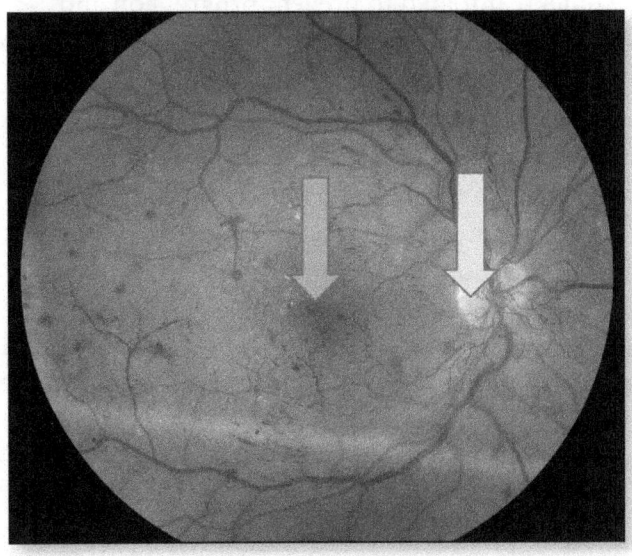

Diabetic retinopathy is divided into 2 major forms: nonproliferative and proliferative, named for the absence or presence of abnormal new blood vessels emanating from the retina. Nonproliferative diabetic retinopathy consists of a variable display of nerve-fiber layer infarcts (cotton wool spots), intraretinal hemorrhages, and hard exudates and microvascular abnormalities (including microaneurysms, occluded vessels, and dilated or tortuous vessels) primarily in the macula and posterior retina. Vision loss in nonproliferative diabetic retinopathy is mainly due to the development of macular edema. Proliferative diabetic retinopathy is marked by the presence of neovascularization arising from the disc and/or retinal vessels and the consequences of this neovascularization, including preretinal and vitreous hemorrhage, subsequent fibrosis, and traction retinal detachment. The severity of proliferative diabetic retinopathy can be classified as early, high risk, and severe. In early proliferative diabetic retinopathy, new vessels are present as fine loops or networks, but they do not meet the criteria for the high-risk category. There is a 75% 5-year risk of progression from early- to high-risk stages. Untreated high-risk proliferative diabetic retinopathy results in a 60% risk of severe vision loss at 5 years. Macular edema can be present with any degree of proliferative diabetic retinopathy and should be addressed as part of the overall treatment strategy.

Treatment for proliferative retinopathy must be quickly initiated to prevent progression and vision loss. Both panretinal photocoagulation and anti-VEGF agents (intravitreal once-a-month injection) have been shown to be effective in preventing progression of proliferative diabetic retinopathy and subsequent vision loss. Five-year data comparing initial treatment of proliferative diabetic retinopathy with ranibizumab vs panretinal photocoagulation show equivalent visual acuity outcomes. Although anti-VEGF agents are more effective in the short term, delays in treatment (missed appointments) can lead to significant progression of disease, whereas panretinal photocoagulation is a more durable treatment than anti-VEGF inhibitors to prevent severe vision loss. Therefore, in this patient who is not adherent to her treatment regimen and will most likely miss appointments, panretinal laser photocoagulation (Answer D) is the better option. Anti-VEGF agents (Answer B) would be incorrect because there is a significant risk of proliferative diabetic retinopathy recurrence and/or progression with loss to follow-up after treatment with these agents. Focal laser photocoagulation (Answer A) is incorrect because this is an established treatment for macular edema alone, not for proliferative retinopathy. Vitrectomy (Answer C) is incorrect, as this technique is used in proliferative retinopathy that progresses to vitreous hemorrhage that is nonclearing (or prevents photocoagulation) or traction retinal detachment (not the case with this patient). Intravitreal glucocorticoid monotherapy (Answer E) may have some benefit in patients with refractory macular edema, but not proliferative retinopathy. However, these benefits are counterbalanced by an often transient response and an increased risk of adverse effects, including glaucoma and cataract.

EDUCATIONAL OBJECTIVE
Diagnose and manage proliferative diabetic retinopathy

REFERENCE(S)

Sabanayagam C, Banu R, Chee ML, et al. Incidence and progression of diabetic retinopathy: a systematic review. *Lancet Diabetes Endocrinol.* 2019;7(2):140-149. PMID: 30005958

Wubben TJ, Johnson MW; Anti-VEGF Treatment Interruption Study Group. Anti-vascular endothelial growth factor therapy for diabetic retinopathy: consequences of inadvertent treatment interruptions. *Am J Ophthalmol.* 2019;204:13-18. PMID: 30878488

Gross JG, Glassman AR, Liu D, et al; Diabetic Retinopathy Clinical Research Network. Five-year outcomes of panretinal photocoagulation vs intravitreous ranibizumab for proliferative diabetic retinopathy: a randomized clinical trial. *JAMA Ophthalmol.* 2018;136(10):1138-1148. PMID: 30043039

El Rami H, Barham R, Sun JK, Silva PS. Evidence-based treatment of diabetic retinopathy. *Semin Ophthalmol.* 2017;32(1):67-74. PMID: 27700224

Stitt AW, Curtis TM, Chen M, et al. The progress in understanding and treatment of diabetic retinopathy. *Prog Retin Eye Res.* 2016;51:156-186. PMID: 26297071

6   ANSWER: C) Morning detemir, 12 units; evening detemir, 10 units; insulin-to-carbohydrate ratio, 1:12; insulin sensitivity factor, 1:40

In general, specific risks of diabetes in pregnancy include spontaneous abortion, fetal anomalies, preeclampsia, fetal demise, macrosomia, neonatal hypoglycemia, hyperbilirubinemia, and neonatal respiratory distress syndrome, among others. In addition, diabetes in pregnancy may increase the risk of obesity, hypertension, and type 2 diabetes in offspring later in life. All women of childbearing age with diabetes should be informed about the importance of achieving and maintaining as near euglycemia as is safely possible before conception and throughout pregnancy. Observational studies show an increased risk of diabetic embryopathy, especially anencephaly, microcephaly, congenital heart disease, renal anomalies, and caudal regression, directly proportional to elevations in hemoglobin A_{1c} during the first 10 weeks of pregnancy. Although observational studies are confounded by the association between elevated periconceptional hemoglobin A_{1c} and other poor self-care behavior, the quantity and consistency of data are convincing and support the recommendation to optimize glycemia before conception, given that organogenesis occurs primarily between 5 and 8 weeks' gestation, and a hemoglobin A_{1c} level less than 6.5% (<48 mmol/mol) (if safely achieved without hypoglycemia) is associated with the lowest risk of congenital anomalies.

The American Diabetes Association recommends that the mother's hemoglobin A_{1c} level be less than 6.0% to 6.5% (<42-48 mmol/mol) during early pregnancy, with a lower target (<6.0% [<42 mmol/mol]) by the second and third trimesters. The American Diabetes Association and American College of Obstetricians and Gynecologists recommend the following blood glucose targets:

- Fasting blood glucose concentration <95 mg/dL (<5.3 mmol/L)
- One-hour postprandial blood glucose concentration <140 mg/dL (<7.8 mmol/L)
- Two-hour postprandial glucose concentration <120 mg/dL (<6.7 mmol/L)

This patient's fasting, 1-hour postprandial, and 2-hour postprandial glucose values are all above target, necessitating an increase in the evening insulin detemir dose from 8 units to 10 units and an increase in the insulin-to-carbohydrate ratio from 1:15 to 1:12 (Answer C). Her blood glucose values before dinner are not provided, so a decision cannot be made regarding the morning detemir dose. Her sensitivity factor should remain the same, as no data are provided showing that a correctional insulin dose does not bring her blood glucose down to goal.

EDUCATIONAL OBJECTIVE
Manage diabetes during pregnancy.

REFERENCE(S)

American Diabetes Association. Management of diabetes in pregnancy: standards of medical care in diabetes-2021. *Diabetes Care.* 2021;44(Suppl 1):S200-S210. PMID: 33298425

Battarbee AN, Venkatesh KK, Aliaga S, Boggess KA. The association of pregestational and gestational diabetes with severe neonatal morbidity and mortality. *J Perinatol.* 2020;40(2):232-239. PMID: 31591489

McCance DR, Casey C. Type 1 diabetes in pregnancy. *Endocrinol Metab Clin North Am.* 2019;48(3):495-509. PMID: 31345519

Murphy HR, Bell R, Dornhorst A, Forde R, Lewis-Barned N. Pregnancy in diabetes: challenges and opportunities for improving pregnancy outcomes. *Diabet Med.* 2018;35(3):292-299. PMID: 29337383

Feghali MN, Umans JG, Catalano PM. Drugs to control diabetes during pregnancy. *Clin Perinatol.* 2019;46(2):257-272. PMID: 31010559

7 ANSWER: E) Repeat measurement of the urinary albumin-to-creatinine ratio

A normal urinary albumin-to-creatinine ratio is less than 30 mg/g of creat; persistently elevated values between 30 and 300 mg/g creat are characterized as moderately increased albuminuria (the new terminology for what was formerly called "microalbuminuria"). A ratio above 300 mg/g creat is considered to represent severely increased albuminuria (the new terminology for what was formerly called "macroalbuminuria," overt albuminuria, or dipstick-positive albuminuria).

However, the urinary albumin-to-creatinine ratio is a continuous measurement, and differences within the normal and abnormal ranges are associated with renal and cardiovascular outcomes. Furthermore, because of high biologic variability of more than 20% between measurements in urinary albumin excretion, 2 of 3 specimens collected within a 3- to 6-month period should be abnormal before considering a patient to have a high albuminuria. In addition, exercise within 24 hours, infection, fever, congestive heart failure, marked hyperglycemia, menstruation, and marked hypertension may elevate the urinary albumin-to-creatinine ratio independently of kidney damage.

This patient with excellent glycemic control (hemoglobin A_{1c} <7.0% [<53 mmol/mol]) suddenly has a urinary albumin-to-creatinine ratio greater than 300 mg/g creat, while 3 months ago, it was normal. This is suspicious for menstruation causing a high ratio. Therefore, the urinary albumin-to-creatinine ratio measurement must be repeated (Answer E), and the patient should be given instructions not to provide a urine sample during her menses.

Lowering the patient's hemoglobin A_{1c} level to less than 6.5% (Answer A) is incorrect because the increase in her hemoglobin A_{1c} from 6.4% to 6.9% would not increase the urinary albumin-to-creatinine ratio to greater than 300 mg/g creat. At a hemoglobin A_{1c} value of 6.9%, she is still at goal and there is no need to intensify her insulin regimen. Treatment with an ACE inhibitor (Answer B) or angiotensin receptor blocker (Answer C) should not be initiated based on a single abnormal urinary albumin-to-creatinine ratio measurement. Adding canagliflozin (Answer D) is incorrect because it is not indicated for type 1 diabetes. Canagliflozin has a renal indication only in type 2 diabetes when the urinary albumin-to-creatinine ratio is greater than 300 mg/g creat.

EDUCATIONAL OBJECTIVE
Interpret the urinary albumin-to-creatinine ratio in a patient with diabetes mellitus.

REFERENCE(S)

American Diabetes Association. Microvascular complications and foot care: standards of medical care in diabetes-2020. *Diabetes Care.* 2020;43(Suppl 1):S135-S151. PMID: 31862754

Persson F, Rossing P. Diagnosis of diabetic kidney disease: state of the art and future perspective. *Kidney Int Suppl.* 2018;8(1):2-7. PMID: 30675433

Tankeu AT, Kaze FF, Noubiap JJ, Chelo D, Dehayem MY, Sobngwi E. Exercise-induced albuminuria and circadian blood pressure abnormalities in type 2 diabetes. *World J Nephrol.* 2017;6(4):209-216. PMID: 28729969

Kidney Disease: Improving Global Outcomes (KDIGO) Diabetes Work Group. KDIGO 2020 clinical practice guideline for diabetes management in chronic kidney disease. *Kidney Int.* 2020;98(45): S1-S115. PMID: 32998798

8 ANSWER: B) Add 20 units of regular insulin to TPN bag and 20 units of subcutaneous insulin glargine daily

In patients receiving TPN, insulin may be administered as part of the nutritional solution, if allowed by the hospital pharmacy. To determine the correct dose of insulin to add to the TPN fluid, a separate infusion of regular insulin can be used initially. When blood glucose values have reached goal, the total daily dose of regular insulin provided by the insulin drip is calculated; 80% of this amount is added to the TPN fluid as regular insulin to be delivered over 24 hours. For example, if the intravenous insulin infusion at steady state was set at 2 units per hour (or 48 units per day), 80% of this amount (~40 units) should be added to the TPN solution by the pharmacy to be given over the course of the day. The amount of insulin can then be titrated every 1 to 2 days, based on glucose monitoring. Since more frequent adjustments are impractical and costly, the concurrent use of rapid- or short-acting insulin as correction every 6 hours will help to fine-tune control.

If TPN is interrupted, most patients with type 2 diabetes can be followed with careful glucose monitoring. Insulin should be administered if hyperglycemia occurs. If all insulin is withheld in patients with type 1 diabetes, such as in the patient in this vignette, hyperglycemia will occur and can result in ketosis. Thus, patients with type 1 diabetes require insulin when TPN is interrupted. The amount and type of insulin depend on the anticipated duration of the interruption. Because of the potential for inadvertent discontinuation of insulin therapy if TPN is interrupted, clinicians recommend giving a portion of the basal insulin as an injection (eg, 50%) in patients with type 1 diabetes. In the example above (patient receiving 48 units of regular insulin daily, 80% of this amount would be ~40 units), approximately 20 units of regular insulin can be added to the TPN solution and 20 units of NPH, glargine, or detemir can be administered as a basal injection. This approach can also be used in insulin-requiring patients with type 2 diabetes, but it is essential in type 1 diabetes in order to prevent diabetic ketoacidosis. In this patient with type 1 diabetes, recent diabetic ketoacidosis, and a very difficult venous access with potential TPN interruption, it is best to split the insulin needs into regular insulin in the TPN bag and a basal insulin injection (Answer B).

Answer A is incorrect as it carries a risk of diabetic ketoacidosis in the event that the TPN is interrupted. Starting subcutaneous regular insulin sliding scale (Answer D) is incorrect because a patient with type 1 diabetes needs daily basal insulin; ketosis can occur if only a sliding scale is used. Lispro insulin is not used intravenously (in a TPN bag) (Answer C), and when it is used subcutaneously in a patient with type 1 diabetes without basal insulin, it should be given every 4 hours (not every 6 hours [Answer E]) to avoid low insulin levels that could lead to hyperglycemia and ketosis.

EDUCATIONAL OBJECTIVE
Manage insulin and total parenteral nutrition in hospitalized patients with type 1 diabetes mellitus.

REFERENCE(S)

Olveira G, Abuin J, Lopez R, et al. Regular insulin added to total parenteral nutrition vs subcutaneous glargine in non-critically ill diabetic inpatients, a multicenter randomized clinical trial: INSUPAR trial. *Clin Nutr.* 2020;39(2):388-394. PMID: 30930133

American Diabetes Association. 15. Diabetes care in the hospital: standards of medical care in diabetes-2021. *Diabetes Care.* 2021;44(Suppl 1):S211-S220. PMID: 33298426

Vennard KC, Selen DJ, Gilbert MP. The management of hyperglycemia in noncritically ill hospitalized patients treated with continuous enteral or parenteral nutrition. *Endocr Pract.* 2018;24(10):900-906. PMID: 30035626

Limonta A, Gastaldi G, Heidegger CP, Pichard C. Insulin therapy and parenteral nutrition in intensive care: practical aspects. *Rev Med Suisse.* 2015;11(467):728-730,732-733. PMID: 26027204

Laesser CA, Cumming P, Reber E, Stanga Z, Muka T, Bally L. Management of glucose control in non-critically ill, hospitalized patients receiving parenteral and/or enteral nutrition: a systematic review. *J Clin Med.* 2019;8(7):935. PMID: 31261760

9 **ANSWER: D) Lifestyle intervention**
Lifestyle intervention (Answer D) is preferred over metformin (Answer C) on the basis of findings from available studies, mainly the landmark Diabetes Prevention Program. In the Diabetes Prevention Program, 3234 patients with obesity (average BMI, 34 kg/m^2) aged 25 to 85 years (average age, 51 years) at high risk for diabetes (based on BMI ≥24 kg/m^2 and fasting and 2-hour plasma glucose concentrations of 96 to 125 mg/dL [5.3-6.9 mmol/L] and 140 to 199 mg/dL [7.8-11.1 mmol/L], respectively) were randomly assigned to one of the following groups:

- Intensive lifestyle changes with the aim of reducing weight by 7% through a behavioral modification program aimed at a low-fat diet and exercise for 150 minutes per week
- Treatment with metformin (850 mg twice daily) plus information on diet and exercise
- Placebo plus information on diet and exercise

After an average follow-up of 3 years, fewer patients in the intensive lifestyle group developed diabetes, as diagnosed by fasting plasma glucose and 2-hour postload glucose concentrations (14% vs 22% and 29% in the metformin and placebo groups, respectively). The intensive lifestyle and metformin interventions reduced the cumulative incidence of diabetes by 58% and 31%, respectively. Lifestyle intervention was effective in men and women in all age groups and in all ethnic groups.

In a follow-up observational study (the Diabetes Prevention Program Outcomes Study), the benefit of the lifestyle intervention was shown to persist more than 10 years. In this study, 85% of patients originally enrolled in the Diabetes Prevention Program joined the long-term follow-up and were offered group-implemented lifestyle intervention. Patients originally assigned to metformin continued receiving it (unblinded). During a cumulative 10 years of follow-up, the incidence of diabetes in the lifestyle and metformin groups was significantly reduced by 34% and 18%, respectively, compared with placebo. In older individuals (≥60 years of age at baseline), the lifestyle intervention was particularly effective (72% reduction in diabetes compared with placebo), while metformin was relatively less effective. Conversely, metformin was particularly effective in individuals who were younger (<60 years), had a higher BMI (>35 kg/m^2), and were at highest risk for developing diabetes.

The Actos Now for Prevention of Diabetes study assessed the ability of pioglitazone (Answer E) (30 to 45 mg daily) to reduce the risk of developing diabetes in 600 patients with impaired glucose tolerance and 1 or more components of the metabolic syndrome. After a median follow-up period of 2.4 years, fewer patients randomly assigned to pioglitazone developed diabetes (5.0% vs 16.7% with placebo; hazard ratio, 0.28; 95% CI, 0.16-0.49). Weight gain was significantly greater with pioglitazone (3.9 vs 0.77 kg), and edema was more common (12.9% vs 6.4%). Pioglitazone should not be used for diabetes prevention in this patient because of potential adverse effects (fluid retention, weight gain, heart failure), especially since she already has 2+ edema on examination.

There are no studies on empagliflozin (Answer B) or dulaglutide (Answer A) with respect to diabetes prevention.

EDUCATIONAL OBJECTIVE
Identify prediabetes (impaired fasting glucose and impaired glucose tolerance) and recommend the best way to prevent progression to diabetes.

REFERENCE(S)

Dunkley AJ, Bodicoat DH, Greaves CJ, et al. Diabetes prevention in the real world: effectiveness of pragmatic lifestyle interventions for the prevention of type 2 diabetes and of the impact of adherence to guideline recommendations: a systematic review and meta-analysis. *Diabetes Care.* 2014;37(4):922-933. PMID: 24652723

Knowler WC, Barrett-Connor E, Fowler SE, et al; Diabetes Prevention Program Research Group. Reduction in the incidence of type 2 diabetes with lifestyle intervention or metformin. *N Engl J Med.* 2002;346(6):393-403. PMID: 11832527

Diabetes Prevention Program Research Group, Knowler WC, Fowler SE, et al. 10-year follow-up of diabetes incidence and weight loss in the Diabetes Prevention Program Outcomes Study [published correction appears in *Lancet.* 2009;374(9707):2054]. *Lancet.* 2009;374(9702): 1677-1686. PMID: 19878986

DeFronzo RA, Tripathy D, Schwenke DC, et al; ACT NOW Study. Pioglitazone for diabetes prevention in impaired glucose tolerance [published corrections appear in *N Engl J Med.* 2011;365(2):189 and *N Engl J Med.* 2011;365(9):869]. *N Engl J Med.* 2011;364(12):1104-1115. PMID: 21428766

Diabetes Prevention Program Research Group. Long-term effects of lifestyle intervention or metformin on diabetes development and microvascular complications over 15-year follow-up: the Diabetes Prevention Program Outcomes Study. *Lancet Diabetes Endocrinol.* 2015;3(11):866-875. PMID: 26377054

10 ANSWER: A) Iron deficiency

Although the international standardization of the hemoglobin A_{1c} assay has decreased potential technical errors in interpreting results, a number of biologic and patient-specific factors can cause misleading values.

Hemoglobin A_{1c} values are influenced by red blood cell survival. Thus, falsely high values in relation to mean blood glucose values can be obtained when red blood cell turnover is low, resulting in a disproportionate number of older red cells. This problem can occur in patients with iron, vitamin B_{12}, or folate deficiency anemia (Answer A).

In contrast, rapid red blood cell turnover leads to a greater proportion of younger red cells and falsely low hemoglobin A_{1c} values. Examples include patients with hemolysis (Answer C); patients treated for iron, vitamin B_{12}, or folate deficiency; and patients treated with erythropoietin.

Laboratory error (Answer B) is unlikely to happen twice—both of the patient's hemoglobin A_{1c} values were high at 7.8% (62 mmol/mol) and 8.2% (66 mmol/mol).

Albuminuria (Answer D) does not affect hemoglobin A_{1c}. However, heavy proteinuria can affect fructosamine measurement.

High nighttime blood glucose values (Answer E) do not typically occur suddenly and without a rise in fasting blood glucose.

EDUCATIONAL OBJECTIVE
Diagnose iron deficiency anemia as a cause of falsely high hemoglobin A_{1c} values.

REFERENCE(S)
National Glycohemoglobin Standardization Program (NGSP) Web site. Factors that interfere with HbA1c test results. Available at: http://www.ngsp.org/factors.asp. Accessed for verification April 2021

Lundholm MD, Emanuele MA, Ashraf A, Nadeem S. Applications and pitfalls of hemoglobin Axand alternative methods of glycemic monitoring. *J Diabetes Complications.* 2020;34(8):107585. PMID: 32553575

Krhac M, Lovrencic MV. Update on biomarkers of glycemic control. *World J Diabetes.* 2019;10(1):1-15. PMID: 30697366

Ahmad J, Rafat D. HbA1c and iron deficiency: a review. *Diabetes Metab Syndr.* 2013;7(2):118-122. PMID: 23680254

Silva JF, Pimentel AL, Camargo JL. Effect of iron deficiency anaemia on HbA1c levels is dependent on the degree of anaemia. *Clin Biochem.* 2016;49(1-2):117-120. PMID: 26365695

11 ANSWER: E) Proteinuria

The turnover of serum proteins, mainly albumin, is more rapid than that of hemoglobin; thus, serum fructosamine values (glycated proteins, mostly albumin) reflect mean blood glucose values over a much shorter period (1 to 2 weeks). There is generally a good correlation between serum fructosamine and hemoglobin A_{1c} values. Fructosamine responds more rapidly to changes in blood glucose control than does hemoglobin A_{1c}. Falsely low fructosamine values in relation to mean blood glucose values occur with rapid albumin turnover, for example, in patients with protein-losing enteropathy or nephrotic syndrome (Answer E).

Biotin (Answer B), hemolysis (Answer C), and hypothyroidism (Answer D) do not falsely lower fructosamine. Laboratory errors (Answer A) do rarely occur, but in this case, the heavy proteinuria explains the normal fructosamine value.

EDUCATIONAL OBJECTIVE
Diagnose nephrotic syndrome as a cause of falsely low fructosamine values.

REFERENCE(S)

Danese E, Montagnana M, Nouvenne A, Lippi G. Advantages and pitfalls of fructosamine and glycated albumin in the diagnosis and treatment of diabetes. *J Diabetes Sci Technol.* 2015;9(2):169-176. PMID: 25591856

Copur S, Onal EM, Afsar B, et al. Diabetes mellitus in chronic kidney disease: biomarkers beyond HbA1c to estimate glycemic control and diabetes-dependent morbidity and mortality. *J Diabetes Complications.* 2020;34(11):107707. PMID: 32861562

Vetter SW. Glycated serum albumin and AGE receptors. *Adv Clin Chem.* 2015;72:205-275. PMID: 26471084

Koga M. Glycated albumin; clinical usefulness. *Clin Chim Acta.* 2014;433:96-104. PMID: 24631132

Parrinello CM, Selvin E. Beyond HbA1c and glucose: the role of nontraditional glycemic markers in diabetes diagnosis, prognosis, and management. *Curr Diab Rep.* 2014;14(11):548. PMID: 25249070

12 ANSWER: B) Zinc transporter 8 (ZnT8) antibody testing

In first-degree relatives of individuals with type 1 diabetes, screening before overt clinical symptoms develop, as occurred in this patient, can detect the disease in a clinically silent phase. Multiple positive antibodies are highly predictive of future disease development, while positivity for only 1 autoantibody may not indicate high risk. Several serum antibodies can be detected before the manifestation of autoimmune hyperglycemia, including islet-cell antibodies, insulin autoantibodies, glutamic acid decarboxylase antibodies, and antibodies to tyrosine phosphatase-like proteins. Analysis of zinc transporter 8 (ZnT8) antibodies (Answer B) increases the diagnostic sensitivity of islet autoantibodies for type 1 diabetes, as 26% of patients with antibody-negative type 1 diabetes (negative for insulin, glutamic acid decarboxylase, tyrosine phosphatase-like proteins, and islet-cell antibodies) have ZnT8 autoantibodies.

This patient's hemoglobin A_{1c} value is consistent with the high self-monitored blood glucose values. Measurement of fructosamine (Answer A) or 1,5-anhydroglucitol (Answer E) would not add any useful information. Both measurements would be high, similar to her hemoglobin A_{1c}. This patient is much more likely to have type 1 diabetes than maturity-onset diabetes of the young (MODY), both statistically and because of the family history, and testing for pathogenic variants in the *GCK* gene (Answer C) or the *HNF1A* gene (Answer D) would only be indicated if the ZnT8 antibody measurement is negative.

EDUCATIONAL OBJECTIVE

Select the best test to confirm the diagnosis of type 1 diabetes mellitus.

REFERENCE(S)

Broome DT, Pantalone KM, Kashyap S, Philipson LH. Approach to the patient with MODY-monogenic diabetes. *J Clin Endocrinol Metab.* 2021;106(1):237-250. PMID: 33034350

Rochmah N, Faizi M, Windarti SW. Zinc transporter 8 autoantibody in the diagnosis of type 1 diabetes in children. *Clin Exp Pediatr.* 2020;63(10):402-405. PMID: 33050689

Williams CL, Long AE. What has zinc transporter 8 autoimmunity taught us about type 1 diabetes? *Diabetologia.* 2019;62(11):1969-1976. PMID: 31444530

Mrena S, Virtanen SM, Laippala P, et al. Models for predicting type 1 diabetes in siblings of affected children. *Diabetes Care.* 2006;29(3):662-667. PMID: 16505523

Greenbaum CJ, Cuthbertson D, Krischer JP; Disease Prevention Trial of Type 1 Diabetes Study Group. Type 1 diabetes manifested solely by 2-h oral glucose tolerance test criteria. *Diabetes.* 2001;50(2):470-476. PMID: 11272162

Andersson C, Vaziri-Sani F, Delli A, et al; BDD Study Group. Triple specificity of ZnT8 autoantibodies in relation to HLA and other islet autoantibodies in childhood and adolescent type 1 diabetes. *Pediatr Diabetes.* 2013;14(2):97-105. PMID: 22957668

Vaziri-Sani F, Delli AJ, Elding-Larsson H, et al. A novel triple mix radiobinding assay for the three ZnT8 (ZnT8-RWQ) autoantibody variants in children with newly diagnosed diabetes. *J Immunol Methods.* 2011;371(1-2):25-37. PMID: 21708156

Vermeulen I, Weets I, Asanghanwa M, et al; Belgian Diabetes Registry. Contribution of antibodies against IA-2β and zinc transporter 8 to classification of diabetes under 40 years of age. *Diabetes Care.* 2011;34(8):1760-1765. PMID: 21715527

Gorus FK, Balti EV, Vermeulen I, et al. Screening for insulinoma antigen 2 and zinc transporter 8 autoantibodies: a cost-effective and age-dependent strategy to identify rapid progressors to clinical onset among relatives of type 1 diabetic patients. *Clin Exp Immunol.* 2013;171(1):82-90. PMID: 23199327

13 **ANSWER: C) Assessment for ketones**
In patients with type 1 diabetes, the urine should be tested for ketones (Answer C) if the blood glucose concentration is above 300 mg/dL (>16.7 mmol/L) for unexplained reasons, especially if the person feels unwell at the time. Testing for ketonuria should also be performed during periods of illness or stress or if there are symptoms compatible with ketoacidosis such as nausea, vomiting, and abdominal pain. If ketonuria is present in the setting of hyperglycemia, diabetic ketoacidosis should be suspected and the patient should be ideally sent to the emergency department for more testing (serum ketones, electrolytes, bicarbonate, pH, etc) and treated accordingly with intravenous fluids and insulin drip if diabetic ketoacidosis is indeed present.

While basal rate testing (Answer A), diabetes education (Answer B), and a continuous glucose sensor (Answer D) are all needed to help this patient achieve a lower hemoglobin A_{1c}, none of these options is the best immediate step to take now. These steps can be done over weeks to months. Therapy for stress management (Answer E) is appropriate if she is willing to explore it, but again, this is not immediately necessary.

EDUCATIONAL OBJECTIVE
Determine when urine ketones should be measured in a patient with type 1 diabetes mellitus.

REFERENCE(S)
Albanese-O'Neill A, Wu M, Miller KM, et al; T1D Exchange Clinic Network. *Diabetes Care.* 2017;40(4):e38-e39. PMID: 28100607

Marks BE, Wolfsdorf JI. Monitoring of pediatric type 1 diabetes. *Front Endocrinol (Lausanne).* 2020;11:128. PMID: 32256447

Cao X, Zhang X, Xian Y, Wu J, et al. The diagnosis of diabetic acute complications using the glucose-ketone meter in outpatients at endocrinology department. *Int J Clin Exp Med.* 2014;7(12):5701-5705. PMID: 25664094

Weber C, Kocher S, Neeser K, Joshi SR. Prevention of diabetic ketoacidosis and self-monitoring of ketone bodies: an overview. *Curr Med Res Opin.* 2009;25(5):1197-1207. PMID: 19327102

Goldstein DE, Little RR, Lorenz RA, et al. Tests of glycemia in diabetes. *Diabetes Care.* 2004;27(7):1761-1773. PMID: 15220264

14 **ANSWER: E) TPO antibodies**
Fifteen to thirty percent of patients with type 1 diabetes mellitus have positive antithyroid antibodies (TPO and/or thyroglobulin antibodies) (Answer E). Patients with circulating antibodies may be euthyroid, or they may develop autoimmune hypothyroidism, with a prevalence of about 2% to 5% in patients with type 1 diabetes. Rarely, children and adolescents with type 1 diabetes are hyperthyroid, with a reported prevalence of about 1%, with circulating thyroid-stimulating immunoglobulins.

Testing for autoantibodies to intrinsic factor (Answer B) is used to identify pernicious anemia, an autoimmune condition that leads to severely impaired vitamin B_{12} absorption. Five to ten percent of patients with type 1 diabetes are diagnosed with autoimmune gastritis and/or pernicious anemia.

About 5% of patients with type 1 diabetes develop celiac disease (gluten-sensitive enteropathy diagnosed by a positive small-bowel biopsy sample), and 7% to 10% have tissue transglutaminase antibodies (Answer A). Traditional gliadin antibody tests (Answer D) have lower diagnostic accuracy than other serologic tests for celiac disease and are no longer recommended because they yield false-positive results in 15% to 20% of patients tested.

Less than 1% to 2% of children and adolescents with type 1 diabetes have autoimmune adrenalitis with circulating antibodies to steroid 21-hydroxylase (Answer C).

EDUCATIONAL OBJECTIVE
List the prevalence of various autoimmune conditions (mostly Hashimoto thyroiditis) in patients with type 1 diabetes mellitus.

REFERENCE(S)
Kahaly GJ, Hansen MP. Type 1 diabetes associated autoimmunity. *Autoimmun Rev.* 2016;15(7):644-648. PMID: 26903475

Kakleas K, Soldatou A, Karachaliou F, Karavanaki K. Associated autoimmune diseases in children and adolescents with type 1 diabetes mellitus (T1DM). *Autoimmun Rev.* 2015;14(9):781-797. PMID: 26001590

Ruggeri RM, Giuffrida G, Campenni A. Autoimmune endocrine diseases. *Minerva Endocrinol.* 2018;43(3):305-322. PMID: 28990742

Warncke K, Fröhlich-Reiterer EE, Thon A, et al; DPV Initiative of the German Working Group for Pediatric Diabetology; German BMBF Competence Network for Diabetes Mellitus. Polyendocrinopathy in children, adolescents, and young adults with type 1 diabetes: a multicenter analysis of 28,671 patients from the German/Austrian DPV-Wiss database. *Diabetes Care.* 2010;33(9):2010-2012. PMID: 20551013

Van den Driessche A, Eenkhoorn V, Van Gaal L, De Block C. Type 1 diabetes and autoimmune polyglandular syndrome: a clinical review. *Neth J Med.* 2009;67(11):376-387. PMID: 20009114

Dost A, Rohrer TR, Fröhlich-Reiterer E, et al; DPV Initiative and the German Competence Network Diabetes Mellitus. Hyperthyroidism in 276 children and adolescents with type 1 diabetes from Germany and Austria. *Horm Res Paediatr.* 2015;84(3):190-198. PMID: 26202175

Likhari T, Magzoub S, Griffiths MJ, Buch HN, Gama R. Screening for Addison's disease in patients with type 1 diabetes mellitus and recurrent hypoglycaemia. *Postgrad Med J.* 2007;83(980):420-421. PMID: 17551075

15 ANSWER: D) Refer for psychological evaluation

Eating disorders are relatively common in patients with diabetes, especially in female adolescents and young adults with type 1 diabetes. Eating disorders have a deleterious effect on glycemic control and on long-term outcomes in these patients. One study evaluated 91 female patients with type 1 diabetes (mean age, 15 years) at baseline and at follow-up 4 to 5 years later. The following findings were noted:

- Twenty-six (29%) had a self-reported eating disorder at baseline, which persisted in 16 (18%) at follow-up.
- Among the patients with normal eating patterns at baseline, 15% had disordered eating at follow-up.
- Dieting or omission of insulin for weight loss and bulimia nervosa were the most common eating disorders. Bulimia nervosa is characterized by recurrent episodes of binge eating and inappropriate compensatory behaviors (such as self-induced vomiting), as well as frequent comorbid psychopathology. Insulin omission leading to weight loss is a unique purging behavior available to patients with type 1 diabetes, observed mainly in female patients.

Eating disorders are suspected in a patient with type 1 diabetes when there is suboptimal glycemic control associated with recurrent episodes of diabetic ketoacidosis (due to omission of insulin) and recurrent hypoglycemia (deliberately inducing hypoglycemia through intentional insulin overdosing to justify eating sweets and high-carbohydrate meals, often followed by self-induced vomiting), frequently missed medical appointments, refusal to be weighed, and preoccupation with appearance. It is important to evaluate patients with diabetes, especially young women, for eating disorders (or misreporting of insulin administration) and arrange appropriate psychological counseling and support when indicated (Answer D). Pharmacotherapy can be used at a later stage; first-line treatment is a selective serotonin reuptake inhibitor.

Switching to insulin pump therapy (Answer A) would not help, as her eating disorder must be addressed first. Her ACTH level, electrolytes, and blood pressure are normal, making Addison disease an extremely unlikely diagnosis. Thus, a cosyntropin-stimulation test (Answer B) is unnecessary. Biotin can lead to falsely low TSH in certain assays. Because this patient's TSH is normal, she is not hyperthyroid and there is no need to measure TSH again after she has stopped biotin (Answer C).

EDUCATIONAL OBJECTIVE
Screen for eating disorders in patients with type 1 diabetes mellitus.

REFERENCE(S)

Winston AP. Eating disorders and diabetes. *Curr Diab Rep.* 2020;20(8):32. PMID: 32537669

Wagner G, Karwautz A. Eating disorders in adolescents with type 1 diabetes mellitus. *Curr Opin Psychiatry.* 2020;33(6):602-610. PMID: 32858602

Cecilia-Costa R, Volkening LK, Laffel LM. Factors associated with disordered eating behaviours in adolescents with type 1 diabetes. *Diabet Med.* 2019;36(8):1020-1027. PMID: 30582670

Pinhas-Hamiel O, Hamiel U, Levy-Shraga Y. Eating disorders in adolescents with type 1 diabetes: challenges in diagnosis and treatment. *World J Diabetes.* 2015;6(3):517-526. PMID: 25897361

Mannucci E, Rotella F, Ricca V, Moretti S, Placidi GF, Rotella CM. Eating disorders in patients with type 1 diabetes: a meta-analysis. *J Endocrinol Invest.* 2005;28(5):417-419. PMID: 16075924

Ardabilygazir A, Afshariyamchlou S, Mir D, Sachmechi I. Effect of high-dose biotin on thyroid function tests: case report and literature review. *Cureus.* 2018;10(6):e2845. PMID: 30140596

16 ANSWER: E) Hepatic glucose output and β-cell dysfunction

GLP-1 is an incretin produced from the proglucagon gene in the L cells of the small intestine and is secreted in response to nutrients. GLP-1 is deficient in persons with type 2 diabetes. DPP-4 inhibitors are a class of oral diabetes drugs that inhibit the enzyme DPP-4. This is a ubiquitous enzyme expressed on the surface of most cell types that deactivates GLP-1; therefore, its inhibition could potentially affect glucose regulation through multiple effects.

Incretin-based therapies include DPP-4 inhibitors and GLP-1 receptor agonists. DPP-4 inhibitors, through increasing endogenous GLP-1, can stimulate glucose-dependent insulin secretion from the β cells and can lower glucagon secretion, thereby lowering hepatic glucose output (Answer E). GLP-1 receptor agonists exert the same effects and, in addition, slow gastric emptying and decrease food intake.

DPP-4 inhibitors have no effect on insulin action (Answers A and D) or satiety (Answers B and C).

EDUCATIONAL OBJECTIVE
Summarize the pathogenesis of type 2 diabetes mellitus and the mechanism of action of incretin therapies.

REFERENCE(S)

Kerru N, Singh-Pillay A, Awolade P, Singh P. Current anti-diabetic agents and their molecular targets: a review. *Eur J Med Chem.* 2018;152:436-488. PMID: 29751237

Andersen ES, Deacon CF, Holst JJ. Do we know the true mechanism of action of the DPP-4 inhibitors? *Diabetes Obes Metab.* 2018;20(1):34-41. PMID: 28544214

DeFronzo RA, Eldor R, Abdul-Ghani M. Pathophysiologic approach to therapy in patients with newly diagnosed type 2 diabetes. *Diabetes Care.* 2013;36(Suppl 2):S127-S138. PMID: 23882037

Demuth HU, McIntosh CH, Pederson RA. Type 2 diabetes--therapy with dipeptidyl peptidase IV inhibitors. *Biochim Biophys Acta.* 2005;1751(1):33-44. PMID: 15978877

Koliaki C, Doupis J. Incretin-based therapy: a powerful and promising weapon in the treatment of type 2 diabetes mellitus. *Diabetes Ther.* 2011;2(2):101-121. PMID: 22127804

17 ANSWER: D) Switch insulin glargine and lispro to U500 regular insulin

This patient has markedly uncontrolled, symptomatic hyperglycemia. She has insulin resistance as evidenced by her lack of responsiveness to a total daily dose of more than 200 units of U100 insulin.

In patients requiring more than 200 units of insulin daily, the volume of insulin given becomes a problem, both in terms of patient comfort and pharmacokinetics. Large-volume insulin injections are poorly absorbed. Also, adherence is challenging with 4 to 5 daily injections of U100 insulins. In such cases, U500 regular insulin should be considered (Answer D). There is increasing evidence of more reliable delivery of insulin and successful outcomes with the use of U500 regular insulin in patients such as the one in this vignette. Although the formulation of U500 regular insulin is similar to that of regular insulin, the duration of action is up to 13 to 24 hours, permitting adequate delivery with 2 or 3 injections per day. Fortunately, U500 regular insulin pens are now available, and patients with severe insulin resistance are good candidates for U500 regular insulin.

Recommendations for the conversion from U100 to U500 insulin generally incorporate the baseline U100 insulin doses, as well as the hemoglobin A_{1c} level, to determine appropriate doses of the concentrated insulin. One randomized titration-to-target trial provided a clear and specific recommendation on how to convert from U100 to U500 insulin:

- If hemoglobin A_{1c} is >8.0% at the time of conversion, use 100% of the U100 insulin total dose
- If hemoglobin A_{1c} ≤8.0% at the time of conversion, use 80% of the U100 insulin total dose

Split of the U500 regular insulin can be done either as twice daily (60% 30 minutes before breakfast and 40% 30 minutes before dinner) or 3 times daily (40% 30 minutes before breakfast, 30% 30 minutes before lunch, and 30% 30 minutes before dinner).

In this trial, regimens of dosing twice daily and 3 times daily led to similar hemoglobin A_{1c} reductions. The only difference was the incidence and rate of documented symptomatic, nonsevere hypoglycemia (glucose ≤70 mg/dL [≤3.9 mmol/L]), which were lower for participants on the twice-daily regimen vs patients on the thrice-daily regimen.

Switching insulin glargine to insulin degludec (Answer A) would not lower the patient's hemoglobin A_{1c} to goal. In meta-analyses of phase 3 trials, compared with insulin glargine, insulin degludec is associated with equivalent hemoglobin A_{1c} control.

Increasing her insulin doses by 20% (Answer B) is unlikely to sufficiently overcome insulin resistance to improve her glycemic control, and it would not address the challenge of multiple daily insulin injections (5+ in this case).

SGLT-2 inhibitors such as ertugliflozin (Answer C) would not lower her hemoglobin A_{1c} to goal at an estimated glomerular filtration rate of 48 mL/min per 1.73 m^2, especially as her hemoglobin A_{1c} level is 9.0% (75 mmol/mol) despite a high insulin dose and treatment with a GLP-1 receptor agonist.

This patient is already on a GLP-1 receptor agonist (oral semaglutide) and adding dulaglutide (Answer E) is incorrect. Even switching between various GLP-1 receptor agonists would not significantly affect her hemoglobin A_{1c}.

EDUCATIONAL OBJECTIVE

Determine when to prescribe a concentrated insulin.

REFERENCE(S)

Heinemann L, Beals JM, Malone J, Anderson J, Jacobson JG, Sinha V, Corrigan SM. Concentrated insulins: History and critical reappraisal. *J Diabetes.* 2018;11(4):292-300. PMID: 30264527

Davies MJ, D'Alessio DA, Fradkin J, et al. Management of hyperglycemia in type 2 diabetes, 2018. A consensus report by the American Diabetes Association (ADA) and the European Association for the Study of Diabetes (EASD). *Diabetes Care.* 2018;41(12):2669-2701. PMID: 30291106

American Diabetes Association. Pharmacologic approaches to glycemic treatment: standards of medical care in diabetes-2020. *Diabetes Care.* 2020;43(Suppl 1):S98-S110. PMID: 31862752

Wysham C, Hood RC, Warren ML, Wang T, Morwick TM, Jackson JA. Effect of total daily dose on efficacy, dosing, and safety of 2 dose titration regimens of human regular U-500 insulin in severely insulin-resistant patients with type 2 diabetes. *Endocr Pract.* 2016;22(6):653-665. PMID: 26789342

Hood RC, Arakaki RF, Wysham C, Li YG, Settles JA, Jackson JA. Two treatment approaches for human regular U-500 insulin in patients with type 2 diabetes not achieving adequate glycemic control on high-dose U-100 insulin therapy with or without oral agents: a randomized, titration-to-target clinical trial. *Endocr Pract.* 2015;21(7):782-793. PMID: 25813411

Vora J, Christensen T, Rana A, Bain SC. Insulin degludec versus insulin glargine in type 1 and type 2 diabetes mellitus: a meta-analysis of endpoints in phase 3a trials. *Diabetes Ther.* 2014;5(2):435-446. PMID: 25081590

18 **ANSWER: B) Decrease insulin degludec to 40 units at bedtime; discontinue nateglinide; continue alogliptin**

Individuals with severely insulin-deficient type 2 diabetes can experience hypoglycemia unawareness or hypoglycemia-associated autonomic failure. Hypoglycemia unawareness is characterized by a reduction in the sympathoadrenal and autonomic responses and is more common in those with longer duration of type 2 diabetes and in older adults. This syndrome can lead to a prolonged exposure to hypoglycemia, resulting in loss of consciousness, seizures, or brain damage. However, it is possible to improve the control of glycemia and reduce the frequency of hypoglycemia with short-term relaxation of glycemic targets. This hypoglycemia avoidance includes reducing insulin therapy for several weeks to allow the patient's blood glucose levels to run a little higher, thereby increasing sensitivity to symptoms. In addition, the glycemic targets in older patients are more relaxed, with a hemoglobin A_{1c} goal between 7.0% and 8.0% (53-64 mmol/mol). Accordingly, this patient's insulin dosage should be decreased by 10% to 20% and insulin secretagogues (like nateglinide, which is a meglitinide) should be discontinued (Answer B). Although approaches that discontinue the insulin secretagogue are preferred, replacing degludec with the same dose of insulin detemir (Answer C) or NPH (Answer D) would not resolve the issue. An approach that continues the use of an insulin secretagogue (Answer A) should be avoided. Alogliptin is a DPP-4 inhibitor that enhances glucose-dependent insulin secretion (as opposed to meglitinides and sulfonylureas) and it does not increase the risk of hypoglycemia.

EDUCATIONAL OBJECTIVE
Manage hypoglycemia in patients with type 2 diabetes mellitus.

REFERENCE(S)
Freeman J. Management of hypoglycemia in older adults with type 2 diabetes. *Postgrad Med.* 2019;131(4):241-250. PMID: 30724638

Sircar M, Bhatia A, Munshi M. Review of hypoglycemia in the older adult: clinical implications and management. *Can J Diabetes.* 2016;40(1):66-72. PMID: 26752195

American Diabetes Association. Older adults: standards of medical care in diabetes-2020. *Diabetes Care.* 2020;43(Suppl 1):S152-S162

American Diabetes Association. 9. Pharmacologic approaches to glycemic treatment: standards of medical care in diabetes-2020. *Diabetes Care.* 2020;43(Suppl 1):S98-S110. PMID: 31862752

Cryer PE. Diverse causes of hypoglycemia-associated autonomic failure in diabetes. *N Engl J Med.* 2004;350(22):2272-2279. PMID: 15163777

19

ANSWER: A) 1.5 L of 0.9% NaCl over the first hour, and intravenous insulin bolus of 10 units then 10 units per hour

This patient meets the criteria for the hyperosmolar hyperglycemic state (also known as hyperosmotic hyperglycemic nonketotic state). The diagnostic criteria are a plasma glucose concentration greater than 600 mg/dL (>33.3 mmol/L), effective serum osmolality greater than 320 mOsm/kg (>320 mmol/kg), arterial pH greater than 7.30, serum bicarbonate greater than 18 mEq/L (>18 mmol/L), and severe dehydration with absence of or minimal ketoacidosis.

The most common precipitating factors for hyperosmolar hyperglycemic state are infection (often pneumonia or urinary tract infection) and discontinuation of or inadequate insulin therapy. Compromised water intake due to underlying medical conditions, particularly in older patients, can promote the development of severe dehydration and the hyperosmolar hyperglycemic state. Other conditions and factors associated with the hyperosmolar hyperglycemic state include acute major illnesses such as myocardial infarction, cerebrovascular accident, sepsis, or pancreatitis, etc.

The hyperosmolar hyperglycemic state is treated with fluids and insulin. Because of severe dehydration, isotonic 0.9% NaCl is initiated at a rate of 15 to 20 mL/kg over the first hour (thus, Answers C, D, and E are incorrect). A decision is then made as to whether to continue the 0.9% NaCl or switch to 0.45% NaCl depending on volume status and corrected serum sodium. In fact, in this patient, the corrected serum sodium was 145 mEq/L (145 mmol/L) (serum sodium may be corrected by adding 1.6 mg/dL to the measured serum sodium for each 100 mg/dL of glucose above 100 mg/dL [>5.6 mmol/L]). Administration of hypertonic saline at 3.0% (Answer E) might worsen the hypernatremia and hyperosmolarity.

Intravenous insulin treatment can be initiated with an intravenous bolus of regular insulin (0.1 units/kg body weight) followed within 5 minutes by a continuous infusion of regular insulin of 0.1 units/kg per hour (bolus of 10 units and 10 units as a drip in this patient who weighs 220 lb [100 kg]) (thus, Answer B is incorrect).

Alternatively, the bolus dose can be omitted if a higher dose of continuous intravenous regular insulin (0.14 units/kg per hour) is initiated.

The best approach for this patient is to administer 1.5 L of 0.9% NaCl over the first hour, and then an intravenous insulin bolus of 10 units followed by 10 units per hour (Answer A).

EDUCATIONAL OBJECTIVE
Manage the hyperosmolar hyperglycemic state.

REFERENCE(S)

Dhatariya KK, Vellanki P. Treatment of diabetic ketoacidosis (DKA)/hyperglycemic hyperosmolar state (HHS): novel advances in the management of hyperglycemic crises (UK versus USA). *Curr Diab Rep.* 2017;17(5):33. PMID: 28364357

French EK, Donihi AC, Korytkowski MT. Diabetic ketoacidosis and hyperosmolar hyperglycemic syndrome: review of acute decompensated diabetes in adult patients. *BMJ.* 2019;365:l1114. PMID: 31142480

American Diabetes Association. 15. Diabetes care in the hospital: standards of medical care in diabetes-2020. *Diabetes Care.* 2020;43(Suppl 1):S193-S202. PMID: 31862758

Kitabchi AE, Umpierrez GE, Miles JM, Fisher JN. Hyperglycemic crises in adult patients with diabetes. *Diabetes Care.* 2009;32(7):1335-1343. PMID: 19564476

Nyenwe EA, Kitabchi AE. Evidence-based management of hyperglycemic emergencies in diabetes mellitus. *Diabetes Res Clin Pract.* 2011;94(3):340-351. PMID: 21978840

20

ANSWER: D) Liraglutide

The current American Diabetes Association guidelines state that for patients with established atherosclerotic cardiovascular disease (ASCVD) or indicators of high ASCVD risk (eg, patients ≥55 years with coronary, carotid, or lower-extremity artery stenosis greater than 50% or left ventricular hypertrophy), established kidney disease, or heart failure, an SGLT-2 inhibitor or GLP-1 receptor agonist with demonstrated cardiovascular disease benefit is recommended as part of the glucose-lowering regimen independent of hemoglobin A_{1c} and in consideration of patient-specific factors. When heart failure with reduced ejection fraction and/or chronic kidney disease predominate, SGLT-2 inhibitors are the drugs of choice, specifically the one(s) with evidence-based outcomes based on randomized controlled trials.

In this patient with a history of myocardial infarction and ischemic stroke, liraglutide (Answer D) (a GLP-1 receptor agonist) is the best of the listed options. Liraglutide, studied in the LEADER trial (Liraglutide Effect and Action in Diabetes: Evaluation of Cardiovascular Outcome Results), demonstrated an absolute risk reduction of 1.9% with a hazard ratio of 0.87 (95% CI, 0.78-0.97; $P = .01$ for superiority) for the primary composite outcome of cardiovascular death, nonfatal myocardial infarction, and nonfatal stroke (major adverse cardiac events) compared with placebo over 3.8 years. Each component of the composite contributed to the benefit, and the hazard ratio for cardiovascular death was 0.78 (95% CI, 0.66-0.93; $P = .007$; absolute risk reduction, 1.7%). The LEADER trial also demonstrated a hazard ratio of 0.85 (95% CI, 0.74-0.97; $P = .02$; absolute risk reduction, 1.4%) for all-cause mortality.

Overall, cardiovascular outcome trials of DPP-4 inhibitors have demonstrated safety (ie, noninferiority relative to placebo for the primary major adverse cardiovascular events endpoint, but not cardiovascular benefit). The TECOS trial (Trial Evaluating Cardiovascular Outcomes with Sitagliptin) comparing sitagliptin (Answer A) with placebo showed no cardiovascular benefit with sitagliptin.

Overall, second-generation sulfonylureas such as glimepiride (Answer B) appear to be cardiovascular neutral. They will not offer cardiovascular benefit to this patient who has a history of myocardial infarction and ischemic stroke. In a meta-analysis of 47 trials (of at least 1-year duration) comparing second-generation sulfonylureas (glibenclamide, glimepiride, glipizide, and gliclazide) with diet, placebo, or an active comparator, sulfonylureas were not associated with an increased risk of overall mortality, cardiovascular mortality, myocardial infarction, or stroke. The trials in these meta-analyses were not specifically designed to evaluate cardiovascular safety. In a specifically designed cardiovascular outcomes trial comparing linagliptin with glimepiride in 6042 patients with type 2 diabetes and elevated cardiovascular risk (median follow-up of 6.3 years), the occurrence of the composite outcome (cardiovascular death, nonfatal myocardial infarction, or nonfatal stroke) was similar in the 2 groups (11.8% vs 12% with glimepiride, hazard ratio, 0.98; 95% CI, 0.84-1.14). Hospitalization for heart failure did not differ between the 2 groups. Rates of severe hypoglycemia (0.07 vs 0.45 per 100 patient-years) and hospitalization for hypoglycemia (0.01 vs 0.18 per 100 patient-years) were low in both groups, albeit higher in the sulfonylurea group. This trial, along with a similarly designed trial comparing linagliptin with placebo that did not show an increased risk of major adverse cardiovascular events, provides reassurance regarding the cardiovascular safety of glimepiride.

Combination oral agent and insulin glargine therapy (Answer C) does not appear to reduce or increase cardiovascular outcomes compared with oral agent(s) alone, as illustrated by the findings of the Outcome Reduction with Initial Glargine Intervention (ORIGIN) trial. In this trial, more than 12,500 patients with cardiovascular risk factors plus type 2 diabetes or prediabetes were randomly assigned to an evening dose of glargine or to standard care. Approximately 60% of the patients with prior diabetes were using oral glucose-lowering agents (predominantly metformin or sulfonylurea). The glargine was titrated to achieve a fasting glucose concentration less than 95 mg/dL (<5.3 mmol/L). After a median follow-up of 6 years, the achieved median fasting glucose concentrations were 94 and 123 ng/dL (5.2 mmol/L and 6.8 mmol/L), respectively. The rates of incident cardiovascular outcomes were similar in the insulin glargine and standard care groups.

There are no long-term studies of meglitinides (Answer E) regarding cardiovascular outcomes or mortality in patients with type 2 diabetes, although most experts believe they are neutral in terms of cardiovascular disease risk.

EDUCATIONAL OBJECTIVE

Compare and contrast the cardiovascular outcome trials in diabetes mellitus.

REFERENCE(S)

American Diabetes Association. 9. Pharmacologic approaches to glycemic treatment: standards of medical care in diabetes-2021. *Diabetes Care.* 2021;44(Suppl 1):S111-S124. PMID: 33298420

Davies MJ, D'Alessio DA, Fradkin J, et al. Management of hyperglycemia in type 2 diabetes, 2018. A consensus report by the American Diabetes Association (ADA) and the European Association for the Study of Diabetes (EASD). *Diabetes Care.* 2018;41(12):2669-2701. PMID: 30291106

Green JB, Bethel MA, Armstrong PW, et al; TECOS Study Group. Effect of sitagliptin on cardiovascular outcomes in type 2 diabetes. *N Engl J Med.* 2015;373(3):232-242. PMID: 26052984

Marso SP, Daniels GH, Brown-Frandsen K, et al; LEADER Steering Committee; LEADER Trial Investigators. Liraglutide and cardiovascular outcomes in type 2 diabetes. *N Engl J Med.* 2016;375(4):311-322. PMID: 27295427

Rados DV, Pinto LC, Remonti LR, Leitao CB, Gross JL. The association between sulfonylurea use and all-cause and cardiovascular mortality: a meta-analysis with trial sequential analysis of randomized clinical trials. *PLoS Med.* 2016;13(4):e1001992. PMID: 27071029

Rosenstock J, Kahn SE, Johansen OE, et al; CAROLINA Investigators. Effect of linagliptin vs glimepiride on major adverse cardiovascular outcomes in patients with type 2 diabetes: the CAROLINA randomized clinical trial. *JAMA.* 2019;322(12):1155-1166. PMID: 31536101

ORIGIN Trial Investigators; Gerstein HC, Bosch J, Dagenais GR, et al. Basal insulin and cardiovascular and other outcomes in dysglycemia. *N Engl J Med.* 2012;367(4):319-328. PMID: 22686416

21 ANSWER: A) History of previous ulceration

The lifetime risk of developing a foot ulcer in persons with diabetes mellitus is about 25%. Multiple factors are associated with an increased risk of ulceration, including previous ulceration or amputation, the presence of peripheral neuropathy with loss of protective sensation, foot deformity, and suboptimally controlled diabetes. All of the listed options are risk factors for the development of future ulcers, but the strongest predictive factor is a history of previous ulceration (Answer A), with an odds ratio of 56.8 and up to a 10-fold increased risk for amputation. Other factors are absent ankle reflexes (Answer C) associated with neuropathy (odds ratio, 6.48), abnormal monofilament testing (Answer D) (odds ratio, 18.42), and male gender (odds ratio, 2.15). Peripheral vascular disease (Answer B) is an important prognostic factor for delayed wound healing and amputations but not a strong independent predictor of foot ulceration. Callus formation (Answer E) does not predispose to foot ulcers.

EDUCATIONAL OBJECTIVE

Identify predictors of increased risk of foot ulcers.

REFERENCE(S)

Van Netten JJ, Raspovic A, Lavery LA, et al. Prevention of foot ulcers in the at-risk patient with diabetes: a systematic review. *Diabetes Metab Res Rev.* 2020;36(Suppl 1):e3270213

Hicks CW, Canner JK, Mathiousdakis N, Lippincott C, Sherman RL, Abularrage CJ. Incidence and risk factors associated with ulcer recurrence among patients with diabetic foot ulcers treated in a multidisciplinary setting. *J Surg Res.* 2020;246:243-250. PMID: 31610352

Ahmad J. The diabetic foot. *Diabetes Metab Syndr.* 2016;10(1):48-60. PMID: 26072202

Noor S, Zubair M, Ahmad J. Diabetic foot ulcer--a review on pathophysiology, classification and microbial etiology. *Diabetes Metab Syndr.* 2015;9(3):192-199. PMID: 25982677

Moura Neto A, Zantut-Wittmann DE, Fernandes TD, Nery M, Parisi MCR. Risk factors for ulceration and amputation in diabetic foot: study in a cohort of 496 patients. *Endocrine.* 2013;44(1):119-124. PMID: 23124278

Boulton AJ, Armstrong DG, Albert SF, et al;
American Diabetes Association; American
Association of Clinical Endocrinologists.
Comprehensive foot examination and risk assess-
ment: a report of the task force of the foot care
interest group of the American Diabetes
Association, with endorsement by the American
Association of Clinical Endocrinologists. *Diabetes
Care.* 2008;31(8):1679-1685. PMID: 18663232

McNeely MJ, Boyko EJ, Ahroni JH, et al. The independent contributions of diabetic neuropathy and
vasculopathy in foot ulceration. How great are the
risks? *Diabetes Care.* 1995;18(2):216-219.
PMID: 7729300

22 ANSWER: A) Diabetes mellitus

The lesion in the photograph is
necrobiosis lipoidica, which frequently occurs in
association with diabetes mellitus (Answer A), thus
accounting for the past use of the term *necrobiosis
lipoidica diabeticorum* for this condition. Necrobiosis
lipoidica usually begins as asymptomatic, well-
circumscribed, yellow to pink-brown or red-
brown, slightly elevated papules or plaques.
Erythema or a violaceous skin color may be present
at the periphery. Necrobiosis lipoidica is most often
found on the pretibial area, but can involve the
scalp, face, trunk, genitals, or upper extremities.
Biopsy of the lesion shows collagen degeneration
with a granulomatous and inflammatory response,
thickening of blood vessel walls, and fat deposition
in the dermis.

The other listed conditions can have associated
skin manifestations that look different than this
patient's lesion. Glucagonoma (Answer C) is
associated with necrolytic migratory erythema
(biopsy would show superficial necrolysis with
separation of the outer layers of the epidermis and
perivascular infiltration with lymphocytes and
histiocytes). Graves disease (Answer B) is associated
with pretibial myxedema (biopsy would show
mucinous edema and the fragmentation of collagen
fibers with deposition of acid mucopolysaccharides
[hyaluronic acid] in the papillary and reticular
dermis). Pseudohypoparathyroidism (Answer D)
can be associated with subcutaneous calcifications.
Familial hypercholesterolemia (Answer E) can be
associated with xanthomas (biopsy would show
deposition of lipid and associated inflammation in
the skin).

EDUCATIONAL OBJECTIVE
Diagnose necrobiosis lipoidica and recognize its
association with diabetes mellitus.

REFERENCE(S)
Lima AL, Illing T, Schliemann S, Elsner P. Cutaneous
manifestations of diabetes mellitus: a review.
Am J Clin Dermatol. 2017;18(4):541-553.
PMID: 28374407

Marchand L, Villar-Fimbel S. Necrobiosis lipoidica.
Am J Med. 2020;133(3):e112. PMID: 31520619

Mendes AL, Miot HA, Junior VH. Diabetes mellitus
and the skin. *An Bras Dermatol.* 2017;92(1):8-20.
PMID: 28225950

Murphy-Chutorian B, Han G, Cohen SR.
Dermatologic manifestations of diabetes mellitus:
a review. *Endocrinol Metab Clin North Am.*
2013;42(4):869-898. PMID: 24286954

Reid SD, Ladizinski B, Lee K, Baibergenova A, Alavi
A. Update on necrobiosis lipoidica: a review of
etiology, diagnosis, and treatment options. *J Am
Acad Dermatol.* 2013;69(5):783-791.
PMID: 23969033

Jabbour SA. Skin manifestations of hormone-
secreting tumors. *Dermatol Ther.* 2010;23(6):643-
650. PMID: 21054708

23 ANSWER: A) Now

Although the mainstay of diabetes
prevention should always focus on lifestyle
management, including diet and physical activity
counseling, the screening guidelines vary. Current
guidelines (American Diabetes Association, World
Health Organization) suggest a BMI criterion of
23 kg/m^2 for type 2 diabetes screening in Asian
Americans (decreased from 25 kg/m^2 in the general
population) because data demonstrate that Asian
Americans are at greater risk for diabetes at a lower
BMI than non-Asian populations. Therefore, this
patient should be screened for type 2 diabetes now
(Answer A). Delaying screening (Answers B, C, D,
and E) would not serve his best interests.

In asymptomatic adults, diabetes screening should be considered in patients who are overweight or obese who have 1 or more of the following risk factors: first-degree relative with diabetes, high-risk race/ethnicity, history of cardiovascular disease, hypertension, HDL-cholesterol concentration less than 35 mg/dL (<0.90 mmol/L) and/or triglyceride concentration greater than 250 mg/dL (>2.82 mmol/L), polycystic ovary syndrome (in women), and physical inactivity. Patients with prediabetes should have annual testing, and women diagnosed with gestational diabetes should have testing at least every 3 years.

According to the American Diabetes Association guidelines, screening for diabetes should begin at age 45 years regardless of other factors such as ethnicity, family history, BMI, blood pressure, and dyslipidemia.

EDUCATIONAL OBJECTIVE
Select the appropriate criteria for type 2 diabetes mellitus/prediabetes screening in patients of diverse racial/ethnic backgrounds.

REFERENCE(S)
American Diabetes Association. 2. Classification and diagnosis of diabetes: standards of medical care in diabetes-2021. *Diabetes Care.* 2021;44(Suppl 1):S15-S33. PMID: 33298413

Yip WCY, Sequeira IR, Plank LD, Poppitt SD. Prevalence of pre-diabetes across ethnicities: a review of impaired fasting glucose (IFG) and impaired glucose tolerance (IGT) for classification of dysglycaemia. *Nutrients.* 2017;9(11):1273. PMID: 29165385

Pottie K, Jaramillo A, Lewin G, et al; Canadian Task Force on Preventive Health Care. Recommendations on screening for type 2 diabetes in adults [published correction appears in *CMAJ.* 2012;184(16):1815]. *CMAJ.* 2012;184(15):1687-1696. PMID: 23073674

Siu Al; US Preventive Services Task Force. Screening for abnormal blood glucose and type 2 diabetes mellitus: U.S. Preventive Services Task Force Recommendation Statement. *Ann Intern Med.* 2015;163(11):861-868. PMID: 26501513

24 ANSWER: B) Sulfonylurea screen

This patient has severe hypoglycemia due to either an insulinoma or intake of sulfonylurea. Before diagnosing insulinoma and pursuing localizing studies (Answer A), a sulfonylurea screen (Answer B) must be performed because sulfonylureas stimulate β cells to release insulin, C-peptide, and proinsulin; the hypoglycemia panel looks similar to that of insulinoma. Abdominal CT can be misleading in the absence of a definitive diagnosis and after sulfonylureas have been excluded as a cause of hypoglycemia. The patient himself, his wife, or a pharmacy mistake could account for the sulfonylurea intake.

A plasma insulin concentration of 3.0 μIU/mL or higher (≥20.8 pmol/L) by immunochemiluminometric assay when the plasma glucose concentration is below 55 mg/dL (<3.1 mmol/L) indicates insulin excess and is consistent with hyperinsulinemia (either from insulinoma or exogenous insulin or sulfonylurea). Plasma C-peptide distinguishes endogenous from exogenous hyperinsulinemia at a cutoff value of 0.6 ng/mL (0.20 nmol/L). In patients with insulinoma or sulfonylurea intake, the C-peptide concentration is at least 0.6 ng/mL (≥0.20 nmol/L), as opposed to exogenous insulin where the C-peptide concentration is 0.6 ng/mL (0.20 nmol/L). A plasma proinsulin concentration of 44 pg/mL or greater (≥5.0 pmol/L) is seen in the setting of insulinoma or sulfonylurea intake. Because of the antiketogenic effect of insulin, plasma β-hydroxybutyrate concentrations are lower in patients with insulinoma than in those without. All patients with hyperinsulinemia or IGF-mediated hypoglycemia have plasma β-hydroxybutyrate values of 2.7 mmol/L or less. A plasma sulfonylurea screen would reveal the sulfonylurea agent causing the hypoglycemia.

In adrenal insufficiency, the plasma insulin concentration is less than 3.0 μIU/mL (<20.8 pmol/L), plasma C-peptide concentration is less than 0.6 ng/mL (<0.20 nmol/L), plasma proinsulin concentration is less than 44 pg/mL (<5 pmol/L), and plasma β-hydroxybutyrate concentration is greater than 2.7 mmol/L. Thus, there is no need for a cosyntropin-stimulation test (Answer C). In IGF-2–secreting tumors, the plasma insulin is less than 3.0 μIU/mL (<20.8 pmol/L), plasma C-peptide concentration is less than 0.6 ng/mL (<0.20 nmol/L), plasma proinsulin concentration is less than 44 pg/mL (<5 pmol/L), but plasma β-hydroxybutyrate concentration is 2.7 mmol/L or less. Thus, there is no need for IGF-2 measurement (Answer E). There is no role for a supervised fast (Answer D) in this case, as there is already documentation of all the laboratory tests needed during the episode of hypoglycemia in the emergency department.

EDUCATIONAL OBJECTIVE
Guide the appropriate evaluation of hypoglycemia.

REFERENCE(S)
Cryer PE, Axelrod L, Grossman AB, et al; Endocrine Society. Evaluation and management of adult hypoglycemic disorders: an Endocrine Society clinical practice guideline. *J Clin Endocrinol Metab.* 2009;94(3):709-728. PMID: 19088155

Iglesias P, Diez JJ. Management of endocrine disease: a clinical update on tumor-induced hypoglycemia. *Eur J Endocrinol.* 2014;170(4):R147-R157. PMID: 24459236

Service FJ, O'Briend PC. Increasing serum betahydroxybutyrate concentrations during the 72-hour fast: evidence against hyperinsulinemic hypoglycemia. *J Clin Endocrinol Metab.* 2005;90(8):4555-4558. PMID: 15886243

Vezzosi D, Bennet A, Grunenwald S, Caron P. Hypoglycemia in nondiabetic patients: when is the 72-hour-fast test required and how can it be interpreted? *Presse Med.* 2016;45(6 Pt 1):588-594. PMID: 27208915

25 ANSWER: C) Discontinuation of insulin and initiation of glimepiride

Monogenic forms of diabetes comprise a heterogeneous group of disorders. They are caused by single-gene pathogenic variants and are characterized by impaired insulin secretion. Up to 5% of all diabetes cases are monogenic, and affected patients are often undiagnosed or are misclassified as having type 1 or type 2 diabetes.

Accurate diagnosis is important because of the special implications for treatment, prognosis, and familial risk. Monogenic diabetes includes maturity-onset diabetes of the young (MODY), mitochondrial diabetes, and neonatal diabetes. Many pathogenic variants have been identified that cause diabetes by disturbing the coupling of blood glucose concentration and insulin secretion.

The patient in this vignette has MODY, characterized by (1) young age at diagnosis, often under 25 years, (2) a marked family history of diabetes in every generation due to autosomal dominant inheritance, (3) absence of obesity and signs of insulin resistance, (4) commonly mild hyperglycemia without the need for insulin therapy, and (5) negative results for β-cell antibodies. The diagnosis can be confirmed by genetic testing where available. MODY 3 (due to an *HNF1A* pathogenic variant [hepatocyte nuclear factor-1-alpha gene on chromosome 12]), the most prevalent MODY form, presents with early glycosuria and hyperglycemia, which is often postprandial. Optimal treatment of MODY 3 is sulfonylureas (thus, Answer C is correct and Answers A and E are incorrect). One study documented a significantly greater drop in hemoglobin A_{1c} level with a sulfonylurea compared with metformin (Answer D). Almost 70% of patients previously treated with insulin are successfully switched to sulfonylureas once an *HNF1A* pathogenic variant is identified. Patients with MODY 3 are at risk for microvascular and macrovascular complications of type 1 and type 2 diabetes. In addition, individuals with MODY 3 appear to have an increased risk of cardiovascular mortality compared with unaffected family members. There are no data on the use of SGLT-2 inhibitors (Answer B) in patients with MODY.

EDUCATIONAL OBJECTIVE
Diagnose monogenic diabetes mellitus that was initially mischaracterized as type 1 diabetes and assess the treatment implications.

REFERENCE(S)
Valkovicova T, Skopkova M, Stanik J, Gasperikova D. Novel insights into genetics and clinics of the HNF1A-MODY. *Endocr Regul.* 2019;53(2):110-134. PMID: 31517624

Petersmann A, Muller-Wieland D, Muller UA, et al. Definition, classification and diagnosis of diabetes mellitus. *Exp Clin Endocrinol Diabetes.* 2019;127(S 01):S1-S7. PMID: 31860923

Henzen C. Monogenic diabetes mellitus due to defects in insulin secretion. *Swiss Med Wkly.* 2012;142:w13690. PMID: 23037711

Thanabalasingham G, Owen KR. Diagnosis and management of maturity onset diabetes of the young (MODY). *BMJ.* 2011;343:d6044. PMID: 22012810

Wherrett DK, Bundy B, Becker DJ, et al; Type 1 Diabetes TrialNet GAD Study Group. Antigen-based therapy with glutamic acid decarboxylase (GAD) vaccine in patients with recent-onset type 1 diabetes: a randomised double-blind trial. *Lancet.* 2011;378(9788):319-327. PMID: 21714999

Shepherd M, Shields B, Ellard S, Rubio-Cabezas O, Hattersley AT. A genetic diagnosis of HNF1A diabetes alters treatment and improves glycaemic control in the majority of insulin-treated patients. *Diabet Med.* 2009;26(4):437-441. PMID: 19388975

26 **ANSWER: D) Reduced albuminuria**

Following successful pancreas transplant alone, recurrent and de novo diabetic nephropathy is prevented. Pancreas transplant alone may reverse established diabetic lesions in patients with early diabetic nephropathy. Regarding nephropathy 5 to 10 years after successful pancreas transplant, mesangial volume and mesangial matrix volume are significantly decreased as compared with the same measurements at 0 and 5 years. In some patients, the width of the glomerular and tubular basement membranes and the mesangial volumes return to normal, and nodular glomerular lesions disappear. Tubular atrophy appears improved, possibly due to reabsorption of diseased nephrons. In all patients, urine albumin excretion improves significantly. Thus, reduced albuminuria (Answer D) can be expected within 5 years after a successful pancreas transplant.

After pancreas transplant alone, there is stabilization and, in some cases, improvement in peripheral and autonomic diabetic neuropathy. In addition, after successful pancreas transplant, the velocity of motor and sensory nerve conduction, as well as clinical neuropathy, stabilizes but does not regress (Answer B). Abnormalities of gastric motility do not improve (Answer C).

The effect of pancreas transplant on diabetic retinopathy is not clear. While some studies have found no benefit in terms of halting or reversing the progression of advanced retinopathy after pancreas transplant, other reports have noted stabilization or occasional regression of retinal lesions (Answer A) (but not at a proliferative stage like this patient).

After pancreas transplant, serum triglyceride and LDL-cholesterol concentrations tend to fall, and serum HDL-cholesterol concentrations tend to rise.

Quality-of-life studies consistently demonstrate benefits, such as return to work and successful pregnancies, with no notable adverse effects on the fetus or the mother (Answer E).

EDUCATIONAL OBJECTIVE

Describe the potential benefits of pancreas transplant 5 to 10 years after successful transplant.

REFERENCE(S)

Coppelli A, Giannarelli R, Vistoli F, et al. The beneficial effects of pancreas transplant alone on diabetic nephropathy. *Diabetes Care.* 2005;28(6):1366-1370. PMID: 15920053

Jenssen T, Hartmann A, Birkeland KI. Long-term diabetes complications after pancreas transplantation. *Curr Opin Organ Transplant.* 2017;22(4):382-388. PMID: 28598888

Dean PG, Kukla A, Stegall MD, Kudva YC. Pancreas transplantation. *BMJ.* 2017;357:j1321. PMID: 28373161

de Sá JR, Monteagudo PT, Rangel EB, et al. The evolution of diabetic chronic complications after pancreas transplantation. *Diabetol Metab Syndr.* 2009;1(1):11. PMID: 19825148

Boggi U, Rosati CM, Marchetti P. Follow-up of secondary diabetic complications after pancreas transplantation. *Curr Opin Organ Transplant.* 2013;18(1):102-110. PMID: 23283247

27 ANSWER: A) Polysomnography

In both men and women, the strongest risk factor for obstructive sleep apnea is obesity. The prevalence of obstructive sleep apnea progressively increases as BMI and associated markers increase (eg, neck circumference, waist-to-hip ratio). In a prospective study of nearly 700 adults with 4-year longitudinal follow-up, a 10% increase in weight was associated with a 6-fold increase in the risk of incident obstructive sleep apnea. In a population-based study of more than 1000 adults who underwent polysomnography, moderate-to-severe obstructive sleep apnea (apnea-hypopnea index ≥15 events/h) was present in 11% of patients who were normal weight, 21% of those who were overweight (BMI, 25-30 kg/m^2), and 63% of those with obesity (BMI >30 kg/m^2).

Most patients with obstructive sleep apnea first come to the attention of a clinician because of fatigue, daytime sleepiness, or report by the patient's bed partner of loud snoring, gasping, snorting, or interruptions in breathing while sleeping. Diagnostic testing for obstructive sleep apnea should be performed in any patient with unexplained excessive daytime sleepiness, which is the clinically relevant symptom of obstructive sleep apnea that is most responsive to treatment. In the absence of excessive daytime sleepiness, diagnostic testing is pursued if the patient snores and either works in a mission-critical profession (eg, airline pilots, bus drivers, and truck drivers) or has 2 or more additional clinical features of obstructive sleep apnea.

Full-night, attended, in-laboratory polysomnography (Answer A) is considered the gold-standard diagnostic test for obstructive sleep apnea. It involves monitoring the patient during a full night's sleep. Patients in whom obstructive sleep apnea is diagnosed and who choose positive airway pressure therapy are subsequently brought back for another study, during which their positive airway pressure device is titrated. Split-night, attended, in-laboratory polysomnography is similar, except the diagnostic portion of the study is performed during the first part of the night only. Those patients in whom obstructive sleep apnea is diagnosed during the first part of the night and who choose positive airway pressure therapy can have their positive airway pressure device titrated during the second part of the night.

There is no role for a cosyntropin-stimulation test (Answer D) in this case. The patient has no other symptoms suggestive of adrenal insufficiency, and he has normal blood pressure and electrolytes.

Total testosterone can be lower than normal because of obesity. Obesity decreases the serum concentration of SHBG, thereby decreasing the serum total testosterone concentration, usually without lowering the free testosterone concentration. The binding abnormality is proportional to the degree of obesity and is corrected by weight loss. Therefore, before diagnosing hypogonadism, serum free testosterone should be measured by equilibrium dialysis. If it is normal, pituitary MRI (Answer B) and prolactin measurement (Answer C) are not necessary. This patient also has normal libido, which is consistent with a normal gonadal axis; the erectile dysfunction is most likely due to his diabetes and other comorbidities.

Free T$_4$ measurement (Answer E) is incorrect because the normal TSH level excludes primary hypothyroidism unless he has central hypothyroidism. However, there is no indication that he has hypothyroidism (no history of pituitary surgery, no radiation, and no obvious pituitary hormone abnormalities).

EDUCATIONAL OBJECTIVE
Diagnose sleep apnea in patients with obesity and type 2 diabetes mellitus.

REFERENCE(S)

Ralls F, Cutchen L. A contemporary review of obstructive sleep apnea. *Curr Opin Pulm Med.* 2019;25(6):578-593. PMID: 31589188

Muraki I, Wada H, Tanigawa T. Sleep apnea and type 2 diabetes. *J Diabetes Investig.* 2018;9(5):991-997. PMID: 29453905

Reutrakul S, Mokhlesi B. Obstructive sleep apnea and diabetes: a state of the art review. *Chest.* 2017;152(5): 1070-1086. PMID: 28527878

Peppard PE, Young T, Barnet JH, Palta M, Hagen EW, Hla KM. Increased prevalence of sleep-disordered breathing in adults. *Am J Epidemiol.* 2013;177(9):1006-1014. PMID: 23589584

Qaseem A, Dallas P, Owens DK, Starkey M, Holty JE, Shekelle P; Clinical Guidelines Committee of the American College of Physicians. Diagnosis of obstructive sleep apnea in adults: a clinical practice guideline from the American College of Physicians. *Ann Intern Med.* 2014;161(3):210-220. PMID: 25089864

Cooper LA, Page ST, Amory JK, Anawalt BD, Matsumoto AM. The association of obesity with sex hormone-binding globulin is stronger than the association with ageing--implications for the interpretation of total testosterone measurements. *Clin Endocrinol (Oxf).* 2015;83(6):828-833. PMID: 25777143

28 ANSWER: E) Stop vitamin C, as it can interfere with sensor glucose readings

The flash glucose monitoring system was approved by the US FDA in October 2017 and became available by prescription in the United States by the end of 2017. Calibration free, it is a disk worn on the arm for 10 to 14 days, which is designed to largely replace the recommended 4 to 10 painful fingerstick blood glucose readings required each day for the self-management of diabetes. The initial device was designed for 10 days, but in August 2018 the US FDA approved the 14-day version.

In randomized controlled trials, use of the flash glucose monitoring system is associated with reduced hypoglycemia and, in observational studies, with improved hemoglobin A_{1c} levels. User satisfaction is high and adverse events are low. Accuracy of this system in adults, children, and in women during pregnancy is comparable to that of currently available real-time continuous glucose monitors. The cost of the flash glucose monitoring system is lower than that of real-time continuous glucose monitors.

Glucose data can be visualized in multiple devices and platforms and summarized in an ambulatory glucose profile to aid pattern recognition and adjustment of insulin doses. Both users and health care professionals must be appropriately educated to harness the full benefits. Further randomized controlled trials to assess the long-term impact on hemoglobin A_{1c}, particularly in patients with high baseline hemoglobin A_{1c} values and in specific age groups (eg, such as adolescents and young adults), are warranted. The potential effect on diabetes-related complications is yet to be realized.

The manufacturer has undertaken tests to evaluate the flash glucose monitoring system with 16 potentially interfering substances. Testing confirmed no clinically significant interference for the substances tested, with the exception of ascorbic acid and salicylic acid. Taking ascorbic acid may falsely raise glucose readings and salicylic acid may slightly lower glucose readings. The level of inaccuracy depends on the amount of interfering substance.

In this patient, high doses of vitamin C led to falsely high sensor glucose readings. Therefore, vitamin C should be stopped (Answer E). Cinnamon (Answer C) and acetaminophen (Answer D) do not interfere with sensor readings. The patient's diabetes is well-controlled and her normal blood glucose values determined by fingerstick are consistent with her hemoglobin A_{1c} value. Therefore, it would be incorrect to adjust her insulin based on the sensor data (Answer A). Changing the site of the sensor from the arm to the abdomen (Answer B) is incorrect because the arm is the FDA-approved site. One study showed that the accuracy and precision of the flash glucose monitoring system placed on the upper thigh are similar to those when it is worn on the upper arm, but the abdomen performed unacceptably poorly.

The table summarizes the main features of the flash glucose monitoring system (*see table on the following page*).

EDUCATIONAL OBJECTIVE

List the substances known to interfere with glucose readings derived from the flash glucose monitoring system.

Table 1. Overview of Features in the FreeStyle Libre Systems Approved in the United States

This overview is representative of the FreeStyle Libre systems approved in the United States at time of publication.* The FreeStyle Libre system is approved in the European Union (EU) as of September 2014 and in the United States as of November 2017. The FreeStyle Libre 14 day system is approved in the United States as of July 2018. EU and US systems have differences in patient indication and interface options. Refer to the table for features of US approved systems only.

Minimum use age:	≥18 years
Sensor placement:	Back of arm; placement is not approved for other sites
Sensor warm-up period:	▸ FreeStyle Libre system: 12 hours after insertion before able to retrieve glucose data ▸ FreeStyle Libre 14 day system: 1 hour after insertion before able to retrieve glucose data
Sensor wear time:	▸ FreeStyle Libre system: 10 days ▸ FreeStyle Libre 14 day system: 14 days
Calibration:	Factory calibrated; does not require daily calibration
Insulin dosing:	Individuals are able to use sensor glucose reading for treatment decisions without confirmatory fingerstick monitoring. Under the following conditions, sensor glucose readings may not be accurate, and you should conduct a fingerstick: ▸ If inaccurate reading is suspected ▸ If experiencing symptoms that may be due to low or high blood glucose ▸ If experiencing symptoms that do not match sensor glucose readings ▸ During times of rapidly changing glucose of more than 2 mg/dL per minute (i.e., straight up or down trend arrow) ▸ When the sensor glucose reading does not include a current glucose number or trend arrow ▸ To confirm hypoglycemia or impending hypoglycemia as reported by the sensor ▸ When "Check Blood Glucose" symbol appears in the reader ▸ During the first 12 hours of wearing a FreeStyle Libre 14 day Sensor
Cautions and Contraindications:	▸ The system is not approved for use in pregnant women or persons on dialysis and has not been evaluated in these populations. ▸ The system has not been evaluated for use in patients with hypoglycemia unawareness and will not automatically alert to current or impending hypoglycemic event without scanning the sensor. The system will not automatically notify the user when experiencing hypoglycemia or hyperglycemia unless the sensor is scanned.
Potential Interferents:	▸ Salicylic acid (used in aspirin and other pain relievers) at doses ≥650 mg may cause falsely lower glucose values ▸ Ascorbic acid (vitamin C) at doses ≥500 mg may cause falsely higher readings. ▸ At lower doses, salicylic acid and ascorbic acid are known to have minimal effect on sensor glucose readings in the FreeStyle Libre systems.

* For full indications for use and safety information, seek out product information from the manufacturer.

Reprinted from Kudva YC, Ahmann AJ, Bergenstal RM, et al. Approach to using trend arrows in the FreeStyle Libre Flash Glucose Monitoring Systems in adults. J Endocr Soc. 2018;2(12):1320-1337. © Endocrine Society.

REFERENCE(S)

Leelarathna L, Wilmot EG. Flash forward: a review of flash glucose monitoring. *Diabetic Med.* 2018;35(4):472-482. PMID: 29356072

Chen C, Zhao XL, Li ZH, Zhu ZG, Qian SH, Flewitt AJ. Current and emerging technology for continuous glucose monitoring. *Sensors (Basel).* 2017;17(1): pii: E182. PMID: 28106820

Charleer S, Mathieu C, Nobels F, Gillard P. Accuracy and precision of flash glucose monitoring sensors inserted into the abdomen and upper thigh compared with the upper arm. *Diabetes Obes Metab.* 2018;20(6):1503-1507. PMID: 29381253

Kudva YC, Ahmann AJ, Bergenstal RM, et al. Approach to using trend arrows in the FreeStyle Libre Flash Glucose Monitoring Systems in adults. *J Endoc Soc.* 2018;2(12):1320-1337. PMID: 30474069

Diabetes Mellitus, Section 2 Board Review

Marie E. McDonnell, MD

29 **ANSWER: B) Approximately 10% of glucose values at 6 AM are below 50 mg/dL (<2.8 mmol/L)**

In the standard ambulatory glucose profile, glucose values are presented as an aggregate over 7 to 90 days and the display shows the glucose by percentile and time of day. On the right side of the image above, the specific lines are assigned a percentile, which indicates the percentage of values captured that were below the indicator line. If one identifies the 10% line and follows it to 6 AM, the line is at approximately 50 mg/dL (2.8 mmol/L). This indicates that 10% of values obtained in this period were below 50 mg/L (<2.8 mmol/L) (Answer B), an indicator of clinically significant hypoglycemia. One cannot derive a mean, lowest measured value, or time in range from the data presented (thus, Answers A and C are incorrect). The 25th percentile mark indicates that approximately 25% of values are below the indicator line. Accordingly, based on the 25th percentile indicator line, 25% of values are *lower than* 250 mg/dL (<13.9 mmol/L), while the majority are greater than 250 mg/dL (>13.9 mmol/L) (thus, Answer D is incorrect). Although the 10th percentile line at 12 PM is just above 70 mg/dL (3.9 mmol/L), it is not possible to conclude from the data that no glucose values were below 70 mg/dL (<3.9 mmol/L) (thus, Answer E is incorrect).

Hypoglycemia in the fasting and/or overnight state is one of the most significant and problematic glucose patterns in patients with diabetes who take insulin.

EDUCATIONAL OBJECTIVE

Interpret aggregate continuous glucose monitoring data.

REFERENCE(S)

Johnson ML, Martens TW, Criego AB, Carlson AL, Simonson GD, Bergenstal RM. Utilizing the ambulatory glucose profile to standardize and implement continuous glucose monitoring in clinical practice. *Diabetes Technol Ther*. 2019;21(S2):S217-S225. PMID: 31169432

30 **ANSWER: B) Perform CT of the chest, abdomen, and pelvis**

This patient most likely has a tumor producing excess circulating IGF-2 from an undiagnosed malignancy. The suppressed β-hydroxybutyrate and rise in glucose after glucagon suggest an insulin receptor–mediated process. However, the low insulin and C-peptide levels suggest that human insulin is not the culprit. An exploratory CT (Answer B) is a reasonable first step in diagnosing a large solid tumor. This condition is usually confirmed by a combination of imaging to identify the tumor and measuring the ratio of IGF-2 to IGF-1. If the ratio of IGF-2 to IGF-1 is greater than 3, IGF-2 is most likely being secreted by a tumor. Measuring only IGF-1 (Answer C) is incorrect because the IGF-2 level is required to make the diagnosis. As this is a special laboratory test, the result often takes significant time to return. Thus, it is reasonable to move directly to imaging given the history and results of the fast.

Requesting ACTH and cortisol measurement (Answer A) suggests that adrenal insufficiency could have a role, but in this condition the response to glucagon is most often impaired rather than robust as in this case. Factitious hypoglycemia due to surreptitious use of an insulin analogue is possible, and as a veterinarian this patient would potentially have easy access to insulin. However, in that scenario, the levels of both insulin and

C-peptide are typically extremely low or undetectable. Seeking permission to search the patient's room and personal belongings for insulin (Answer D) is not warranted. Performing abdominal ultrasonography (Answer E) is incorrect, as it is not sensitive enough to be used for exploratory imaging when a solid tumor is expected.

EDUCATIONAL OBJECTIVE
Assess a patient presenting with hypoglycemia and correctly interpret the results of laboratory results obtained during a supervised fast.

REFERENCE(S)
Cryer PE, Axelrod L, Grossman AB, et al; Endocrine Society. Evaluation and management of adult hypoglycemic disorders: an Endocrine Society clinical practice guideline. *J Clin Endocrinol Metab.* 2009;94(3):709-728. PMID: 19088155

31 ANSWER: B) Insulinoma

In a person with documented Whipple triad, the combination of inappropriately high plasma insulin, C-peptide, and proinsulin levels; negative oral hypoglycemic agent screen; and negative circulating insulin antibodies in the setting of fasting hypoglycemia is most consistent with unregulated secretion of endogenous insulin. The most likely cause of this condition is insulinoma (Answer B), which is considered to be significantly more common than adult-onset nesidioblastosis (Answer E).

Autoimmune hypoglycemia, or Hirata disease (Answer A), would be expected to have high plasma insulin levels measured during hypoglycemia and high-titer serum insulin antibodies. In adrenal insufficiency (Answer C), severe hypoglycemia may occur due to an insufficient counterregulatory response to hypoglycemia, and both insulin and C-peptide levels would be low. Hypoglycemia due to factitious insulin administration (Answer D) would have yielded either a suppressed or very high insulin level (depending on the specificity of the insulin assay used) along with suppressed C-peptide and proinsulin levels.

EDUCATIONAL OBJECTIVE
Assess a patient presenting with hypoglycemia and correctly interpret the results of laboratory results obtained during a modified supervised fast performed in the office setting.

REFERENCE(S)
Cryer PE, Axelrod L, Grossman AB, et al; Endocrine Society. Evaluation and management of adult hypoglycemic disorders: an Endocrine Society clinical practice guideline. *J Clin Endocrinol Metab.* 2009;94(3):709-728. PMID: 19088155

32 ANSWER: D) Inquire about alcohol intake at the end of the work week

Given the pattern of overnight hypoglycemia occurring on weekend nights and overall poor glycemic control, unhealthy alcohol intake as a key underlying factor should be explored with this patient (Answer D). Given the known fetal risks of maternal alcohol consumption, discussing alcoholic intake with this patient is especially important. The relationship between alcohol use and poor diabetes self-care has been shown by large data sets to be complex, although most of the available data is regarding type 2 diabetes. Numerous factors may underlie this link, including decreased food intake after alcohol intake and impaired attention to diet, medication, or other self-care behaviors such as exercise and glucose self-monitoring. This patient has developed maladaptive behaviors with her insulin pump that increased alcohol intake could influence further, such as allowing her pod pump to run out of insulin before changing it and potentially reusing old sites, causing lipohypertrophy. She reports stress and depression, which increase the risk of alcohol use disorders.

Intermittent alcohol consumption often results in a typical pattern on CGM reports. In 1 small study of 16 free-living patients with type 1 diabetes, the glycemic effect of alcohol (0.85 g/kg) vs orange juice consumed at 7 PM was observed over the subsequent 24 hours. The average interstitial glucose level measured by continuous glucose monitoring (CGM) was about 20 mg/dL (1.1 mmol/L) lower the morning after drinking alcohol, and patients reported more than twice as many hypoglycemic episodes during the subsequent day compared with the number of episodes reported by those who consumed the placebo drink. While the greatest effect was seen within the first 8 hours, there was a persistent risk of hypoglycemia continuing for 24 hours.

Inquiring if she uses her pump's internal dosing tool to arrive at correction doses (Answer A) is incorrect, as she does not use a CGM device that is integrated with her insulin pump to allow for automated correction doses.

While inaccurate CGM readings are more likely to occur on the first day of a new sensor, her pattern of hypoglycemia is recurrent over 2 to 3 days, and hence it is not related to when she changes her site (thus, Answer B is incorrect).

Acetominophen use (Answer C) can lead to falsely elevated glucose on certain CGM devices, which could lead to inadvertent insulin corrections and subsequent hypoglycemia, but this would generally be reported by the patient and would not be expected to occur in a weekly pattern.

As the hypoglycemia events occur both in the overnight and fasting states as well as during the day, bolusing excessive insulin doses before meals (Answer E) would not explain the pattern.

EDUCATIONAL OBJECTIVE

Identify glycemic and behavior patterns concerning for alcohol use disorder in patients with type 1 diabetes mellitus.

REFERENCE(S)

Engler PA, Ramsey SE, Smith RJ. Alcohol use of diabetes patients: the need for assessment and intervention. *Acta Diabetol.* 2013;50(2):93-99. PMID: 20532803

Richardson T, Weiss M, Thomas P, Kerr D. Day after the night before: influence of evening alcohol on risk of hypoglycemia in patients with type 1 diabetes. *Diabetes Care.* 2005;28(7):1801-1802. PMID: 15983341

33 ANSWER: C) PI3 kinase inhibitor

Unlike the other medications listed, PI3 kinase inhibitors (Answer C) can directly cause rapid onset, marked hyperglycemia due to impaired insulin signaling. In the SOLAR-1 trial (Study Assessing the Efficacy and Safety of Alpelisib Plus Fulvestrant in Men and Postmenopausal Women With Advanced Breast Cancer Which Progressed on or After Aromatase Inhibitor Treatment), 572 women with or without diabetes were randomly assigned to either the PI3 kinase inhibitor alpelisib + fulvestrant or placebo + fulvestrant. Treatment with alpelisib-fulvestrant prolonged progression-free survival among patients with *PIK3CA*-mutated, HR-positive, HER2-negative advanced breast cancer who had received endocrine therapy previously. However, alpelisib was associated with 36% rate of grade 3/4 hyperglycemia, or glucose levels greater than 250 mg/dL (>13.9 mmol/L). PI3 kinase is critical in insulin signaling steps that allow for glucose transport, and its blockade can result in dramatic insulin resistance in patients with and without diabetes. As was seen in published studies, as well as in clinical practice, the effect is dose-dependent and is quickly reversed after stopping the drug.

PD-1 and CTLA-4 inhibitors (Answers A and D), often called checkpoint inhibitors, cause a fulminant form of autoimmune diabetes that most resembles type 1 diabetes, which has thus far been found to be irreversible. The mTOR inhibitors (Answer B) commonly cause hyperglycemia that is generally milder, with a slower and less dramatic onset compared with the PI3 kinase inhibitors and checkpoint inhibitors. Platinum-based drugs (Answer E) do not directly cause hyperglycemia, but they are often administered alongside glucocorticoids to prevent severe nausea and the steroids can cause dramatic hyperglycemia.

EDUCATIONAL OBJECTIVE

Identify cancer drug classes that can cause hyperglycemia in a patient with established diabetes and the expected pattern of hyperglycemia.

REFERENCE(S)

André F, Ciruelos E, Rubovszky G, et all; SOLAR-1 Study Group. Alpelisib for *PIK3CA*-mutated, hormone receptor-positive advanced breast cancer. *N Engl J Med*. 2019;380(20):1929-1940. PMID: 31091374

34 ANSWER: A) Pathogenic variant in the *HNF1B* gene

Diabetes due to a pathogenic variant in the hepatic nuclear factor 1 β gene (*HNF1B*) (Answer A), or maturity-onset diabetes of the young type 5 (MODY type 5), represents approximately 5% to 10% of all known monogenic diabetes and is one of the more rare types. Unlike MODY due to pathogenic variants in *HNF1A* or *GCK* (Answer B) (MODY type 3 and MODY type 2, respectively), MODY type 5 is typically not responsive to sulfonylurea therapy for a significant period. Due to progressive decline in β-cell mass, most patients with MODY type 5 require insulin well before middle-age, and often at the time diabetes is diagnosed. *HNF1B*-related diabetes has also been called renal cysts and diabetes syndrome, as it is associated with urogenital malformations, including renal agenesis, renal cysts, and renal hypoplasia. Other conditions associated with *HNF1B* pathogenic variants include hypomagnesemia (which sometimes mimics Gitelman syndrome), gout, and chronically elevated liver enzymes. The most common genetic abnormality is complete deletion of the gene, although multiple point mutations have also been identified, and this most likely explains the variability of the MODY type 5 phenotype.

Pancreatic divisum (Answer C) is a potential cause of recurrent pancreatitis, which over time can lead to diabetes. As this patient does not have a history of pancreatitis, this diagnosis is unlikely. Type 1 diabetes (Answer D) is not the likely etiology because the patient reports not having ketoacidosis despite missing basal insulin for many days in a row, several years after diagnosis. Antibodies to the insulin receptor (Answer E) is the underlying cause of type B insulin resistance, which is a rare condition that causes a brief period of hypoglycemia followed by marked hyperglycemia and severe insulin resistance that is cured only by combination therapy with immunomodulator medications.

EDUCATIONAL OBJECTIVE

Diagnose maturity-onset diabetes of the young type 5 (*HNF1B*-related diabetes).

REFERENCE(S)

Broome DT, Pantalone KM, Kashyap SR, Philipson LH. Approach to the patient with MODY-monogenic diabetes. *J Clin Endocrinol Metab*. 2021;106(1):237-250. PMID: 33034350

Bingham C, Hattersley AT. Renal cysts and diabetes syndrome resulting from mutations in hepatocyte nuclear factor-1beta. *Nephrol Dial Transplant*. 2004;19(11):2703-2708. PMID: 15496559

Verhave JC, Bech AP, Wetzels JFM, Nijenhuis T. Hepatocyte nuclear factor 1β-associated kidney disease: more than renal cysts and diabetes. *J Am Soc Nephrol*. 2016;27(2):345-353. PMID: 26319241

35 ANSWER: C) Perform a cosyntropin-stimulation test

This patient's presenting concern is prediabetes based on a hemoglobin A_{1c} value obtained during the evaluation of a constellation of symptoms, including fatigue and weight loss. However, he exhibits signs and symptoms most concerning for adrenal insufficiency, which is a critical diagnosis to make expeditiously in order to initiate glucocorticoid therapy and, in the case of primary adrenal insufficiency, mineralocorticoid therapy. In this vignette, specific signs of primary adrenal insufficiency, or Addison disease, include the classic pattern observed on this patient's basic metabolic panel, namely low sodium, elevated potassium, and mild metabolic acidosis. Cortisol insufficiency induces the secretion of antidiuretic hormone, resulting in a syndrome of inappropriate secretion of antidiuresis and hence hyponatremia. The metabolic acidosis is due to insufficiency of aldosterone, which causes a decrease in acid secretion in the kidney. Recognizing that he also has glucose intolerance as indicated both by the random blood glucose and the hemoglobin A_{1c} level greater than 5.7% (>39 mmol/mol) is important.

It is now well established that type 1 diabetes presents in stages, as does type 2 diabetes, with a preclinical phase that can be identified by a subclinical elevation in hemoglobin A_{1c}. The concomitant presence of prediabetes, cortisol deficiency, and a TSH value at the upper limit of normal is concerning for Schmidt syndrome (type 1 diabetes, Addison disease, and Hashimoto thyroiditis in the same individual), which can be seen within the constellation of conditions in autoimmune polyglandular syndrome type 2. Diagnosis is critical because other conditions may arise such as primary hypogonadism and nonendocrine autoimmune conditions.

Cosyntropin-stimulation testing (Answer C) is the most sensitive and specific test that can be performed quickly enough to make the diagnosis and begin treatment. If the diagnosis is highly suspected, steroid replacement can begin immediately following the cosyntropin-stimulation test while the result is pending.

Although encouraging fluids and closely following hemoglobin A_{1c} (Answer B) is indicated, as is evaluating for thyroid autoimmunity (Answer D), these are not the most important next steps. Measuring tissue transglutaminase antibodies (Answer A) is also reasonable once the assessment is complete and his condition improves with treatment. Stopping the amphetamine (Answer E) does not directly address the problem and may exacerbate his hypotension. While amphetamines can activate the hypothalamic-pituitary-adrenal axis, they are not known to cause acute adrenal crisis.

EDUCATIONAL OBJECTIVE
Diagnose autoimmune polyglandular syndrome.

REFERENCE(S)
Cutolo M. Autoimmune polyendocrine syndromes. *Autoimmun Rev.* 2014;13(2):85-89. PMID: 24055063

36 ANSWER: A) Provide reassurance
This patient has mononeuritis of the lateral femoral cutaneous nerve, which is a self-limiting condition that does not require specific treatment. Thus, providing reassurance (Answer A) in this setting is correct. Often called meralgia paresthetica, mononeuritis is a compression or entrapment mononeuropathy that is common in diabetes and typically resolves within 12 weeks. It is characterized by tingling, numbness, and burning pain in the outer part of the upper leg. Mononeuritis is caused by compression of the lateral femoral cutaneous nerve. Although no motor symptoms are associated with this condition, the sensory dysfunctions are potentially debilitating and in some patients the condition can be frightening.

MRI (Answer E) would be considered to assess for muscle infarction with or without concurrent infection, which is a rare complication of insulin injection, usually seen in patients with longstanding insulin-dependent diabetes and multiple end-organ microvascular complications. However, muscle infarctions are nearly always tender with palpable swelling and induration of the surrounding tissue, and, for unclear reasons, they occur most often in women. There is a palpable, painful mass, with swelling and induration of the surrounding tissue without systemic symptoms or signs. The painful lesion persists for weeks, occasionally with exacerbations of symptoms, then spontaneously resolves over several weeks to months. A nerve conduction study (Answer C) would not enhance the diagnostic sensitivity or specificity beyond the classic clinical examination and history. Although important to consider given his established cardiovascular disease, the history and physical examination findings are not consistent with a vascular event, so Doppler ultrasonography (Answer D) is not necessary. Herpes zoster, or shingles, presenting without rash or symptoms of malaise would be highly unusual, so treatment with acyclovir (Answer B) is incorrect.

EDUCATIONAL OBJECTIVE
Distinguish entrapment neuropathy/mononeuritis from more serious acute conditions that occur in the setting of diabetes.

REFERENCE(S)
Umpierrez GE, Stiles RG, Kleinbart J, Krendel DA, Watts NB. Diabetic muscle infarction. *Am J Med.* 1996;101(3):245-250. PMID: 8873484

37 **ANSWER: B) Measure fructosamine**
This patient presents with 3 important findings: (1) fasting hyperglycemia following the glucose-based diagnosis of diabetes; (2) hemoglobin A_{1c} level below 5.0% (<31 mmol/mol); and (3) significant anemia. These 3 features are highly consistent with hemolytic anemia and should prompt an evaluation. This patient has hereditary spherocytosis, a familial hemolytic disorder with marked heterogeneity of clinical features, ranging from an asymptomatic condition to fulminant hemolytic anemia. In severe cases, the disorder may be detected in early childhood, but in mild cases it may go unnoticed until later in adult life. On occasion, a low hemoglobin A_{1c} level that is discrepant from glucose levels leads to the identification of hemolysis. Hemoglobin A_{1c} is formed by the nonenzymatic glycation of the N-terminus of the β-chain of hemoglobin A. As blood glucose rises, the increase in nonenzymatic glycation of proteins is proportional to both the level of glucose and the lifespan of the protein in the circulation or tissues. Since the average lifespan of red blood cells is 120 days, hemoglobin A_{1c} reflects the mean daily blood glucose concentration over the preceding 2 to 3 months. In cases where the lifespan is reduced, as in this case, fructosamine (Answer B), a measure of total glycated proteins, can be a useful alternative to assess average glucose. To determine the next step for his diabetes management and to confirm the diagnosis, fructosamine measurement is the best test. It is not affected by anemia and will reflect the average blood glucose over the preceding 2 to 3 weeks.

Discontinuing insulin, continuing metformin, and following up in 3 months (Answer A) or discontinuing insulin and metformin (Answer D) are incorrect strategies, as they do not consider the inaccuracy of the hemoglobin A_{1c} in the assessment. Measuring C-peptide (Answer D) or recommending genetic testing for monogenic diabetes (Answer E) may be useful in the diagnostic evaluation, but they are of low priority, as the most likely diagnosis based on family history and the presence of obesity is type 2 diabetes.

EDUCATIONAL OBJECTIVE
Diagnose hemolytic anemia as a cause of low hemoglobin A_{1c} and describe alternatives to hemoglobin A_{1c} measurement to assess glycemia.

REFERENCE(S)
Ribeiro RT, Macedo MP, Raposo JF. HbA1c, fructosamine, and glycated albumin in the detection of dysglycaemic conditions. *Curr Diabetes Rev.* 2016;12(1):14-19. PMID: 26126638

38 **ANSWER: B) Reduced occurrence of severe hypoglycemia events**
The largest phase 3 clinical trial of cadaveric islet-cell transplant was the Clinical Islet Transplantation Consortium, which was sponsored by the National Institutes of Health. The trial enrolled persons with type 1 diabetes who had problems managing their blood glucose levels, such as severe hypoglycemia and hypoglycemia unawareness. Remarkably, the number of patients reporting a severe hypoglycemia event was reduced from 100% to 10% by 1 year after the first transplant, a finding that persisted for 2 years. Thus, the most likely outcome 1 year after islet-cell transplant is reduced occurrence of severe hypoglycemia events (Answer B). It is for this reason that the main criterion for enrollment in islet-cell transplant clinical trials is recurrent, severe hypoglycemia and/or hypoglycemia unawareness.

The study found that 1 year after islet transplantation, nearly 9 out of 10 transplant recipients had a hemoglobin A_{1c} level below 7.0% (<53 mmol/mol) and did not have episodes of severe hypoglycemia. Nearly half of patients achieved normal hemoglobin A_{1c} (<5.7% [<39 mmol/mol]) (thus, Answer C is incorrect). Approximately half of the recipients did not need to take any insulin after 1 year, which for most required 2 transplants per protocol (thus, Answer A is incorrect). Ongoing research from this study also found that islet-cell transplant recipients experienced significant improvements in their diabetes-related quality of life (thus, Answer D is incorrect) and reported better overall health status after the transplant, and this did not depend on whether the recipient still required insulin.

EDUCATIONAL OBJECTIVE
Explain the currently established benefits of cadaveric islet-cell transplant in patients with type 1 diabetes mellitus.

REFERENCE(S)
Hering BJ, Clarke WR, Bridges ND, et al; Clinical Islet Transplantation Consortium. Phase 3 trial of transplantation of human islets in type 1 diabetes complicated by severe hypoglycemia. *Diabetes Care*. 2016;39(7):1230-1240. PMID: 27208344

39 ANSWER: B) 2-Hour 75-g oral glucose tolerance test

In the 2019 Endocrine Society clinical practice guideline on treating diabetes in older adults, the writing committee determined that for persons aged 65 years and older without known diabetes who meet the criteria for prediabetes by fasting plasma glucose or hemoglobin A_{1c}, a 2-hour oral glucose tolerance test (Answer B) should be performed to rule out diabetes. While standard screening with fasting plasma glucose and hemoglobin A_{1c} (Answer A) categories allow easy identification of both diabetes and prediabetes, many persons older than 60 years who have diabetes and prediabetes are not diagnosed unless an oral glucose tolerance test is performed. In all populations, oral glucose tolerance testing is considered to be the most sensitive and specific screening test. Importantly, the diagnosis of diabetes is most likely to change the management of other cardiovascular risk factors, including lipids and blood pressure.

As acknowledged in the clinical practice guideline, this recommendation is applicable to patients at high risk with any of the following characteristics: overweight or obesity; first-degree relative with diabetes; high-risk race/ethnicity (eg, African American, Latino, Native American, Asian American, Pacific Islander); history of cardiovascular disease; hypertension (≥140/90 mm Hg or on therapy for hypertension); HDL-cholesterol concentration less than 35 mg/dL (<0.90 mmol/L)

and/or a triglyceride concentration greater than 250 mg/dL (2.82 mmol/L); sleep apnea; or physical inactivity. In addition, the recommendation is intended for individuals in overall good health with substantial life expectancy (eg, ≥10 years). Shared decision-making is advised when considering this test in frail older patients or in those for whom it may be overly burdensome.

Both fructosamine measurement (Answer C) and 2-hour postprandial fingerstick glucose measurement (Answer D) are incorrect, as neither is a recommended screening tool for diabetes. In addition, point-of-care glucose measurement using a glucose meter should not be used as a diabetes screening test due to issues with precision and accuracy with this methodology.

EDUCATIONAL OBJECTIVE
Determine when to consider oral glucose tolerance testing when screening older adults for diabetes mellitus.

REFERENCE(S)
LeRoith D, Biessels GJ, Braithwaite SS, et al. Treatment of diabetes in older adults: an Endocrine Society clinical practice guideline. *J Clin Endocrinol Metab*. 2019;104(5):1520-1574. PMID: 30903688

Menke A, Casagrande S, Geiss L, Cowie CC. Prevalence of and trends in diabetes among adults in the United States, 1988-2012. *JAMA*. 2015;314(10):1021-1029. PMID: 26348752

40 ANSWER: D) Type 2 diabetes mellitus

The diagnosis of type 2 diabetes has classically been made on the basis of a fasting plasma glucose value of 126 mg/dL or greater (≥7.0 mmol/L). Mainly used in research settings, an oral glucose tolerance test with a 2-hour cutoff for plasma glucose of 200 mg/dL or greater (≥11.1 mmol/L) can also be used for diagnostic purposes. In 2010, the American Diabetes Association approved hemoglobin A_{1c} measurement as an additional test for diabetes diagnosis, with a threshold of 6.5% or greater (≥48 mmol/mol). According to these guidelines, the diagnosis is confirmed on the basis of 2 positive tests: either a repeat of the originally abnormal test on a separate day or 2 different tests on the same or separate day. For example, if the hemoglobin A_{1c} level is 6.7% (50 mmol/mol) on initial testing and then 6.9% (52 mmol/mol) on confirmatory testing, irrespective of the fasting plasma glucose, diabetes can be diagnosed. The same would apply if 2 fasting plasma glucose measurements are high (eg, 128 and 132 mg/dL [7.1 and 7.3 mmol/L]), regardless of the hemoglobin A_{1c} value. Finally, a high glucose value (eg, 129 mg/dL [7.2 mmol/L]) and high hemoglobin A_{1c} value (eg, 6.6% [49 mmol/mol]) would also be confirmatory.

This patient has type 2 diabetes (Answer D) based on 2 separate hemoglobin A_{1c} measurements that are greater than 6.5% (>48 mmol/mol). Although his impaired fasting glucose value (119 mg/dL [6.6 mmol/L]) is somewhat discordant with his hemoglobin A_{1c} levels, according to the American Diabetes Association guidelines, the diagnosis defaults to the confirmed tests. A normal fasting glucose level is less than 100 mg/dL (<5.6 mmol/L) (thus, Answer A is incorrect). Values between 100 and 125 mg/dL (5.6-6.9 mmol/L) define impaired fasting glucose, the correlate of impaired glucose tolerance by oral glucose tolerance testing (2-hour plasma glucose of 140-199 mg/dL [7.8-11.0 mmol/L]). Both impaired fasting glucose (Answer C) and impaired glucose tolerance (Answer B) are frequently referred to as prediabetes, underscoring their ability to identify a person at significantly increased risk of worsening hyperglycemia over time to the point of developing type 2 diabetes. This transition is typically characterized by progressive β-cell dysfunction. This patient has already progressed to type 2 diabetes.

EDUCATIONAL OBJECTIVE
Define and diagnose type 2 diabetes mellitus on the basis of American Diabetes Association criteria.

REFERENCE(S)
International Expert Committee. International Expert Committee report on the role of the A1C assay in the diagnosis of diabetes. *Diabetes Care.* 2009;32(7):1327-1334. PMID: 19502545

American Diabetes Association. 2. Classification and diagnosis of diabetes: standards of medical care in diabetes-2021. *Diabetes Care.* 2021;44(Suppl 1):S15-S33. PMID: 33298413

41 **ANSWER: C) Reduce basal insulin to 20 units, stop the mealtime insulin, and start linagliptin**

Patients with suboptimally controlled type 2 diabetes may be prescribed multiple daily insulin injections. It is increasingly recognized that this can impose a self-care burden, particularly among older patients. Measuring blood glucose and injecting insulin multiple times daily and, where appropriate, problem solving to adjust insulin doses and/or take correction doses requires complex self-care decision-making skills. The use of rapid- or short-acting insulin also increases hypoglycemia risk, which is of concern in older patients, such as the one presented in this vignette.

Hypoglycemia in elderly patients with diabetes increases the risk of cardiovascular and cerebrovascular events, progression of dementia, injurious falls, emergency department visits, and hospitalization. Hypoglycemic episodes are often difficult to diagnose in this population and are easily missed by intermittent fingerstick blood glucose measurements, as has been shown using continuous glucose monitoring. Munshi et al used continuous glucose monitoring to evaluate hypoglycemia in older patients with type 2 diabetes who had a hemoglobin A_{1c} level greater than 8.0% (>64 mmol/mol). Community-living older patients seen at a diabetes center with a hemoglobin A_{1c} level greater than 8.0% were evaluated with blinded continuous glucose monitoring for a 3-day period while they continued their usual daily activities. Patients checked their blood glucose concentration 4 times daily while wearing the continuous glucose monitor and recorded symptoms suggestive of hypoglycemia. Forty adults aged 75 ± 5 years were evaluated. The mean hemoglobin A_{1c} value was 9.3% ± 1.3%. Most patients (58%) were taking insulin alone. Twenty-six of 40 patients (65%) had at least 1 episode of hypoglycemia (median glucose value of 63 mg/dL (3.5 mmol/L) (range, 42-69 mg/dL [2.3-3.8 mmol/L]) over the 3-day period. Among those with a hemoglobin A_{1c} value between 8.0% and 9.0% (64 to 75 mmol/mol) and greater than 9.0% (>75 mmol/mol), the hypoglycemia rate was 54% and 46%, respectively.

In addition, large studies have shown lack of benefit and higher risk of morbidity and mortality with tight glycemic control. The American Diabetes Association recommends relaxing glycemic control for vulnerable patients, with a goal of less than 7.5% (<58 mmol/mol) in otherwise healthy older adults with few coexisting chronic conditions and intact cognitive and functional status. Among those with multiple coexisting conditions, cognitive impairment or functional dependence goals that are less stringent (eg, <8.0% [<64 mmol/mol] or <8.5% [<69 mmol/mol]), would be considered appropriate.

This patient's basal insulin dose should clearly be reduced, as she becomes hypoglycemic when lunch is late. Her erratic morning blood glucose values suggest that she is also having nocturnal hypoglycemia. Her multiple daily insulin injection regimen requires problem solving, as she must determine when and how to take correction insulin doses. Her C-peptide level indicates that she is still making insulin. She is taking fewer than 10 units of rapid-acting analogue before meals, so it is reasonable to discontinue her mealtime insulin and to add an oral agent that does not independently cause hypoglycemia, such as linagliptin, per national guidelines (Answer C).

Referring her to a diabetes educator (Answer A) is a reasonable adjunctive measure, but it will not lower her risk for hypoglycemia without a concurrent adjustment in her antihyperglycemic medication regimen. Reducing her insulin doses and continuing the multiple daily injection regimen (Answer B) may reduce the frequency of hypoglycemia, but this would still require her to do problem solving, which seems to be challenging for her. Finally, stopping both of her insulins is likely to result in hyperglycemia, as her total daily dose is currently 52 units. The Simplify regimen recommends reducing insulin doses sequentially and replacing mealtime insulin first with an oral agent. Repaglinide with meals (Answer D) might be a reasonable oral agent for this patient, as we

know she is still able to secrete C-peptide; however, it would still require her to take it 3 times daily, so a once-daily agent such as a DPP-4 inhibitor makes more sense for her now.

EDUCATIONAL OBJECTIVE
Simplify the antihyperglycemic regimen in older adults with type 2 diabetes mellitus to prevent hypoglycemia.

REFERENCE(S)
Kirkman MS, Briscoe VJ, Clark N, et al. Diabetes in older adults. *Diabetes Care*. 2012;35(12):2650-2664. PMID: 23100048

Munshi MN, Slyne C, Segal AR, Saul N, Lyons C, Weinger K. Simplification of insulin regimen in older adults and risk of hypoglycemia. *JAMA Intern Med*. 2016;176(7):1023-1025. PMID: 27273335

LeRoith D, Biessels GJ, Braithwaite SS, et al. Treatment of diabetes in older adults: an Endocrine Society clinical practice guideline. *J Clin Endocrinol Metab*. 2019;104(5):1520-1574. PMID: 30903688

42 **ANSWER: E) Refer to a nutritionist**
The American College of Cardiology/American Heart Association and the National Lipid Association blood cholesterol guidelines recommend statin treatment for individuals with diabetes aged 40 to 75 years with LDL-cholesterol levels between 70 and 189 mg/dL (1.81-4.90 mmol/L) who do not have clinical atherosclerotic cardiovascular disease. Thus, starting atorvastatin (Answer B) is incorrect in this case because the patient is 32 years old. The exception is if the patient has had type 1 diabetes for at least 20 years and has complications such as nephropathy (albuminuria, stage 3 chronic kidney disease). Without clinical albuminuria, adding an ACE inhibitor (Answer C) would not be expected to result in a cardiovascular disease benefit in a normotensive, normoalbuminuric patient with type 1 diabetes. For patients with a triglyceride level less than 500 mg/dL (<5.65 mmol/L), treatment with a fibrate (Answer D) or omega-3 fatty acids (Answer A) is not indicated. In addition, in the ASCEND trial, among patients with diabetes

without evidence of cardiovascular disease, there was no significant difference in the risk of serious vascular events between those who were assigned to receive omega-3 fatty acid supplementation and those who were assigned to receive placebo.

Her BMI is elevated and her lipids are abnormal, suggesting a poor diet. She would greatly benefit from seeing a nutritionist (Answer E).

EDUCATIONAL OBJECTIVE

Determine when statin use is appropriate as part of cardiovascular risk reduction in patients with type 1 diabetes mellitus.

REFERENCE(S)

American Diabetes Association. 10. Cardiovascular disease and risk management: standards of medical care in diabetes-2021. *Diabetes Care*. 2021;44(Suppl 1):S125-S150. PMID: 33298421

Jacobson TA, Ito MK, Maki KC, et al. National Lipid Association recommendations for patient-centered management of dyslipidemia: part 1 - executive summary. *J Clin Lipidol*. 2014;8(5):473-488. PMID: 25234560

Nathan DM, Cleary PA, Backlund JY, et al; Diabetes Control and Complications Trial/Epidemiology of Diabetes Interventions and Complications (DCCT/EDIC) Study Research Group. Intensive diabetes treatment and cardiovascular disease in patients with type 1 diabetes. *N Engl J Med*. 2005;353(25):2643-2653. PMID: 16371630

43 ANSWER: A) 2-Hour oral glucose tolerance test

A 2-hour oral glucose tolerance test (Answer A) (with measurement of fasting and 2-hour glucose) is recommended for all women with polycystic ovary syndrome at initial diagnosis. If this is not feasible, fasting glucose should be measured together with hemoglobin A_{1c}. This approach is consistent with a number of professional organizations' guidelines (eg, the American College of Obstetricians and Gynecologists, American Association of Clinical Endocrinologists, the Endocrine Society, the Androgen Excess Society) and with a consensus panel representing the European Society of Human Reproduction and Embryology and the American Society of Reproductive Medicine.

The rationale for an oral glucose tolerance test is that a standard fasting glucose measurement (Answer D) lacks the sensitivity to detect impaired glucose tolerance or early type 2 diabetes that could be identified by an oral glucose tolerance test in a substantial number of women with polycystic ovary syndrome.

Limited studies have shown poor sensitivity of hemoglobin A_{1c} measurement (Answer C) for detecting impaired glucose tolerance.

In a retrospective observational study at an academic tertiary-care medical center, 208 premenopausal women with polycystic ovary syndrome underwent clinical evaluation (Ferriman-Gallwey score, BMI, waist circumference, blood pressure); hormone analyses (testosterone, SHBG, fasting lipids, insulin, glucose, hemoglobin A_{1c}); transvaginal ultrasonography; and 2-hour oral glucose tolerance tests measuring capillary blood glucose at 0 minutes and 120 minutes, insulin, and C-peptide. The main outcome measures were the results of the oral glucose tolerance test and hemoglobin A_{1c} values. Type 2 diabetes was diagnosed in 20 patients based on results of oral glucose tolerance testing. The sensitivity and specificity of a hemoglobin A_{1c} value of 6.5% or greater ($\geq$48 mmol/mol) for the diagnosis of diabetes were 35% and 99%, respectively, compared with the diagnosis established by oral glucose tolerance testing.

Patients with polycystic ovary syndrome and normal glucose tolerance should be rescreened at least once every 2 years or more frequently if additional risk factors are identified. Patients with impaired glucose tolerance should be screened annually for development of type 2 diabetes.

No tests of insulin resistance are necessary to diagnose polycystic ovary syndrome, nor are they needed to select treatments. There is currently no validated test for measuring insulin resistance in a clinical setting, including insulin levels (Answer B) or HOMA-IR (Answer E).

EDUCATIONAL OBJECTIVE

Guide the screening for prediabetes and type 2 diabetes in women with polycystic ovary syndrome.

REFERENCE(S)

American Diabetes Association. 2. Classification and diagnosis of diabetes: standards of medical care in diabetes-2021. *Diabetes Care.* 2021;44(Suppl 1):S15-S33. PMID: 33298413

Legro RS, Arslanian SA, Ehrmann DA, et al; Endocrine Society. Diagnosis and treatment of polycystic ovary syndrome: an Endocrine Society clinical practice guideline. *J Clin Endocrinol Metab.* 2013;98(12):4565-4592. PMID: 24151290

Velling Magnussen L, Mumm H, Andersen M, Glintborg D. Hemoglobin A1c as a tool for the diagnosis of type 2 diabetes in 208 premenopausal women with polycystic ovary syndrome. *Fertil Steril.* 2011;96(5):1275-1280. PMID: 21982282

Salley KES, Wickham EP, Cheang KI, Essah PA, Karjane NW, Nestler JE. Glucose intolerance in polycystic ovary syndrome--a position statement of the Androgen Excess Society. *J Clin Endocrinol Metab.* 2007;92(12):4546-4556. PMID: 18056778

44 ANSWER: A) Advise him to take his insulin bolus 10 to 15 minutes before meals

The time to onset of action of rapid-acting insulin lispro is 10 to 15 minutes. This patient is taking the dose with his meal, which does not allow enough time for it to be physiologically active to prevent the clear postprandial hyperglycemia peaks, as shown in the continuous glucose monitoring report. Moving the timing of insulin lispro administration to before the meal with a sufficient window to allow onset of its action (Answer A) would be expected to attenuate the postmeal glucose peaks.

This patient is already on a low-carbohydrate meal plan, so further restricting his carbohydrates with meals (Answer B) would not be expected to have a significant impact on his postmeal glucose excursions, nor would it be advisable from a nutrition standpoint.

In the absence of food and exercise, basal insulin should hold the blood glucose level steady. His premeal glucose values are within target range, which demonstrates that the basal insulin dose during this 12-hour window is appropriate. Therefore, performing a basal rate test (Answer C) is incorrect. Basal insulin rate testing can be conducted to help determine the appropriateness of basal dosing in cases where it is not clear if they are optimal. It is set up around the usual framework of mealtimes and sleep patterns and is initiated after the action of the most recently taken meal insulin bolus has dissipated for the period to be tested. If blood glucose drops during the test period, the basal rate is too high, and if it goes up, the basal rate may be too low. The basal rate can then be adjusted to move the glucose to the target value.

As automated closed-loop insulin pump and sensor systems are increasingly being used, the need for patients to conduct basal insulin testing will eventually be superseded by automated technology.

Finally, adjusting his insulin-to-carbohydrate ratio from 1:20 to 1:6 (Answer D) would lead to more than doubling his meal boluses, which would predispose him to hypoglycemia. A more modest adjustment in his insulin-to-carbohydrate ratio (eg, to 1:15) would also be expected to improve his postprandial blood glucose levels.

EDUCATIONAL OBJECTIVE

Manage insulin based on blood glucose patterns.

REFERENCE(S)

Walsh J, Roberts R. *Pumping Insulin.* 6th edition. Torrey Pines Press; 2017.

Gary Scheiner. Getting Down to Basals. Diabetes Self-Management. 2006. Available at: https://www.diabetesselfmanagement.com/managing-diabetes/treatment-approaches/getting-down-to-basals/ Accessed for verification May 2019.

45 ANSWER: A) Temporarily relax his tight glucose targets

Up to 30% of patients with type 1 or longstanding type 2 diabetes mellitus have impaired or absent awareness of hypoglycemia. As plasma glucose levels fall, compromised physiologic counterregulatory defenses include failure of an increase in glucagon secretion and attenuated epinephrine secretion. This, together with inability to reduce circulating insulin levels, results in the clinical syndrome of defective counterregulation, which markedly increases the risk of recurrent severe hypoglycemia. Hypoglycemia-attenuating defense against subsequent hypoglycemia is a concept referred to as hypoglycemia-associated autonomic failure (HAAF). The mainstay therapy for HAAF is the scrupulous avoidance of hypoglycemia. Patients with hypoglycemia unawareness and/or severe hypoglycemia and tight control should be advised to relax their glucose targets for a period to allow awareness to potentially return with adrenergic symptoms (Answer A).

While clearly a patient should be advised to carry with them a source of readily absorbed glucose, if he only has neuroglycopenic symptoms, there would be nothing triggering him to use them, so it would be unlikely to prevent his hypoglycemia. Also, carrying a glucagon emergency kit (Answer B) would not help either as this is used by another person, not the patient, and a companion should be aware of the presence of the kit, as well as how to use it. Although an insulin pump (Answer C) may help reduce hypoglycemia, it would not address the underlying cause of the hypoglycemia unawareness (repetitive hypoglycemic episodes) or guarantee its avoidance. There would also be a delay in initiating pump therapy and a learning curve regarding its use. Even a pump with an automatic suspend function is only as good as its integrated continuous glucose sensor, which can be inaccurate. A patient using this type of pump must be reminded that he still must actively treat the hypoglycemia to prevent it from worsening. While a number of educational programs focusing on hypoglycemia detection and avoidance (Answer D) (Dose Adjustment for Normal Eating [DAFNE], Blood Glucose Awareness Training [BGAT], Hypoglycemia Awareness and Avoidance [HAAT]) have demonstrated effectiveness in reducing the occurrence of hypoglycemia, such an education program is not the most immediate fix for the patient, nor would it address the cause. Lastly, as noted above, while raising the continuous glucose monitoring alert to a higher glucose value (Answer E) may assist with early recognition, continuous glucose monitoring can be inaccurate, particularly in the lower and higher glucose ranges. Raising the threshold is an adjunctive measure to loosening glycemic targets in this case. Moreover, there is some concern for "alarm fatigue" with continuous glucose monitor use, and raising the low glucose threshold may generate more alarms without perceived benefit to the patient, causing him to pay less attention to them.

EDUCATIONAL OBJECTIVE

Recommend management for severe hypoglycemia and hypoglycemia unawareness in type 1 diabetes mellitus.

REFERENCE(S)

Little SA, Leelarathna L, Barendse SM, et al. Severe hypoglycaemia in type 1 diabetes mellitus: underlying drivers and potential strategies for successful prevention. *Diabetes Metab Res Rev.* 2014;30(3):175-190. PMID: 24185859

Awoniyi O, Rehman R, Dagogo-Jack S. Hypoglycemia in patients with type 1 diabetes: epidemiology, pathogenesis, and prevention. *Curr Diab Rep.* 2013;13(5):669-678. PMID: 23912765

Oyer DS. The science of hypoglycemia in patients with diabetes. *Curr Diabetes Rev.* 2013;9(3):195-208. PMID: 23506375

Cryer PE. Mechanisms of hypoglycemia-associated autonomic failure in diabetes. *N Engl J Med.* 2013;69(4):362-372. PMID: 23883381

Rodbard D. Continuous glucose monitoring: a review of successes, challenges, and opportunities. *Diabetes Technol Ther.* 2016;18(Suppl 2):S3-S13. PMID: 26784127

46 **ANSWER: C) Rationing his insulin**
Euglycemic diabetic ketoacidosis (DKA) is diagnosed when a patient presents with acidosis and ketosis but has a glucose concentration of 250 mg/dL or less (≤13.9 mmol/L). This condition has become an emerging concern. Causes of euglycemic DKA include recent insulin administration, decreased caloric intake, substantial

alcohol consumption, chronic liver disease, or rarely, glycogen storage issues. In addition, SGLT-2 inhibitors such as canagliflozin (Answer B) can cause euglycemic DKA, although they are not likely to be prescribed to a patient with well-controlled type 1 diabetes. Given his recent change in housing and prior good glycemic control, it is most likely that his social situation has led him to have difficulty affording his insulin. This patient may be rationing his insulin (Answer C). While alcohol intoxication (Answer D) is also an important consideration, typically in this setting the glucose level is even lower due to suppression of gluconeogenesis. With lack of hypotension, adrenal insufficiency (Answer A) is less likely.

Insulin is lifesaving for persons with diabetes and is included on the Model List of Essential Medicines formulated by the World Health Organization. This means it should be available at all times at a price the individual and the community can afford. However, over the past decade, out-of-pocket costs per prescription have doubled. The price of insulin tripled between 2002 and 2013, and since 2008, 3 of the makers have raised the list price of insulin at least 10 times. High costs of medications can contribute to nonadherence, but the prevalence of cost-related insulin underuse is unknown. These issues may apply to any insulin-requiring patient with diabetes who does not have insurance and/or anyone who is underinsured. It is extremely important to discuss access to and affordability of insulin with individuals with diabetes, particularly those with type 1, who are prescribed insulin. Some insulins are less expensive than others for use as basal and bolus choices. These include U100 human regular insulin, U100 human NPH insulin, and premixed 70/30 insulin (NPH/regular). The vial and syringe option is less expensive than prefilled pens.

EDUCATIONAL OBJECTIVE
Recall precipitating factors for euglycemic diabetic ketoacidosis.

REFERENCE(S)
Herkert D, Vijayakumar P, Luo J, et al. Cost-related insulin underuse among patients with diabetes. *JAMA Intern Med.* 2019;179(1):112-114. PMID: 30508012

Rosenthal E. When high prices mean needless death. *JAMA Intern Med.* 2019;179(1):114-115. PMID: 30508014

Fralick M, Schneeweiss S, Patorno E. Risk of diabetic ketoacidosis after initiation of an SGLT2 inhibitor. *N Engl J Med.* 2017;376(23):2300-2302. PMID: 28591538

47 ANSWER: B) Consult with psychiatrist to change olanzapine to aripiprazole

The key features in this case are rapid weight gain and development of hypertriglyceridemia since initiation of olanzapine therapy. Atypical antipsychotic agents, such as olanzapine, are now frequently used to treat thought disorders because of a lower risk of extrapyramidal adverse effects than with traditional antipsychotic drugs. However, several compounds in this drug class have metabolic consequences, including weight gain, hyperlipidemia, insulin resistance, and impaired glucose metabolism. The drugs most frequently implicated are clozapine and olanzapine (thus, switching to clozapine [Answer A] would not make sense). Risperidone and quetiapine have intermediate effects, and aripiprazole (Answer B), ziprasidone, and amisulpride have little or no association with metabolic abnormalities. Although definitive epidemiologic data are not available, up to 30% to 40% of patients treated with clozapine and olanzapine are reported to develop weight gain and associated metabolic disorders. In this patient, the temporal association of olanzapine initiation and the onset of weight gain with subsequent hypertension and hypertriglyceridemia suggests that use of this medication is the proximate cause of his problems. Given that there are other antipsychotic drugs that have lesser metabolic effects, it is important to communicate with the physician treating the schizophrenia, discuss the likely role of olanzapine in this case, and explore alternative treatments.

Cushing syndrome is in the differential diagnosis of rapid weight gain and can be associated with hypertension and disordered lipid and glucose metabolism. However, this patient does not have cushingoid features on examination, making a biochemical workup unnecessary.

Although his triglyceride level is high, it is not in the range that causes concern for spontaneous pancreatitis (>1000 mg/dL [>11.30 mmol/L]). There is no urgency to lower his triglycerides with a fibrate (Answer C) as a means of primary prevention of coronary artery disease.

Although metformin (Answer D) effectively prevents the progression to diabetes in persons with prediabetes, a more direct solution to his impaired fasting glucose level is changing his psychotropic medication.

The combination of phentermine/topiramate (Answer E) has been approved to treat obesity. This medication has been reported to induce 5% to 10% weight loss, and this would most likely improve both the lipid disorder and impaired fasting glucose. However, the 2 components of this agent are centrally acting drugs and it has not been formally studied in persons with psychiatric disease. Trying to reduce body weight by other means is more prudent.

EDUCATIONAL OBJECTIVE
Manage the metabolic complications of atypical antipsychotic medications.

REFERENCE(S)

Newcomer JW. Metabolic considerations in the use of antipsychotic medications: a review of recent evidence. *J Clin Psychiatry*. 2007;68(Suppl 1):20-27. PMID: 17286524

48   ANSWER: B) U200 basal insulin degludec once daily plus mealtime insulin

The new ultralong-acting basal insulins (U100 degludec, U200 degludec, and U300 glargine) have a longer duration of action than the long-acting insulins U100 detemir and U100 glargine. An ultralong-acting basal insulin, such as U200 degludec (Answer B), which has a duration of action of up to 42 hours, would offer this patient increased dosing flexibility and reduce the likelihood of developing diabetic ketoacidosis when he misses an insulin dose. Importantly, it would be necessary to obtain preauthorization from his Medicaid plan to provide him with this new insulin analogue.

While a recently released hybrid closed-loop continuous subcutaneous insulin infusion pump with a sensor system (Answer A) would be ideal for this patient in terms of autoregulation of his insulin dosing, there are several major hurdles to this possibility from a practical perspective. These obstacles include the fact that he is homeless (access to supplies issues), he has severe mental illness that would most likely interfere with his ability to use such a pump when an exacerbation occurs, and preauthorization for payment would likely be a challenge to obtain.

A tubeless insulin pump (Answer C) might also be considered as an option for this patient. However, insulin pump therapy requires substantial patient engagement and organization to ensure timely pump changes every 2 to 3 days in order to avoid ketoacidosis. This would likely introduce a new challenge for this patient rather than improve his current situation.

U500 regular human insulin (Answer D) has delayed onset and longer duration of action than U100 regular human insulin as it has both basal and prandial properties. It may be given 2 or 3 times daily, which would be convenient for this patient; however, its niche is for patients with insulin resistance who require high total daily doses of insulin (typically in excess of 200 units daily), which is not the case in this young man with type 1 diabetes.

EDUCATIONAL OBJECTIVE
Appropriately prescribe the new ultralong-acting insulin analogues.

REFERENCE(S)

American Diabetes Association. 9. Pharmacologic approaches to glycemic treatment: standards of medical care in diabetes-2021. *Diabetes Care*. 2021;44(Suppl 1):S111-S124. PMID: 33298420

Riddle MC, Bolli GB, Home PD, et al. Efficacy and safety of flexible versus fixed dosing intervals of insulin glargine 300 U/mL in people with type 2 diabetes. *Diabetes Technol Ther.* 2016;18(4):252-257. PMID: 26840338

Meneghini L, Atkin SL, Gough SCL, et al; NN1250-3668 (BEGIN FLEX) Trial Investigators. The efficacy and safety of insulin degludec given in variable once-daily dosing intervals compared with insulin glargine and insulin degludec dosed at the same time daily: a 26-week, randomized, open-label, parallel-group, treat-to-target trial in individuals with type 2 diabetes. *Diabetes Care.* 2013;36(4):858-864. PMID: 23340894

REFERENCE(S)

Vermeersch P, Geboes K, Marien G, Hoffman I, Hiele M, Bossuyt X. Serological diagnosis of celiac disease: comparative analysis of different strategies. *Clin Chim Acta.* 2012;413(21-22):1761-1767. PMID: 22771970

Barker JM. Clinical review: type 1 diabetes-associated autoimmunity: natural history, genetic associations, and screening. *J Clin Endocrinol Metab.* 2006;91(4):1210-1217. PMID: 16403820

Acerini CL, Ahmed ML, Ross KM, Sullivan PB, Bird G, Dunger DB. Coeliac disease in children and adolescents with IDDM: clinical characteristics and response to gluten-free diet. *Diabetic Med.* 1998;15(1):38-44. PMID: 9472862

49 ANSWER: B) Measurement of tissue transglutaminase antibodies

The incidence of celiac disease in individuals with type 1 diabetes mellitus is 5% to 7%. Affected patients may report typical symptoms of celiac sprue (bloating, diarrhea, abdominal pain, weight loss) or be relatively asymptomatic. Sometimes a chronic inflammatory rash (dermatitis herpetiformis) develops suddenly, lasts for weeks to months, and may also be associated with other gastrointestinal diseases. The best initial test is measurement of tissue transglutaminase antibodies (Answer B).

Colonoscopy (Answer A) would not be diagnostic. An upper gastrointestinal series with small-bowel follow-through (Answer D) would probably show nonspecific small-bowel findings but would also not be diagnostic. TPO antibody measurement (Answer C) is irrelevant to this case. A skin biopsy (Answer E) should diagnose the rash as dermatitis herpetiformis, but it would not identify the specific associated gastrointestinal condition—in this case, celiac disease.

EDUCATIONAL OBJECTIVE

Recognize the signs and symptoms of celiac disease and initiate appropriate evaluation.

50 ANSWER: C) Empagliflozin

Cardiovascular disease and heart failure are major causes of morbidity and mortality in type 2 diabetes. Once congestive heart failure is present, mortality is increased 10-fold and 5-year survival is only 12.5%. Several diabetes drugs have been associated with an unexpected increase in heart failure risk during clinical trials and postmarketing surveillance, raising concerns about overall risks and benefits.

Recently completed cardiovascular outcome trials for type 2 diabetes drugs for patients with or at high risk of cardiovascular disease have provided new evidence that can be factored in when making choices about which antihyperglycemic agents to use. On the basis of proven cardiovascular and renal benefit, the antihyperglycemic drugs empagliflozin (Empa-Reg Outcomes study), liraglutide (LEADER study), and semaglutide (SUSTAIN study) may be preferentially used as second-line treatments in these patient populations, typically in addition to metformin (semaglutide is still under review by the US FDA). However, neither metformin (Answer A) nor the GLP-1 receptor agonist liraglutide (Answer E) has been shown to affect heart failure hospitalization.

Relevant specifically to heart failure risk, which is high in this patient, use of empagliflozin (Answer C) in the EMPA-Reg Outcomes study resulted in a hazard ratio for hospital admissions due to congestive heart failure of 0.64 (95% CI, 0.50-0.85; *P* = .002). Empagliflozin is therefore the best choice.

The US FDA has added a warning to the drug labels for saxagliptin (Answer B) and alogliptin regarding increased risk of heart failure, particularly in those who have heart disease or kidney disease. In the SAVOR-TIMI 53 trial, saxagliptin was associated with an unexpected 27% increase in heart failure hospital admissions, representing 3.5% of patients who received the drug. In the EXAMINE trial, 3.9% of alogliptin-treated patients were hospitalized for heart failure vs 3.3% in the placebo group.

Thiazolidinediones such as pioglitazone have long been associated with increased risk for heart failure, and insulin glargine (Answer D) in the ORIGIN study had a neutral effect on cardiovascular outcomes, including risk for hospitalizations for heart failure.

EDUCATIONAL OBJECTIVE
Select empagliflozin over other antihyperglycemic agents for patients at high risk for heart failure.

REFERENCE(S)

Standl E, Schnell O, McGuire DK, Ceriello A, Ryden L. Integration of recent evidence into management of patients with atherosclerotic cardiovascular disease and type 2 diabetes. *Lancet Diabetes Endocrinol.* 2017;5(5):391-402. PMID: 28131656

Zinman B, Wanner C, Lachin JM, et al; EMPA-REG OUTCOME Investigators. Empagliflozin, cardio-vascular outcomes, and mortality in type 2 diabetes. *N Engl J Med.* 2015;373(22):2117-2128. PMID: 26378978

McGuire DK, Van de Werf F, Armstrong PW, et al; Trial Evaluating Cardiovascular Outcomes With Sitagliptin (TECOS) Study Group. Association between sitagliptin use and heart failure hospital-ization and related outcomes in type 2 diabetes mellitus: secondary analysis of a randomized clinical trial. *JAMA Cardiol.* 2016;1(2):126-135. PMID: 27437883

Green JB, Bethel MA, Armstrong PW, et al; TECOS Study Group. Effect of sitagliptin on cardiovascu-lar outcomes in type 2 diabetes. *N Engl J Med.* 2015;373(3):232-242. PMID: 26052984

ORIGIN Trial Investigators; Gerstein HC, Bosch J, et al. Basal insulin and cardiovascular and other outcomes in dysglycemia. *N Engl J Med.* 2012;367(4):319-328. PMID: 22686416

51   ANSWER: D) Indeterminate

Given the increased risk of type 2 diabetes mellitus in women with a history of gestational diabetes, the American Diabetes Association guidelines recommend screening for undiagnosed type 2 diabetes at the time that pregnancy is established in patients such as this one. Screening is done using the established criteria for the diagnosis of diabetes in adults.

Hemoglobin A_{1c}, fasting plasma glucose, and the 75-g oral glucose tolerance test may all be used as screening tests for type 2 diabetes. The oral glucose tolerance test is the most sensitive modality. However, in this vignette, the patient's hemoglobin A_{1c} level is less than 6.5% (<48 mmol/mol)—the diagnostic threshold for diabetes—but her 2-hour plasma glucose value is greater than 200 mg/dL (>11.1 mmol/L) during the 75-g oral glucose tolerance test, which meets the criteria for type 2 diabetes. In the absence of unequivocal hyperglycemia, discordant results should be confirmed by repeated testing. Thus, the best assessment of this woman's current glycemic status is indeterminate (Answer D).

Establishing a diagnosis of type 2 diabetes that has not previously been recognized in the first trimester of pregnancy is important. If diabetes was preexisting, glycemic control before and during the pregnancy has implications for the health of both the mother and the baby. Management targeting glycemic control throughout the pregnancy is required for optimal outcomes.

If type 2 diabetes is not present, the oral glucose tolerance test should be repeated at 24 to 28 weeks' gestation to screen for gestational diabetes. This could consist of a 2-step process (50-g oral glucose tolerance test and then, depending on threshold criteria, the 100-g oral glucose tolerance test) or a 1-step process (75-g oral glucose tolerance test). The 1-step process has significantly increased the number of women identified with gestational diabetes because it requires only 1 abnormal value rather than 2. However, because this increased identification has not clearly translated into improved maternal or neonatal outcomes, the 2-step approach to diagnosing gestational diabetes is still supported by several organizations, including the American College of Obstetrics and Gynecology.

EDUCATIONAL OBJECTIVE
Recommend a screening protocol for early pregnancy in a patient with a history of gestational diabetes.

REFERENCE(S)
American Diabetes Association. 2. Classification and diagnosis of diabetes: standards of medical care in diabetes. *Diabetes Care.* 2021;44(Suppl 1):S15-S33. PMID: 33298413

ACOG practice bulletin No. 190: gestational diabetes mellitus. *Obstet Gynecol.* 2018;131(2):e49-e64. PMID: 29370047

52 ANSWER: C) Mononeuritis affecting the third cranial nerve

In oculomotor (third) nerve palsy, the involved eye is deviated "down and out" (ie, infraducted and abducted). Diabetic mononeuropathy (Answer C) is one of the less common forms of neuropathy. Patients with diabetes can develop diplopia from isolated oculomotor (third), trochlear (fourth), or abducens (sixth) nerve palsies. Ophthalmoplegia, despite being a rare entity in diabetes mellitus, is associated with anxiety for the patient and is a diagnosis that is made after other pathologies have been excluded. In a 10-year series of more than 6000 patients hospitalized with diabetes, 0.4% were diagnosed with ophthalmoplegia, among whom isolated third nerve palsies accounted for most (59.3%), with sixth nerve palsies and multiple palsies accounting for the remainder. The mean age in this series was 65 ± 10 years, mean duration of diabetes was 16 ± 10 years, and most patients had type 2 diabetes. Most had suboptimally controlled diabetes with a mean hemoglobin A_{1c} level of 8.8% ± 2.5%. Those with sixth nerve palsies had higher rates of coexistent diabetic retinopathy and cardiovascular disease risk factors.

Among all cases of ocular misalignment from cranial nerve palsies, third nerve palsies are important because a subset is caused by life-threatening aneurysms. In a recent series of 145 patients from the Rochester Epidemiology Project, the most common causes of acquired third nerve palsy were presumed microvascular (42%), trauma (12%), compression from neoplasm (11%), postneurosurgery (10%), and compression from aneurysm (6%).

No specific treatment of nerve palsy–induced diplopia in patients with diabetes has been established. Management is expectant and the patient should be reassured.

Unilateral endocrine ophthalmopathy (Answer A) with entrapment of ocular muscles can cause diplopia, but one would not expect its onset to be sudden, and other features such as proptosis, chemosis, and conjunctival injection are common accompaniments. In addition, a characteristic appearance of the extraocular muscles on CT (enlargement of the *extraocular muscle* bellies with sparing of their tendinous insertions [frequently: inferior rectus > medial rectus > superior rectus]) associated with endocrine ophthalmopathy was not seen in this patient. It is not typical for pituitary adenomas (Answer B) to cause isolated third nerve impingement. As these neoplasms grow, they are more likely to cause visual field defects due to pressure on the optic nerve, rather than impinging on the oculomotor nerves. This patient does not have loss of vision due to optic nerve compression, just isolated third cranial nerve oculomotor deficits. He also does not have a reversible ischemic neurologic deficit (Answer D) as an etiology for his oculomotor palsy by definition because the deficit is still persistent after several days. Macular edema (Answer E) would not be expected to cause diplopia.

EDUCATIONAL OBJECTIVE
Diagnose third cranial nerve palsy.

REFERENCE(S)
Fang C, Leavitt JA, Hodge DO, et al. Incidence and etiologies of acquired third nerve palsy using a population-based method. *JAMA Ophthalmol.* 2017;135(1):23-28. PMID: 27893002

Greco D, Gambina F, Maggio F. Ophthalmoplegia in diabetes mellitus: a retrospective study. *Acta Diabetol.* 2009;46(1):23-26. PMID: 18758685

53 ANSWER: B) Change the insulin bolus to extended for high-fat meals

Food contains 3 different fuels (carbohydrate, fat, and proteins) that affect glycemia through different mechanisms. The fat in certain foods such as ice cream may delay the absorption of carbohydrates from the gastrointestinal tract and reduce the expected rise in blood glucose, leading to early hypoglycemia from the insulin bolus. Certain high-fat meals such as pizza create rapid temporary insulin resistance (high free fatty acids from high-fat meals cause insulin resistance) for up to 6 to 12 hours after a meal, making blood glucose rise later after the insulin bolus effect is gone. Also, excess free fatty acids contribute to gluconeogenesis.

In addition, large quantities of protein, such as a 12-ounce steak, can cause a rise in blood glucose. Almost 50% of protein calories are slowly converted to glucose (amino acids contribute to gluconeogenesis) over a period of several hours (4-12 hours). Excessive amino acid availability can interfere with insulin action.

In this case of a high-fat meal, the only solution is to change the bolus to extended (Answer B) where the percentage of each component varies depending on the meal and the patient. It could start with 50%/50% split where the extended bolus is given over 2 hours. Then, depending on results, the percentage and duration of the extended bolus could be changed accordingly.

Changing his insulin-to-carbohydrate ratio to 1 unit per 12 g for high-fat meals (Answer A) is incorrect because less insulin would make the late hyperglycemia worse. Aspart-niacinamide (Answer D) is faster acting than aspart and would exacerbate the early hypoglycemia. Eating more carbohydrates (Answer C) would lead to more weight gain and his BMI is already higher than normal. Metoclopramide (Answer E) is used to treat gastroparesis, which the patient does not have.

EDUCATIONAL OBJECTIVE

Explain the benefit of extended insulin bolus with high-fat meals.

REFERENCE(S)

Lopez PE, Smart CE, McElduff P, et al. Optimizing the combination insulin bolus split for a high-fat, high-protein meal in children and adolescents using insulin pump therapy. *Diabet Med.* 2017;34(10):1380-1384. PMID: 28574182

van der Hoogt M, van Dyk JC, Doman RC, Pieters M. Protein and fat meal content increase insulin requirement in children with type 1 diabetes – role of duration of diabetes. *J Clin Transl Endocrinol.* 2017;10:15-21. PMID: 29204367

Bell KJ, Toschi E, Steil GM, Wolpert HA. Optimized mealtime insulin dosing for fat and protein in type 1 diabetes: application of a model-based approach to derive insulin doses for open-loop diabetes management. *Diabetes Care.* 2016;39(9):1631-1634. PMID: 27388474

54 ANSWER: D) Rapid-acting insulin

Cystic fibrosis–related diabetes (CFRD) is the result of a primary defect of insulin secretion due in part to nonautoimmune destruction of β cells (mainly) and also α cells in the pancreas, so both insulin and glucagon secretion are defective. However, histologic studies have reported variability in the degree of islet-cell destruction. This indicates there are other factors contributing to the insulin deficiency in CFRD, perhaps "collateral damage" from fibrosis and fatty infiltration or islet amyloid. The presence of CFRD strongly correlates with poorer clinical status, reflected by reduced pulmonary function and nutritional status, increased frequency of acute pulmonary exacerbations, and significant sputum pathogens. Annual screening for CFRD in all patients with cystic fibrosis is recommended beginning by 10 years of age, consistent with guidelines from the American Diabetes Association, Cystic Fibrosis Foundation, Pediatric Endocrine Society, and International Society for Pediatric and Adolescent Diabetes (ISPAD). The best test for screening and diagnosis of CFRD is the oral glucose tolerance test.

The recommended treatment of CFRD is insulin (Answer D), as this clearly has beneficial nutritional effects and probably improves pulmonary function and survival. Although hemoglobin A_{1c} is not recommended as a screening test for CFRD, it is helpful in monitoring treatment, and it should be measured every 3 months in patients on insulin therapy. For patients with CFRD, experts suggest trying to maintain hemoglobin A_{1c} as low as possible, ideally in the lower part of the normal range (eg, <5.5% [<37 mmol/mol]). This target is designed to optimize lung function and reduce pulmonary exacerbations.

Use of oral hypoglycemic agents (Answer B) to augment insulin production is largely unsuccessful. No data exist regarding treatment of CFRD with SGLT-2 inhibitors, GLP-1 receptor agonists (Answer C), or DPP-4 inhibitors. Metformin (Answer A) is not expected to work either, and it might not be safe because cystic fibrosis is affecting this patient's liver function. While referral to a nutritionist (Answer E) will be an important part of her treatment, with her degree of postmeal hyperglycemia in the setting of insulin deficiency, insulin therapy is the best next step.

EDUCATIONAL OBJECTIVE
Recommend the best treatment for cystic fibrosis–related diabetes mellitus.

REFERENCE(S)
Moran A, Pillay K, Becker DJ, Acerini CL; International Society for Pediatric and Adolescent Diabetes. ISPAD Clinical Practice Consensus Guidelines 2014. Management of cystic fibrosis-related diabetes in children and adolescents. *Pediatr Diabetes.* 2014;15(Suppl 20):65-76. PMID: 25182308

O'Shea D, O'Connell J. Cystic fibrosis related diabetes. *Curr Diab Rep.* 2014;14(8):511. PMID: 24915888

Kelly A, Moran A. Update on cystic fibrosis-related diabetes [published correction appears in *J Cyst Fibros.* 2014;13(1):119]. *J Cyst Fibros.* 2013;12(4): 318-331. PMID: 23562217

55 ANSWER: C) Dumping syndrome
Bariatric surgery is a useful treatment for patients with type 2 diabetes and morbid obesity. Observational studies and randomized controlled trials have shown that these procedures, including Roux-en-Y gastric bypass, sleeve gastrectomy, gastric banding, and biliopancreatic diversion, significantly improve glycemic control and favorably affect cardiovascular risk factors.

Hypoglycemia following gastric bypass surgery procedures may be complicated by early or late hypoglycemia, and it may occur in patients with or without diabetes. Hyperinsulinemic (or reactive) hypoglycemia, which is seen within an hour of eating (early dumping), is attributed to concentrated nutrients and carbohydrates rapidly entering the small bowel. This disorder is seen early in the postoperative course. It is controlled by dietary intervention and most likely represents a different pathophysiology than late post–gastric bypass hypoglycemia. This patient had surgery several months ago, so her episode is consistent with early dumping syndrome (Answer C).

Hypoglycemia (Answer E) is recognized as a late sequela of gastric bypass surgery and thus it would not be a likely explanation in this vignette given the timeframe. Affected patients present with hypoglycemia associated with neuroglycopenic symptoms (including confusion, syncope, and seizures). This disorder presents 2 to 4 years after surgery. The potential mechanisms are hypothesized to be nesidioblastosis that is most likely due to the trophic effects of gastric inhibitory polypeptide and GLP-1 on pancreatic islet cells, increased insulin sensitivity (Answer D), and/or increased islet functional activity, none of which is at play in dumping syndrome. Risk is not increased with vertical banded gastroplasty or gastric banding. The clinical syndrome is seen only in patients who have Roux-en-Y bypass procedures, and it occurs in 0.2% of patients. Treatment for late postbypass hypoglycemia involves a low-carbohydrate diet. Diazoxide, octreotide, or calcium-channel blockers may be required. If necessary, surgical treatment involves consideration of a restrictive bariatric procedure, with or without reconstitution of gastrointestinal continuity. Insulinoma (Answer A) is rare and atypically presents as primarily postprandial hypoglycemia. Noninsulinoma pancreatogenous hypoglycemia syndrome (Answer B) is very rare and is a diagnosis of exclusion after all other diagnoses are considered.

EDUCATIONAL OBJECTIVE
Distinguish between early and late development of hypoglycemia after gastric bypass surgery.

REFERENCE(S)

Cui Y, Elahi D, Anderson DK. Advances in the etiology and management of hyperinsulinemic hypoglycemia after Roux-en-Y gastric bypass. *J Gastrointest Surg.* 2011;15(10):1879-1888. PMID: 21671112

Marsk R, Jonas E, Rasmussen F, Naslund E. Nationwide cohort study of post-gastric bypass hypoglycaemia including 5,040 patients undergoing surgery in for obesity in 1986-2006 in Sweden. *Diabetologia.* 2010;53(11):2307-2311. PMID: 20495972

Schauer PR, Bhatt DL, Kirwan JP, et al; STAMPEDE Investigators. Bariatric surgery versus intensive medical therapy for diabetes--3-year outcomes. *N Engl J Med.* 2014;370(21):2002-2013. PMID: 24679060

Schauer PR, Bhatt DL, Kirwan JP, et al; STAMPEDE Investigators. Bariatric surgery versus intensive medical therapy for diabetes - 5-year outcomes. *N Engl J Med.* 2017;376(7):641-651. PMID: 28199805

De León DD, Stanley CA. Determination of insulin for the diagnosis of hyperinsulinemic hypoglycemia. *Best Pract Res Clin Endocrinol Metab.* 2013;27(6):763-769. PMID: 24275188

56 ANSWER: A) Sitagliptin

In general, in the hospital setting for noncritically ill patients, a basal-bolus insulin regimen correction dose when blood glucose is high is preferred for glycemic management for individuals with good nutritional intake. In contrast, a single dose of long-acting insulin plus correction insulin is preferred for patients with poor or no oral intake. When a patient with type 2 diabetes has mild to moderate hyperglycemia and is otherwise clinically stable, the addition of an oral agent to the regimen—to prepare for discharge—may be considered. The Sita-Hospital Study was conducted in 5 US hospitals among 18- to 80-year-old adults with type 2 diabetes who had random blood glucose concentrations ranging from 140 to 400 mg/dL (7.8-22.2 mmol/L). For inclusion, patients needed to be eating and taking less than 0.6 units/kg per day of insulin. They were randomly assigned to sitagliptin (Answer A) plus basal insulin (n = 138) or a basal-bolus insulin regimen (n = 139).

Glycemic control between the groups assessed as the mean percentage of blood glucose values ranging from 70 to 180 mg/dL (3.9-10 mmol/L) did not differ at 57% for the sitagliptin plus basal insulin group and 59.6% for the basal-bolus group ($P = .58$). A relatively small percentage from each group experienced treatment failure (16% vs 19%, $P = .54$), which was recognized 2 to 3 days following randomization. There was no severe hypoglycemia (blood glucose <40 mg/dL [<2.2 mmol/L]). The only significant difference between groups was in the total daily insulin dose requirement (units/kg), which was lower at 0.2 (±0.1) for patients receiving sitagliptin compared with 0.3 (±0.2) basal-bolus alone ($P < .0001$).

The researchers concluded that treatment with sitagliptin plus basal insulin is as effective and safe as (and a convenient alternative to) a labor-intensive basal-bolus insulin regimen for the management of hyperglycemia in patients with type 2 diabetes admitted to nonintensive care unit general medicine and surgery services.

Metformin (Answer B) in this patient is contraindicated because he has advanced heart failure. Pioglitazone (Answer C) could lead to fluid retention and exacerbation of congestive heart failure. Also, as its time to onset of action is in the range of 2 to 3 weeks, pioglitazone would not lead to short-term improvement in glycemic control during the current hospital stay. Use of an SGLT-2 inhibitor (Answer D) is associated with risk for ketoacidosis, urosepsis, urinary tract infections, and renal injury. Thus, SGLT-2 inhibitors cannot be recommended in the hospital setting, as their safety and effectiveness have not been established.

EDUCATIONAL OBJECTIVE

Manage type 2 diabetes mellitus in the hospital on general medicine and surgery units.

REFERENCE(S)

Lansang MC, Umpierrez GE. Inpatient hyperglycemia management: a practical review for primary medical and surgical teams. *Cleve Clin J Med.* 2016;83(Suppl 1):S34-S43. PMID: 27176681

Pasquel FJ, Gianchandani R, Rubin DJ, et al. Efficacy of sitagliptin for the hospital management of general medicine and surgery patients with type 2 diabetes (Sita-Hospital): a multicentre, prospective, open-label, non-inferiority randomised trial. *Lancet Diabetes Endocrinol.* 2017;5(2):125-133. PMID: 27964837

Female Reproduction Board Review

Kathryn A. Martin, MD

1 ANSWER: C) Luteomas of pregnancy

This patient has gestational hyperandrogenism, with bilateral solid ovarian masses, which makes luteomas of pregnancy (Answer C) the most likely diagnosis. Luteomas are unilateral or bilateral nonneoplastic ovarian masses associated with pregnancy that regress in the post partum period. Serum androgens rise during normal pregnancy (serum total testosterone increases up to about 120 ng/dL), but it is uncommon for women to experience worsening or new hyperandrogenic symptoms and very rare for them to become virilized. This is because they are protected by both the pregnancy-associated rise in SHBG and by placental aromatase, the enzyme that converts androgen precursors to estrogens. Luteomas are usually asymptomatic. However, in approximately 30% to 35% of cases, affected women have extremely high androgen concentrations and present with virilizing signs. However, serum androgen concentrations are not a reliable predictor of virilization. If the mother becomes virilized, there is an 80% chance that a female fetus will also be virilized. If the mother is not virilized, then the fetus will not virilize. Fetal virilization was not observed in this case.

Theca lutein cysts (Answer A) are benign cysts without solid components, which distinguishes them from luteomas or malignancy. Ovaries that contain theca lutein cysts can cause pressure symptoms, as they can be as large as 10 to 15 cm. Approximately 30% of pregnant women with theca lutein cysts develop hirsutism or become virilized; however, female fetuses do not virilize. Women with polycystic ovary syndrome (Answer B) may experience higher serum androgens than women without polycystic ovary syndrome during pregnancy, but they do not experience levels high enough to cause virilization. Dietary supplements (Answer D) would not cause this clinical picture unless they contained significant doses of androgens. Nonclassic congenital adrenal hyperplasia (Answer E) has not been associated with gestational hyperandrogenism.

EDUCATIONAL OBJECTIVE

Determine the most likely cause of virilization in a pregnant woman.

REFERENCE(S)

Wang YC, Su HY, Liu JY, Chang FW, Chen CH. Maternal and female fetal virilization caused by pregnancy luteomas. *Fertil Steril.* 2005;84(2):509. PMID: 16086574

Wadzinski TL, Altowaireb Y, Gupta R, Conroy R, Shoukri K. Luteoma of pregnancy associated with nearly complete virilization of genetically female twins. *Endocr Pract.* 2014;20(2):e18-e23. PMID: 24126228

Kuijper EA, Ket JC, Caanen MR, Lambalk CB. Reproductive hormone concentrations in pregnancy and neonates: a systematic review. *Reprod Biomed Online.* 2013;27(1):33-63. PMID: 23669015

2 ANSWER: B) Anxiety and depression

Sleep disturbances are common in perimenopausal and postmenopausal women. A bothersome feature of hot flashes is that they are more common at night than during the day and are typically associated with arousal from sleep. However, some women experience insomnia even in the absence of hot flashes. Anxiety and depression symptoms (Answer B) also contribute to sleep disturbances, particularly during perimenopause, when there is a high rate of new-onset or recurrent mood disorders. Primary sleep disorders such as restless legs syndrome (Answer C) are also common in this population. Normal aging (Answer A) is associated with sleep disturbances, but this patient has symptoms that are suggestive of anxiety and depression (difficulty falling asleep and midcycle awakening). Progestin therapy (Answer D), such as micronized progesterone, is more typically associated with drowsiness, not insomnia. Metformin therapy (Answer E) is not associated with nocturnal hypoglycemia, and it is not a very effective drug for weight loss. Thus, in perimenopausal or postmenopausal women who report sleep disturbances, treating the vasomotor symptoms may decrease arousals from sleep, but this may not resolve all sleep problems, as there are many other things that can cause insomnia, such as primary sleep disorders, anxiety, and depression.

EDUCATIONAL OBJECTIVE
Construct a differential diagnosis for sleep disturbances in menopausal women.

REFERENCE(S)
Caretto M, Giannini A, Simoncini T. An integrated approach to diagnosing and managing sleep disorders in menopausal women. *Maturitas.* 2019;128:1-3. PMID: 31561815

Bonanni E, Schirru A, Di Perri MC, Bonuccelli U, Maestri M. Insomnia and hot flashes. *Maturitas.* 2019;126:51-54. PMID: 31239118

3 **ANSWER: A) Absent uterus**
This patient has uterine agenesis; terms for this disorder include mullerian agenesis, vaginal agenesis, and Mayer-Rokitansky-Kuster-Hauser syndrome [MKRH]). On pelvic ultrasonography, no uterus is visualized (Answer A). She had normal adrenarche and pubertal development but presented with primary amenorrhea. Her endocrine profile and external genitalia are normal, as one would expect. On examination, she would have a blind vaginal pouch and no palpable uterus, but ovaries would be present. Mullerian agenesis is the second most common cause of primary amenorrhea after gonadal dysgenesis.

Streak ovaries on ultrasonography (Answer B) would be seen with Turner syndrome or other types of gonadal dysgenesis, which this patient does not have given her normal secondary sex characteristics and normal serum FSH level. She has no risk factors for intrauterine adhesions (Answer C), also known as Asherman syndrome, which is seen in the setting of uterine instrumentation/trauma. On ultrasonography, Asherman syndrome is characterized by absence of an endometrial stripe. Absent uterus and ovaries (Answer D) cannot be the answer, as she has ovarian function (she developed normal secondary sexual characteristics). Absence of uterus and ovaries would be seen in a patient with complete androgen insensitivity syndrome. Transverse vaginal septum (Answer E) is incorrect, as she would experience cyclic pelvic pain related to her menstrual cycles.

EDUCATIONAL OBJECTIVE
Differentiate mullerian agenesis from other structural causes of primary amenorrhea by a normal endocrine profile but absent uterus on examination and ultrasonography.

REFERENCE(S)
Herlin M, Bjørn AMB, Rasmussen M, Trolle B, Petersen MB. Prevalence and patient characteristics of Mayer-Rokitansky-Küster-Hauser syndrome: a nationwide registry-based study. *Hum Reprod.* 2016;31(10):2384-2390. PMID: 27609979

Fedele L, Bianchi S, Frontino G, Ciappina N, Fontana E, Borruto F. Laparoscopic findings and pelvic anatomy in Mayer-Rokitansky-Küster-Hauser syndrome. *Obstet Gynecol.* 2007;109(5):1111-1115. PMID: 17470591

Grimbizis GF, Gordts S, Di Spiezio Sardo A, et al. The ESHRE/ESGE consensus on the classification of female genital tract congenital anomalies. *Hum Reprod.* 2013;28(8):2032-2044. PMID: 23771171

4 **ANSWER: D) Unscheduled bleeding (breakthrough bleeding)**
Unscheduled bleeding (also referred to as breakthrough bleeding) (Answer D) is the most

common early adverse effect that women experience with combined estrogen-progestin oral contraceptives (COCs), and the most common reason for COC discontinuation. Unscheduled bleeding is more common with lower-dosage estrogen COCs (10 mcg, 20 mcg ethinyl estradiol) and with continuous administration of COCs. The bleeding typically decreases and resolves over subsequent months. If pills have not been missed, the patient can be reassured that unscheduled bleeding does not indicate a lack of contraceptive efficacy. The cause of the bleeding is progressive endometrial atrophy, as low-dosage COCs and continuous regimens are progestin-dominant regimens.

Although many women have concerns that COCs are associated with weight gain (Answer A), most evidence now suggests that the lower-dosage COCs currently used (20 to 35 mcg ethinyl estradiol) are weight neutral. Sexual dysfunction (decline in libido) (Answer B) is another common concern, given that COCs suppress ovarian androgen secretion. However, available evidence has not shown a consistent negative impact of COCs on sexual function. Data on the risk of developing depression (Answer C) on COCs are mixed; in a large observational study, the absolute rates of first antidepressant use on COCs was 2.2 per 100 woman-years in hormonal contraceptive users compared with 1.7 per 100 woman-years in nonusers (difference of 0.5 per 100 women-years). Although COCs may cause a small increase in systolic blood pressure in some women, they have not been associated with new-onset hypertension (Answer E).

EDUCATIONAL OBJECTIVE

Describe the early adverse effects of combined estrogen-progestin oral contraceptives.

REFERENCE(S)

Gallo MF, Nanda K, Grimes DA, Schulz KF. 20 mcg versus >20 mcg estrogen combined oral contraceptives for contraception. *Cochrane Database Syst Rev.* 2005;(2):CD003989. PMID: 15846690

Skovlund CW, Mørch LS, Kessing LV, Lidegaard Ø. Association of hormonal contraception with depression. *JAMA Psychiatry.* 2016;73(11):1154-1162. PMID: 27680324

Hickey M, Agarwal S. Unscheduled bleeding in combined oral contraceptive users: focus on extended-cycle and continuous-use regimens. *J Fam Plann Reprod Health Care.* 2009;35(4):245-248. PMID: 19849921

Hee L, Kettner LO, Vejtorp M. Continuous use of oral contraceptives: an overview of effects and side-effects. *Acta Obstet Gynecol Scand.* 2013;92(2):125-136. PMID: 23083413

Boozalis A, Tutlam NT, Chrisman Robbins C, Peipert JF. Sexual desire and hormonal contraception. *Obstet Gynecol.* 2016;127(3):563-572. PMID 26855094

5   ANSWER: C) Transdermal 17β-estradiol, 0.025 mg twice weekly, with micronized progesterone, 100 mg daily

Many women with migraines experience worsening of their symptoms during the menopausal transition. The wide fluctuations in serum estradiol concentrations are thought to be associated with more frequent episodes of estrogen-withdrawal migraines (estrogen-associated migraines). Therapies based on maintaining a more stable estrogen environment are associated with reduced migraine frequency, as well as relief of vasomotor symptoms, if present. Estrogen-associated migraines (without aura) are often treated with continuous low-dosage oral contraceptives (COCs) (Answer A) in younger premenopausal women, but after age 35 years, COCs are discouraged for women with migraines without aura and contraindicated in those with aura. However, physiologic dosages of estrogen (menopausal dosages) are a reasonable option, particularly if given transdermally, as these preparations have not been associated with an excess risk of stroke. Transdermal estradiol with daily micronized progesterone (Answer C) would be the treatment of choice in this patient. Of note, however, the continuous progestin administration may be associated with unscheduled bleeding until the patient is postmenopausal.

Low dosages of oral estradiol with cyclic progesterone (Answer B) would not be optimal because transdermal estrogens carry less vascular risk, and cyclic progesterone could worsen her migraines. A levonorgestrel-releasing intrauterine device (Answer D) would provide no relief for her headaches, as ovarian function with estrogen fluctuations would continue. Although bedtime doses of gabapentin (Answer E) are helpful for nocturnal hot flashes, a benefit for migraines has not been demonstrated.

EDUCATIONAL OBJECTIVE
Recommend the best management of estrogen-sensitive migraines during the menopausal transition.

REFERENCE(S)
MacGregor, AE. Migraine, menopause and hormone replacement therapy. *Post Reprod Health*. 2018;24(1):11-18. PMID: 28994639

Ibrahimi K, Couturier EG, MassenVanDenBrink A. Migraine and perimenopause. *Maturitas*. 2014;78(4):277-280. PMID: 24954701

Canonico M, Carcaillon L, Plu-Bureau G, et al. Postmenopausal hormone therapy and risk of stroke: impact of the route of estrogen administration and type of progestogen. *Stroke*. 2016;47(7):1734-1741. PMID: 27256671

6 ANSWER: C) Erythrocytosis
The most common adverse effect of testosterone therapy in transgender men is erythrocytosis (Answer C). Testosterone administration at pharmacologic levels in transgender men causes increased hematocrit and risk of polycythemia. This is a greater concern with parenteral testosterone administration, but it can be seen with testosterone gel as well. Therefore, the current Endocrine Society guideline on treatment of gender-dysphoric/gender-incongruent persons suggests that hematocrit or hemoglobin be measured at baseline and every 3 months for the first year, and then 1 to 2 times per year with a goal of maintaining the hematocrit at less than 50%.

Prostate cancer (Answer B) is not a concern in this population, as there is no prostate tissue. The risk of venous thromboembolism (Answer A) has been a greater concern in transgender women receiving pharmacologic dosages of oral estrogen. Data on the impact of testosterone therapy on insulin resistance in transgender men are conflicting, and there is no evidence to date that the risk of type 2 diabetes (Answer E) is increased. Although cardiovascular risk factors should be monitored in transgender men on testosterone therapy, the risk of cardiovascular disease and myocardial infarction (Answer D) remains unclear.

EDUCATIONAL OBJECTIVE
Identify the most common adverse effect seen with testosterone therapy in transgender men.

REFERENCE(S)
Hembree WC, Cohen-Kettenis PT, Gooren L, et al. Endocrine treatment of gender-dysphoric/gender-incongruent persons: an Endocrine Society clinical practice guideline. *J Clin Endocrinol Metab*. 2017;102(11):3869-3903. PMID: 28945902

Wierckx K, Van Caenegem E, Schreiner T, et al. Cross-sex hormone therapy in trans persons is safe and effective at short-time follow-up: results from the European network for the investigation of gender incongruence. *J Sex Med*. 2014;11(8):1999-2011. PMID: 24828032

Elamin MB, Garcia MZ, Murad MH, Erwin PJ, Montori VM. Effect of sex steroid use on cardio-vascular risk in transsexual individuals: a systematic review and meta-analyses. *Clin Endocrinol (Oxf)*. 2010;72(1):1-10. PMID: 19473174

7 ANSWER: D) Recommend progestin intrauterine device and spironolactone
This patient's deep venous thrombosis is a contraindication to continuing estrogen-progestin contraception, even with a lower estrogen dose (20 mcg) (Answer C) or transdermal route (Answer A). Oral progestin-only contraception (Answer E) might be an option, but the safest method would be a nonoral route such as the progestin intrauterine device (Answer D), which would manage her bleeding, prevent endometrial

hyperplasia, and provide contraception. She could then add spironolactone to manage hirsutism. While metformin (Answer B) might help restore normal cycles, it is unlikely to benefit her hirsutism.

EDUCATIONAL OBJECTIVE
Choose the optimal therapy for irregular menstrual cycles, hyperandrogenic symptoms, and contraception in a woman with polycystic ovary syndrome and a history of deep venous thrombosis.

REFERENCE(S)
Legro RS, Arslanian SA, Ehrmann DA, et al; Endocrine Society. Diagnosis and treatment of polycystic ovary syndrome: an Endocrine Society clinical practice guideline. *J Clin Endocriol Metab.* 2013;98(12):4565-4592. PMID: 24151290

Martin KA, Anderson RR, Chang RJ, et al. Evaluation and treatment of hirsutism in premenopausal women: an Endocrine Society clinical practice guideline. *J Clin Endocrinol Metab.* 2018;103(4):1233-1257. PMID: 29522147

Practice Committee of the American Society for Reproductive Medicine. Combined hormonal contraception and the risk of venous thromboembolism: a guideline. *Fertil Steril.* 2017;107(1):43-51. PMID: 27793376

8 **ANSWER: B) Ovarian hyperthecosis**
Ovarian hyperthecosis or androgen-secreting ovarian or adrenal tumors can cause manifestations ranging from postmenopausal hirsutism to frank virilization. One distinguishing feature between the 2 is the pace of worsening, with hyperthecosis progressing at a slower rate than tumors. Ovarian hyperthecosis (Answer B) occurs when high gonadotropin levels drive androgen production from the theca cells. Although it can occur in premenopausal women, it occurs most often in postmenopausal women. Whether women with hyperthecosis have polycystic ovary syndrome before menopause has not been clarified.

An adrenal virilizing tumor (Answer A) would present with a more rapid onset and more severe symptoms and signs. Androgen-secreting adrenal tumors are usually malignant, but benign tumors have also been described in women. Approximately 60% of adrenocortical carcinomas present with hormone excess (most with Cushing syndrome only, 25% with both Cushing syndrome and virilization, and 10% with virilization alone). A granulosa tumor of the ovary (Answer C) would present with high estrogen levels and endometrial hyperplasia and would not cause virilization. Obesity (Answer D) can cause hirsutism. Adipose tissue can have increased 5α-reductase activity, as well as local aromatase activity, which can cause androgenic and estrogenic effects. However, it does not usually result in such high testosterone levels or virilization. Weight loss and suppression of androgens are the goals with obesity-induced hyperandrogenism. Ovarian tumors that cause hyperandrogenism include Sertoli-Leydig–cell tumors (Answer E), arrhenoblastomas, or hilus-cell tumors that secrete testosterone in the male normal range (>240 ng/dL [>8.3 nmol/L]) and cause virilization. Because these tumors are rare, more common causes of postmenopausal hirsutism and virilization should be considered.

EDUCATIONAL OBJECTIVE
Outline the differential diagnosis of severe hyperandrogenism in a postmenopausal woman.

REFERENCE(S)
Mamoojee Y, Ganguri M, Taylor N, Quinton R. Clinical case seminar: postmenopausal androgen excess-challenges in diagnostic work-up and management of ovarian thecosis. *Clin Endocrinol (Oxf).* 2018;88(1):13-20. PMID: 28980338

Pugeat M, Déchaud H, Raverot V, Denuzière A, Cohen R, Boudou P; French Endocrine Society. Recommendations for investigation of hyperandrogenism. *Ann Endocrinol (Paris).* 2010;71(1):2-7. PMID: 20096825

9 **ANSWER: D) Letrozole**
Women with polycystic ovary syndrome can have intermittent ovulation or anovulation, hyperandrogenism, and insulin resistance. Before planning for fertility, lifestyle should be optimized with diet and exercise. A relatively small amount of weight loss sometimes restores ovulatory cycles.

Addition of metformin as an insulin sensitizer can help regulate cycles and suppress androgens, and it may make lifestyle intervention more effective.

Historically, if fertility was desired, clomiphene citrate (Answer A) (50 mg on cycle days 5 through 9) was prescribed to induce ovulation. Clomiphene citrate is more effective than metformin therapy (Answer C) to achieve live births. Although clomiphene citrate is a potential approach to induce ovulation, the Reproductive Network Trial comparing the second-generation aromatase inhibitor letrozole (Answer D) with clomiphene citrate demonstrated a convincingly higher rate of ovulation induction and live births with letrozole, particularly in women with obesity and polycystic ovary syndrome.

Progesterone suppositories (Answer B) are sometimes prescribed for women with hypothalamic amenorrhea—not for women with polycystic ovary syndrome. They improve menstrual cyclicity, but they have not been shown to increase rates of ovulation induction. Gonadotropin therapy with recombinant FSH (Answer E) is not used as first-line therapy for ovulation induction in women with polycystic ovary syndrome, as it has a greater risk of multiple gestation and ovarian hyperstimulation syndrome. It is typically used in women who have not responded to letrozole and clomiphene.

EDUCATIONAL OBJECTIVE

Compare treatment effectiveness of clomiphene citrate with that of aromatase inhibitors for ovulation induction in women with polycystic ovary syndrome who would like to become pregnant.

REFERENCE(S)

Palomba S. Aromatase inhibitors for ovulation induction. *J Clin Endocrinol Metab.* 2015;100(5):1742-1747. PMID: 25710566

Legro RS, Brzyski RG, Diamond MP, et al; NICHD Reproductive Medicine Network. Letrozole versus clomiphene for infertility in the polycystic ovary syndrome [published correction appears in *N Engl J Med.* 2014;317(15):1465]. *N Engl J Med.* 2014;371(2):119-129. PMID: 25006718

Franik S, Kremer JA, Nelen WL, Farquhar C, Marjoribanks J. Aromatase inhibitors for subfertile women with polycystic ovary syndrome: summary of a Cochrane review. *Fertil Steril.* 2015;103(2):353-355. PMID: 25455536

Legro RS, Arslanian SA, Ehrmann DA, et al; Endocrine Society. Diagnosis and treatment of polycystic ovary syndrome: An Endocrine Society clinical practice guideline. *J Clin Endocriol Metab.* 2013;98(12):4565-4592. PMID: 24151290

10 ANSWER: B) *FMR1* genetic testing

Fragile X premutation screening should be performed in women with primary ovarian insufficiency (menopause before age 40 years). Screening should be recommended for women who have a family history of primary ovarian insufficiency; male relatives with learning disorders, autism, or intellectual disability; or family members with ataxia and/or dementia (suggestive of fragile X–related ataxia). The screening is accomplished by *FMR1* genetic testing (Answer B). In fragile X carriers, CGG repeats are in the premutation range.

Karyotype analysis (Answer A) is now performed in all women with primary ovarian insufficiency to rule out mosaic Turner syndrome. Patients with mosaicism typically have a milder reproductive phenotype, as some girls have breast development followed by pubertal arrest, or puberty followed by secondary amenorrhea. A very small percentage of girls with Turner syndrome have normal pubertal development and regular menses. Positive 21-hydroxylase antibodies (Answer C) are seen in women with autoimmune oophoritis, and they predict future risk of adrenal insufficiency as well. However, this patient does not have typical features of autoimmune oophoritis. Thyroid antibodies (Answer D) may be positive in patients with autoimmune thyroid disease and concomitant autoimmune premature ovarian insufficiency, but an autoimmune etiology would not explain the family history of learning disability and early menopause in relatives. There is no indication for measurement of antimullerian hormone (Answer E), which is an indicator of follicle number and is low in premature ovarian insufficiency and high in polycystic ovary syndrome.

EDUCATIONAL OBJECTIVE
Explain the differential diagnosis of premature ovarian insufficiency and appropriately recommend fragile X carrier testing.

REFERENCE(S)
Welt CK. Primary ovarian insufficiency: a more accurate term for premature ovarian failure. *Clin Endocrinol (Oxf)*. 2008;68(4):499-509. PMID: 17970776

Wang T, Bray SM, Warren ST. New perspectives on the biology of fragile X syndrome. *Curr Opin Genet Dev*. 2012;22(3):256-263. PMID: 22382129

Hoyos LR, Thakur M. Fragile X premutation in women: recognizing the health challenges beyond primary ovarian insufficiency. *J Assist Reprod Genet*. 2017;34(3):315-332. PMID: 27995424

Hipp HS, Charen KH, Spencer JB, Allen EG, Sherman SL. Reproductive and gynecologic care of women with fragile X primary ovarian insufficiency (FXPOI). *Menopause*. 2016;23(9):993-999. PMID: 27552334

11 ANSWER: C) Hematocrit or hemoglobin measurement every 3 months

Testosterone administration at pharmacologic levels in women (or men) causes increased hematocrit and risk of polycythemia. This is a greater concern with parenteral testosterone administration, but it can be seen with testosterone gel as well. Therefore, the current Endocrine Society guideline suggests that hematocrit or hemoglobin be measured at baseline and every 3 months for the first year, and then 1 to 2 times per year.

Serum testosterone measurements (Answer A) are also essential, but they should ideally be drawn midway between injections or at least 2 hours after application of a transdermal preparation. Hemoglobin A_{1c} measurement (Answer B) is not a component of the routine monitoring of hormone therapy for transgender men. Pap smears (Answer E) are performed if cervical tissue is present (many patients undergo hysterectomy and thus do not have cervical tissue). The schedule for cervical screening is the same as for cisgender women (every 3 years). Bone density monitoring at 1 year (Answer D) is not essential, as bone mineral density is expected to be maintained on testosterone therapy. Testosterone is converted peripherally to estradiol, and estradiol maintains bone.

EDUCATIONAL OBJECTIVE
Identify the most important components of monitoring transgender men taking gender-affirming hormone therapy.

REFERENCE(S)
Hembree WC, Cohen-Kettenis PT, Gooren L, et al. Endocrine treatment of gender dysphoric/gender-incongruent persons: an Endocrine Society clinical practice guideline. *J Clin Endocrinol Metab*. 2017;102(11):3869-3903. PMID: 28945902

Gorton RN, Erickson-Schroth L. Hormonal and surgical treatment options for transgender men (female-to-male). *Psychiatr Clin North Am*. 2017;40(1):79-97. PMID: 28159147

Spack NP. Management of transgenderism. *JAMA*. 2013;309(5):478-484. PMID: 23385274

Deutsch MB, Feldman JL. Updated recommendations from the world professional association for transgender health standards of care. *Am Fam Physician*. 2013;87(2):89-93. PMID: 23317072

Fernandez JD, Tannock LR. Metabolic effects of hormone therapy in transgender patients. *Endocr Pract*. 2016;22(4):383-388. PMID: 26574790

12 ANSWER: C) Combination estrogen-progestin oral contraceptive

Contraception in women with polycystic ovary syndrome should be targeted not only to protect against unplanned pregnancy, but also to control the metabolic and hyperandrogenic phenotype (eg, an estrogen-progestin oral contraceptive [Answer C]). An intrauterine device is a consideration, but the levonorgestrel-releasing intrauterine device (Answer A) would not help her hyperandrogenism. There have been case reports of hair loss with this intrauterine device that are reversible with removal of the device. Increasing the metformin dosage would not provide any additional benefit for hirsutism, as no dosage has been found to be beneficial.

Oral contraceptives with a progestin associated with low venous thromboembolic risk such as norethindrone or levonorgestrel are preferred over those that may be associated with higher risk (such as third-generation progestins [eg, desogestrel, gestodene]). All oral contraceptives have an equivalent beneficial effect on hirsutism, using Ferriman-Gallwey scores as the patient-important outcome. Adding spironolactone (Answer B), finasteride (Answer D), or flutamide (Answer E) to the regimen of a patient who is using barrier contraception is not optimal. All 3 drugs, if given inadvertently during early pregnancy, can cause feminization of a male fetus. Barrier contraception does not provide adequate pregnancy protection compared with an oral contraceptive. Flutamide is not recommended for hirsutism, as it has been associated with hepatotoxicity.

EDUCATIONAL OBJECTIVE
Differentiate among contraceptive options for women with polycystic ovary syndrome.

REFERENCE(S)
Martin KA, Anderson RR, Chang RJ, et al. Evaluation and treatment of hirsutism in premenopausal women: an Endocrine Society clinical practice guideline. *J Clin Endocrinol Metab*. 2018;103(4):1233-1257. PMID: 29522147

Buzney E, Sheu J, Buzney C, Reynolds RV. Polycystic ovary syndrome: a review for dermatologists: Part II. Treatment. *J Am Acad Dermatol*. 2014;71(5):859.e1-859.e15. PMID: 25437978

Legro RS, Arslanian SA, Ehrmann DA, et al; Endocrine Society. Diagnosis and treatment of polycystic ovary syndrome: an Endocrine Society clinical practice guideline. *J Clin Endocrinol Metab*. 2013;98(12):4565-4592. PMID: 24151290

13 ANSWER: A) Menopausal transition (perimenopause)

This woman is experiencing some of the typical symptoms of the menopausal transition or perimenopause (change in menstrual cycles and new sleep disturbance, likely due to hot flashes) (Answer A). Many cycles during the transition are anovulatory and serum estradiol levels are extremely high at times, followed by a rapid drop. FSH concentrations vary depending on estradiol levels and whether there has been recent ovulation.

Obesity alone (Answer C) can be associated with a change in menstrual cycles, but it would not explain her high serum estradiol or vasomotor symptoms. Symptoms during the menopausal transition may include breast soreness when estradiol levels are extremely high, and hot flashes/night sweats when estradiol levels fall. Serum progesterone concentrations would be much higher with pregnancy (Answer B). The high estradiol value is not enough to raise suspicion for a granulosa-cell tumor (Answer D). Women with such tumors often have abdominal pain (the tumors are large), and present with bleeding and endometrial hyperplasia. Women with polycystic ovary syndrome (Answer E) typically have a history of irregular menses that began during adolescence. Serum LH is usually greater than FSH in women with polycystic ovary syndrome, while this patient's picture is more consistent with ovarian insufficiency (FSH > LH).

EDUCATIONAL OBJECTIVE
Identify the characteristic clinical and biochemical findings of the menopausal transition.

REFERENCE(S)
Harlow SD, Gass M, Hall JE, et al; STRAW + 10 Collaborative Group. Executive summary of the Stages of Reproductive Aging Workshop + 10: addressing the unfinished agenda of staging reproductive aging. *J Clin Endocrinol Metab*. 2012;97(4):1159-1168. PMID: 22344196

Burger HG, Hale GE, Robertson DM, Dennerstein L. A review of hormonal changes during the menopausal transition: focus on findings from the Melbourne Women's Midlife Health Project. *Hum Reprod Update*. 2007;13(6):559-565. PMID: 17630397

14

ANSWER: B) Start a selective serotonin reuptake inhibitor

Women with premenstrual syndrome experience a wide variety of cyclic and recurrent physical, emotional, behavioral, and cognitive symptoms that start in the luteal phase and diminish and stop after the onset of menses. The most severe form of premenstrual syndrome is known as premenstrual dysphoric disorder. Major symptoms include affective symptoms such as depression, angry outbursts, irritability, and anxiety and somatic symptoms such as breast pain, bloating, swelling, and headache. Initiation of a selective serotonin reuptake inhibitor (Answer B) that targets mood directly is currently the treatment of choice. Controlled studies confirm that abrogation of ovulation with oral contraceptives administered continuously or with a 4-day pill-free interval are also effective.

A cyclic estrogen-progestin oral contraceptive (Answer D) refers to those with a 7-day pill-free interval. Although they may be effective for premenstrual dysphoric disorder, they have not yet been well studied in this setting. Referral for psychotherapy (Answer A) may be helpful, but this has not been shown to be beneficial for this symptom complex. Antidepressants such as amitriptyline (Answer C) have been supplanted by newer targeted drugs and thus a tricyclic antidepressant is not the best option. Benzodiazepines, in particular alprazolam (Answer E), have been used in the past as adjunctive therapy for women with premenstrual dysphoric disorder. However, this approach is no longer used, as the risks of potential misuse outweigh the benefits.

EDUCATIONAL OBJECTIVE

Recommend treatment options for women with premenstrual dysphoric disorder.

REFERENCE(S)

Schmidt PJ, Martinez PE, Nieman LK, et al. Premenstrual dysphoric disorder symptoms following ovarian suppression: triggered by change in ovarian steroid levels but not continuous stable levels. *Am J Psychiatry.* 2017;174(10):980-989. PMID: 28427285

Management of premenstrual syndrome: green-top guideline No. 48. *BJOG.* 2017;124(3):e73-e105. PMID: 27900828

Brown J, O'Brien PM, Marjoribanks J, Wyatt K. Selective serotonin reuptake inhibitors for premenstrual syndrome. *Cochrane Database Syst Rev.* 2009:CD001396. PMID: 19370564

Jarvis CI, Lynch AM, Morin AK. Management strategies for premenstrual syndrome/premenstrual dysphoric disorder. *Ann Pharmacother.* 2008;42(7):967-978. PMID: 18559957

15

ANSWER: B) FSH, estradiol, and prolactin

Functional hypothalamic amenorrhea is a diagnosis of exclusion. Excessive stress, exercise, low weight, and eating disorders may alter the GnRH pulse generator, thereby altering the necessary switch of pulse frequency and amplitude across the menstrual cycle to induce ovulation and ensure regular periods. Hyperprolactinemia due to mild thyroid dysfunction, medications, or prolactin-secreting pituitary tumors can turn off the GnRH pulse generator and present as hypothalamic amenorrhea. Estrogen is low in the settings of hypothalamic amenorrhea and hyperprolactinemia, but it would be high if the patient were pregnant. The best laboratory tests to order next are measurements of FSH, estradiol, and prolactin (Answer B).

Androgens (Answer A) should be measured in a patient who has acne and hirsutism. A stimulated 17-hydroxyprogesterone measurement (Answer C) is the best test to assess for congenital adrenal hyperplasia, but there is no reason to suspect that diagnosis in this vignette because the patient did not describe hyperandrogenic symptoms or early pubic hair. Progesterone (Answer D) is measured to assess ovulation and luteal-phase function in women attempting fertility. Cushing syndrome may result in amenorrhea due to inhibition of gonadotropin secretion by excess cortisol. However, an evaluation for hypercortisolism (Answer E) is not indicated in this case.

EDUCATIONAL OBJECTIVE
Recommend appropriate hormone testing on the basis of the history, examination findings, and presentation in amenorrheic women.

REFERENCE(S)
Gordon CM, Ackerman KE, Berga SL, et al. Functional hypothalamic amenorrhea: an Endocrine Society clinical practice guideline. *J Clin Endocrinol Metab.* 2017;102(5):1413-1439. PMID: 28368518

Gordon CM. Clinical practice. Functional hypothalamic amenorrhea. *N Engl J Med.* 2010;363(4):365-371. PMID: 20660404

Caronia LM, Martin C, Welt CK, et al. A genetic basis for functional hypothalamic amenorrhea. *N Engl J Med.* 2011;364(3):215-225. PMID: 21247312

Melmed S, Casanueva FF, Hoffman AR, et al; Endocrine Society. Diagnosis and treatment of hyperprolactinemia: an Endocrine Society clinical practice guideline. *J Clin Endocrinol Metab.* 2011;96(2):273-288. PMID: 21296991

16 ANSWER: D) Primary ovarian insufficiency

Antimullerian hormone is a marker of ovarian reserve and follicular number. Infertility specialists have used it extensively in clinical practice to evaluate older women with borderline elevated FSH levels to predict response to in vitro fertilization and to diagnose primary ovarian insufficiency (or in its early stages, diminished ovarian reserve/occult ovarian insufficiency). Antimullerian hormone levels are lower in women with impending primary ovarian insufficiency (with higher FSH levels) (Answer D). Another feature suggesting primary ovarian insufficiency in this patient is her short cycles (25 to 26 days) rather than the more typical 28 days.

A woman with polycystic ovary syndrome (Answer A) would have a high antimullerian hormone level and low FSH level. An FSH-secreting pituitary adenoma (Answer B) would be unusual in this age group and would be more likely to present with neurologic symptoms (headache and vision loss) than with infertility and shorter cycles. Importantly, women with hypothalamic amenorrhea (Answer C) also have low antimullerian hormone levels but low-normal FSH levels. Although this patient has autoimmune hypothyroidism, it is unlikely that she has autoimmune oophoritis (Answer E), an uncommon etiology for primary ovarian insufficiency. Serum LH is higher than FSH in this disorder.

EDUCATIONAL OBJECTIVE
Explain the utility of measuring antimullerian hormone in women with amenorrhea.

REFERENCE(S)
Welt CK. Primary ovarian insufficiency: a more accurate term for premature ovarian failure. *Clin Endocrinol (Oxf).* 2008;68(4):499-509. PMID: 17970776

Meczekalski B, Czyzyk A, Kunicki M, et al. Fertility in women of late reproductive age: the role of serum anti-Müllerian hormone (AMH) levels in its assessment. *J Endocrinol Invest.* 2016;39(11):1259-1265. PMID: 27300031

La Marca A, Ferraretti AP, Palermo R, Ubaldi FM. The use of ovarian reserve markers in IVF clinical practice: a national consensus. *Gynecol Endocrinol.* 2016;32(1):1-5. PMID: 26531067

Iliodromiti S, Anderson RA, Nelson SM. Technical and performance characteristics of anti-müllerian hormone and antral follicle count as biomarkers of ovarian response. *Hum Reprod Update.* 2015;21(6):698-710. PMID: 25489055

17 ANSWER: B) Thyroid function tests, hemoglobin A_{1c} measurement, liver enzymes

Turner syndrome occurs in 1 in 2500 live births and is associated with growth failure, pubertal delay, and cardiac abnormalities. In addition, affected patients are at risk for a number of comorbidities, including type 2 diabetes, elevated liver enzymes, autoimmune thyroid disease, celiac disease, hearing loss, orthodontic problems, and psychosocial disorders. Cardiac MRI is the most important test because congenital cardiac abnormalities are present in up to 50% of patients and include coarctation of the aorta, bicuspid aortic valve, and partial anomalous pulmonary venous return. Echocardiography is also sometimes used as part of the routine follow-up of women with Turner syndrome (but it is not performed annually).

Current practice guidelines recommend annual visits for women with Turner syndrome. In addition to measuring blood pressure, calculating BMI, and performing a full skin examination, the following assessments are recommended: thyroid function tests, hemoglobin A_{1c} measurement, and liver enzymes (AST, ALT, γ-glutamyl transferase, alkaline phosphatase) (Answer B). Screening for other comorbidities (eg, celiac disease [Answer C] or kidney disorders [Answer A]) is performed at less frequent intervals. Complete blood cell count (Answer D) is not recommended routinely. Serum antimullerian hormone (a marker of ovarian reserve) and transvaginal ultrasonography (Answer E) are not needed. Her diagnosis of hypogonadism due to Turner syndrome is already established, and she has no current indications for pelvic imaging.

EDUCATIONAL OBJECTIVE
Recommend appropriate evaluation for girls with gonadal dysgenesis.

REFERENCE(S)
Gravholt CH, Andersen NH, Conway GS, et al; International Turner Syndrome Consensus Group. Clinical practice guidelines for the care of girls and women with Turner syndrome: proceedings from the 2016 Cincinnati International Turner Syndrome Meeting. *Eur J Endocrinol.* 2017;177(3):G1-G70. PMID: 28705803

Davenport ML. Approach to the patient with Turner syndrome. *J Clin Endocrinol Metab.* 2010;95(4):1487-1495. PMID: 20375216

Pinsker JE. Clinical review: Turner syndrome: updating the paradigm of clinical care. *J Clin Endocrinol Metab.* 2012;97(6):994-1003. PMID: 22472565

18 **ANSWER: D) Depression and anxiety**
Polycystic ovary syndrome is a common disorder that occurs in 6% to 8% of women. Affected patients usually present with hirsutism, acne, and irregular menses. They are also at increased risk for type 2 diabetes mellitus, dyslipidemia, and hypertension. Despite an increase in metabolic syndrome and cardiac risk factors, studies have not yet shown an increased risk of coronary heart disease (Answer B) in women with polycystic ovary syndrome. Therefore, routine screening for coronary heart disease is not recommended. Women with polycystic ovary syndrome are more likely to have mood disorders (eg, depression and anxiety [Answer D]) than weight-matched women without polycystic ovary syndrome. They are also at risk for eating disorders (binge eating). A number of expert societies, including the Endocrine Society, suggest screening all women with polycystic ovary syndrome for depression and anxiety. One approach is to use validated screening tools such as the Patient Health Questionnaire (PHQ-9) for depression and the Generalized Anxiety Disorder 7 (GAD-7) scale for anxiety disorders.

Neither celiac disease (Answer A) nor autoimmune thyroid disease (Answer C) has been associated with polycystic ovary syndrome, so screening for these comorbidities is not indicated. Polycystic ovary syndrome is associated with an increased risk of endometrial hyperplasia and carcinoma, but this patient should have a reduced risk because of her combined estrogen-progestin oral contraceptive.

EDUCATIONAL OBJECTIVE
Recommend screening for depression and anxiety in women with polycystic ovary syndrome.

REFERENCE(S)
McCartney CR, Marshall JC. Clinical Practice. Polycystic ovary syndrome. *N Engl J Med.* 2016;375(1):54-64. PMID: 27406348

Legro RS, Arslanian SA, Ehrmann DA, et al; Endocrine Society. Diagnosis and treatment of polycystic ovary syndrome: an Endocrine Society Clinical Practice Guideline. *J Clin Endocrinol Metab.* 2013;98(12):4565-4592. PMID: 24151290

Teede HJ, Misso ML, Costello MH, et al; International PCOS Network. Recommendations from the international evidence-based guideline for the assessment and management of polycystic ovary syndrome. *Fertil Steril.* 2018;110(3):364-379. PMID: 30033227

Male Reproduction Board Review

Frances J. Hayes, MB BCh, BAO

1 **ANSWER: B) Blood pressure**

In May 2019, the US FDA approved an oral formulation of testosterone undecanoate for the treatment of male hypogonadism. This testosterone formulation contains a boxed warning on its labeling stating that the drug can cause blood pressure to rise. As a result, it is recommended that health care providers consider a patient's individual heart disease risks and ensure that blood pressure is adequately controlled before prescribing this agent. Providers should also periodically monitor patient blood pressure (Answer B) during treatment. In the case described, the patient's baseline blood pressure is elevated and he has additional risk factors for hypertension, including obesity and obstructive sleep apnea. Thus, he would certainly need close blood pressure monitoring if this formulation were prescribed.

Oral androgens (eg, methyltestosterone), which are designed to resist first-pass metabolism by the liver by being alkylated at the C17 position, are well known to cause hepatoxicity, cholestasis, and peliosis hepatis. However, testosterone undecanoate is absorbed by the lymphatics rather than the blood stream and it therefore bypasses the liver. Thus, monitoring liver function (Answer C) is not indicated.

The Endocrine Society clinical practice guidelines do not advocate screening all hypogonadal men for prostate cancer. Men younger than 40 years, as the patient in this vignette, do not need prostate monitoring with PSA (Answer A) because the risk of prostate cancer is very low in this population. The guidelines recommend that clinicians consider screening and monitoring all men with hypogonadism who are 55 to 69 years of age for whom testosterone replacement therapy is being considered if they are in excellent health and have a life expectancy of more than 10 years. This screening and monitoring should start at age 40 years in men who are at increased risk for high-grade cancers, such as Black men and men with a first-degree male relative with diagnosed prostate cancer.

All androgens, including testosterone undecanoate, can have a modest impact on levels of thyroxine-binding globulin, but they do not cause overt thyroid dysfunction, so close monitoring of TSH levels (Answer D) is not indicated.

EDUCATIONAL OBJECTIVE

Counsel patients about potential adverse effects of the oral formulation of testosterone undecanoate.

REFERENCE(S)

Swerdloff RS, Wang C, White WB, et al. A new oral testosterone undecanoate formulation restores testosterone to normal concentrations in hypogonadal men. *J Clin Endocrinol Metab.* 2020;105(8): 2515-2531. PMID: 32382745

Westaby D, Ogle SJ, Paradinas FJ, Randell JB, Murray-Lyon IM. Liver damage from long-term methyltestosterone. *Lancet.* 1977;2(8032):262-263. PMID: 69876

Bhasin S, Brito JP, Cunningham GR, et al. Testosterone therapy in men with hypogonadism: an Endocrine Society clinical practice guideline. *J Clin Endocrinol Metab.* 2018;103(5):1715-1744. PMID: 29562364

2 **ANSWER: A) Start testosterone replacement therapy**

The diagnosis of hypogonadism made by the patient's primary care physician is correct based on the presence of symptoms of hypogonadism in association with 2 low morning testosterone measurements. While the patient is eager to initiate testosterone therapy in the hope of improving his symptoms, it is the physician's responsibility to ensure that he is an appropriate candidate and that the risk-to-benefit ratio favors treatment.

Starting a phosphodiesterase inhibitor (Answer B) would help his erectile dysfunction, but it would not address his fatigue or decreased libido and would not correct his hypogonadism. This patient is healthy apart from hypogonadism, and he has no contraindication to testosterone therapy. Therefore, starting testosterone replacement (Answer A) is reasonable.

An important objective of the baseline evaluation in men being considered for testosterone replacement therapy is to identify and exclude those who have a history of prostate cancer or are at high risk for developing prostate cancer. Given this patient's age, normal prostate examination, and absence of risk factors for prostate cancer such as Black/African American heritage or having a first-degree relative with prostate cancer, his risk of prostate cancer is low and screening by measuring PSA (Answer C) is not recommended.

Most organizations that provide prostate cancer screening guidelines strongly encourage informing the patient of the potential benefits and risks and engaging him in shared decision-making regarding screening with PSA measurement and digital rectal examination. The Endocrine Society clinical practice guidelines recommend that clinicians consider screening and monitoring for all men with hypogonadism who are 55 to 69 years of age for whom testosterone replacement therapy is being considered if they are in excellent health and have a life expectancy of more than 10 years. Screening should start at age 40 years in men who are at increased risk for high-grade cancers, such as those of Black/African American ancestry and men with a first-degree male relative with diagnosed prostate cancer. Men younger than 40 years do not need prostate monitoring because the risk of prostate cancer is very low in this population. The risk of death due to prostate cancer in men diagnosed when they are older than 70 years is not considered high enough to warrant monitoring. The baseline assessment of prostate cancer risk should consider risk factors such as age, family history (increased risk in men who have a first-degree relative with prostate cancer), race/ethnicity (increased risk in men of Black/African American ancestry), biopsy history, elevated PSA levels, and abnormal prostate examination results.

As a general rule, patients who have a palpable prostate nodule or induration or a PSA level greater than 4.0 ng/mL (>4.0 µg/L) need further urologic evaluation before testosterone therapy is initiated. However, in subgroups of men considered to be at increased risk for prostate cancer, such as Black/African American patients or men with a first-degree relative with prostate cancer, the baseline PSA level at which referral to a urologist is recommended is greater than 3.0 ng/mL (>3.0 µg/L).

The question of when pituitary imaging (Answer D) is indicated for a patient with hypogonadism and low gonadotropin levels is one commonly faced by clinicians. Given that an MRI of the pituitary is an expensive test with a low yield of positive results, the Endocrine Society clinical practice guidelines recommend MRI in the following circumstances: (1) total testosterone concentration <150 ng/dL [<5.0 nmol/L]; (2) presence of hyperprolactinemia; (3) headache or visual field disturbance; and (4) presence of another anterior pituitary hormone deficiency. Therefore, in the patient described who meets none of these criteria, obtaining a pituitary MRI is not the best next step in his management.

EDUCATIONAL OBJECTIVE
Determine whether a patient is an appropriate candidate for testosterone replacement therapy.

REFERENCE(S)
Bhasin S, Brito JP, Cunningham GR, et al. Testosterone therapy in men with hypogonadism: an Endocrine Society clinical practice guideline. *J Clin Endocrinol Metab*. 2018;103(5):1715-1744. PMID: 29562364

3 ANSWER: B) Measure testosterone 2 to 8 hours after the gel has been applied

Gel delivery systems are the preferred form of testosterone replacement therapy for many hypogonadal patients because they provide an easy and convenient way to restore and maintain testosterone levels in the physiologic range, have minimal adverse effects, and have favorable pharmacokinetics. Endocrine Society guidelines recommend that when monitoring patients being treated with a testosterone gel, the testosterone concentration should be assessed 2 to 8 hours after gel application (Answer B). Many patients apply the gel at home and then arrive in the lab early in the day to have their blood drawn before to going to work, which has the potential to give an erroneously high testosterone reading. Therefore, reducing the dosage (Answer A) in this patient who was previously stable on this dosage is not appropriate without first rechecking the testosterone level and ensuring that the sample was drawn under the right conditions. The fact that the patient's hematocrit has not increased is reassuring and suggests that his testosterone level is not chronically elevated. Switching to alternate-day administration of the gel (Answer D) would not be appropriate given the known pharmacokinetics of the gel.

This patient expressed a clear preference for a transdermal route of testosterone administration when treatment options were initially discussed. Switching to an intramuscular preparation (Answer C) at this point would offer no advantage and would most likely have a negative effect on adherence.

EDUCATIONAL OBJECTIVE
Appropriately monitor hypogonadal patients receiving replacement with a testosterone gel.

REFERENCE(S)

Bhasin S, Brito JP, Cunningham GR, et al. Testosterone therapy in men with hypogonadism: an Endocrine Society clinical practice guideline. *J Clin Endocrinol Metab.* 2018;103(5):1715-1744. PMID: 29562364

4 ANSWER: C) Hypothyroidism

Several factors are known to affect the levels of circulating SHBG and therefore testosterone levels in men. This patient has an SHBG level at the lower end of the normal range. Of the answer options listed, only hypothyroidism (Answer C) causes a low SHBG level. Topiramate (Answer A) (an enzyme inducer), liver disease (Answer B), HIV infection (Answer D), and age (Answer E) all tend to increase SHBG levels, in which case total testosterone levels are often in the mid-normal to high range, while free testosterone levels are low-normal or low.

EDUCATIONAL OBJECTIVE
Explain the effect of hypothyroidism on SHBG levels when evaluating men for hypogonadism.

REFERENCE(S)

Dumoulin SC, Perret BP, Bennet AP, Caron PJ. Opposite effects of thyroid hormones on binding proteins for steroid hormones (sex hormone-binding globulin and corticosteroid-binding globulin) in humans. *Eur J Endocrinol.* 1995;132(5):594-598. PMID: 7749500

Bhasin S, Brito JP, Cunningham GR, et al. Testosterone therapy in men with hypogonadism: an Endocrine Society clinical practice guideline. *J Clin Endocrinol Metab.* 2018;103(5):1715-1744. PMID: 29562364

5 ANSWER: D) Recheck his PSA level

Although this patient's PSA level remains within the reference range and he has no lower urinary tract symptoms, the magnitude of its change is higher than one would expect. However, PSA levels are known to fluctuate in an individual and also have considerable test-retest variability. Therefore, the most appropriate next step is to confirm that there has been a significant increase by rechecking his PSA level (Answer D). If the repeated PSA value is normal, testosterone therapy can be continued and a urology referral is not necessary. However, a confirmed increase in PSA of greater than 1.4 ng/mL (>1.4 µg/L) over the course of a year in a man on testosterone therapy cannot be attributed to random variation alone and should therefore prompt referral to a urologist for consideration of prostate biopsy (Answer C). A systematic review of prostate risk during testosterone therapy found that the average PSA increase after initiation of testosterone therapy is 0.3 ng/mL and 0.44 ng/mL in young and old men, respectively. A cutoff of 1.4 ng/mL has been adopted on the basis of the findings of a clinical trial that evaluated the effectiveness of finasteride vs placebo on lower urinary tract symptoms and prostate volume in men with benign prostatic hyperplasia. In that study, the upper limit of the 90% confidence interval for the change in PSA level in the placebo arm was 1.4 ng/mL (1.4 µg/L). Hence, on the basis of the findings of the finasteride study and the fact that the average increase in PSA levels on testosterone therapy is less than 0.5 ng/mL (<0.5 µg/L) (regardless of patient age), the Endocrine Society's clinical practice guidelines recommend that patients with a PSA increase of greater than 1.4 ng/mL (>1.4 µg/L) during testosterone therapy should be referred for urologic consultation. It is important to understand that this increase of 1.4 ng/mL (1.4 µg/L) in PSA concentration does not indicate prostate cancer, but only serves as a trigger for further evaluation.

This patient has experienced symptomatic improvement on his current testosterone dosage, and his on-treatment testosterone concentration is normal. Therefore, discontinuing treatment (Answer A) is not indicated now. Similarly, given that his testosterone level is in the mid-normal range, there is no indication to reduce the dosage (Answer B). Although this patient's PSA level has increased, he does not have lower urinary tract symptoms. Therefore, treatment with a 5α-reductase inhibitor (Answer E) is not warranted.

EDUCATIONAL OBJECTIVE
Outline appropriate prostate monitoring for middle-aged and older patients receiving testosterone replacement.

REFERENCE(S)
Bhasin S, Brito JP, Cunningham GR, et al. Testosterone therapy in men with hypogonadism: an Endocrine Society clinical practice guideline. *J Clin Endocrinol Metab.* 2018;103(5):1715-1744. PMID: 29562364

6 ANSWER: C) Functional hypogonadotropic hypogonadism

Men who exercise excessively and/or restrict calories can develop functional hypogonadotropic hypogonadism (Answer C). This is caused by suppression of GnRH secretion and is analogous to functional hypogonadotropic hypogonadism seen in women with hypothalamic amenorrhea. Leptin has an important role in GnRH signaling, and the low levels in patients with such energy deficits are thought to mediate the suppression of the reproductive axis.

Congenital leptin deficiency (Answer A) is a rare condition due to pathogenic variants in the *LEP* gene. It is characterized by onset of severe obesity in early childhood, as well as hypogonadotropic hypogonadism resulting in absent or delayed puberty. While this patient has a very low leptin level, the fact that he is slim and well virilized indicates that his low leptin level is an acquired, rather than congenital, deficiency.

Kallmann syndrome (Answer B) is a cause of congenital hypogonadotropic hypogonadism with anosmia, and it would not explain low testosterone levels in a patient who had gone through puberty and has normal-sized testes.

A hydrocele (Answer D) is a collection of fluid between the testis and the tunica albuginea. While it can cause scrotal swelling and discomfort, it does not interfere with Leydig-cell secretion of testosterone.

Use of anabolic steroids (Answer E) could explain this patient's muscular appearance. However, patients taking anabolic steroids have undetectable LH levels due to suppression of their hypothalamic-pituitary-gonadal axis. They also tend to have hematocrit levels that are significantly higher than those in this vignette. Anabolic steroid use would also not explain the patient's low leptin level.

EDUCATIONAL OBJECTIVE

Identify stress and low body fat as causes of suppression of the hypothalamic-pituitary-gonadal axis in men.

REFERENCE(S)

Dwyer AA, Chavan NR, Lewkowitz-Shpuntoff H, et al. Functional hypogonadotropic hypogonadism in men: underlying neuroendocrine mechanisms and natural history. *J Clin Endocrinol Metab.* 2019;104(8):3403-3414. PMID: 31220265

Young J. Approach to the male patient with hypogonadotropic hypogonadism. *J Clin Endocrinol Metab.* 2012;97(3):707-718. PMID: 22392951

Montague CT, Farooqi IS, Whitehead JP, et al. Congenital leptin deficiency is associated with severe early-onset obesity in humans. *Nature.* 1997;387(6636):903-908. PMID: 9202122

7 ANSWER: B) Synkinesia

In the last decade, considerable advances have been made in unraveling the genetic basis of congenital hypogonadotropic hypogonadism, and to date, pathogenic variants have been identified in approximately 40% of cases. In familial cases such as the one described in this vignette, the mode of inheritance can be used to guide genetic testing. This pedigree is consistent with an X-linked mode of inheritance and thus a pathogenic variant in *ANOS1*. In an analysis of 219 patients with congenital hypogonadotropic hypogonadism, the following clinical features were highly associated with specific gene defects: synkinesia (*ANOS1*), dental agenesis (*FGF8/FGFR1*), digital bony abnormalities (*FGF8/FGFR1*), and hearing loss (*CHD7*). Thus, in the case described, the physical finding most likely to be encountered is synkinesia (Answer B). In addition to the important role of anosmin 1 in the neuronal migration of both the GnRH neurons and the olfactory structures, it is also important for the crossing of the neurons in the developing brain across the midline, and this accounts for the mirror movements seen in patients with pathogenic variants in *ANOS1*.

Bony abnormalities, including syndactyly (Answer A), are typically encountered in patients with pathogenic variants in genes involved in the FGF pathway such as *FGF8* or *FGFR1*. Coloboma (Answer C) is one of the characteristic features of CHARGE syndrome due to a pathogenic variant in the *CHD7* gene. Axillary freckling (Answer D) is a cutaneous manifestation of neurofibromatosis type 1, while a shortened fourth metacarpal (Answer E) is seen in patients with pseudohypoparathyroidism.

EDUCATIONAL OBJECTIVE

Identify synkinesia as a phenotypic feature of Kallmann syndrome due to a pathogenic variant in the *ANOS1* gene.

REFERENCE(S)

Costa-Barbosa FA, Balasubramanian R, Keefe KW, et al. Prioritizing genetic testing in patients with Kallmann syndrome using clinical phenotypes. *J Clin Endocrinol Metab.* 2013;98(5):E943-E953. PMID: 23533228

Young J, Xu C, Papadakis GE, et al. Clinical management of congenital hypogonadotropic hypogonadism. *Endocr Rev.* 2019;40(2):669-710. PMID: 30698671

8 ANSWER: B) Congenital hypogonadotropic hypogonadism

This patient had prepubertal onset of hypogonadism as evidenced by his failure to develop secondary sexual characteristics or an increase in testicular size and eunuchoidal proportions (arm span >5 cm above height). Laboratory tests show profound secondary hypogonadism with otherwise normal pituitary function and prolactin levels. His presentation is thus consistent with congenital hypogonadotropic hypogonadism (Answer B). Distinguishing between constitutional delay of growth and puberty (Answer A) and congenital hypogonadotropic hypogonadism can be challenging in younger adolescent boys. The fact that this patient's father was a late bloomer might lead one to suspect constitutional delay of growth and puberty. However, the absence of any signs of puberty by age 18 years, by definition, rules this out. It is important to recognize that delayed, but otherwise normal, puberty is seen in up to 12% of families with congenital hypogonadotropic hypogonadism.

Pathogenic variants in the *PROP1* gene (Answer C) are one of the most common causes of both familial and sporadic congenital combined pituitary hormone deficiency (GH, TSH, LH, FSH). Thus, the fact that the patient's pituitary hormone profile is normal apart from gonadotropin deficiency rules out an abnormality in *PROP1*.

Similarly, pathogenic variants in the *POU1F1* gene (Answer D), which were first described in 1992, cause combined pituitary hormone deficiency and are associated with GH, prolactin, and TSH deficiencies, with variable pituitary hypoplasia. Deficiencies of GH and prolactin are generally complete, but TSH deficiency is more variable. Gonadotropin deficiency is not seen in patients with *POU1F1* pathogenic variants, so it would not explain this patient's phenotype.

EDUCATIONAL OBJECTIVE
Construct the differential diagnosis of a patient with congenital hypogonadotropic hypogonadism.

REFERENCE(S)
Palmert MR, Dunkel L. Clinical practice. Delayed puberty. *N Engl J Med.* 2012;366(5):443-453. PMID: 22296078

Hayes FJ, Seminara SB, Crowley WF Jr. Hypogonadotropic hypogonadism. *Endocrinol Metab Clin North Am.* 1998;27(4):739-763. PMID: 9922906

Young J. Approach to the male patient with hypogo-nadotropic hypogonadism. *J Clin Endocrinol Metab.* 2012;97(3):707-718. PMID: 22392951

Costa-Barbosa FA, Balasubramanian R, Keefe KW, et al. Prioritizing genetic testing in patients with Kallmann syndrome using clinical phenotypes. *J Clin Endocrinol Metab.* 2013;98(5):E943-E953. PMID: 23533228

Turton JP, Reynaud R, Mehta A, et al. Novel muta-tions within the *POU1F1* gene associated with variable combined pituitary hormone deficiency. *J Clin Endocrinol Metab.* 2005;90(8):4762-4770. PMID: 15928241

9 ANSWER: B) Hereditary hemochromatosis

This patient has secondary hypogonadism (symptoms and/or signs of hypogonadism, low serum testosterone, and low or inappropriately normal gonadotropin levels). Considering that his testes are adult sized and he is normally virilized, one can conclude he has acquired secondary hypogonadism after the onset of puberty. The differential diagnosis of postpubertal, acquired secondary hypogonadism includes pituitary macroadenoma, Cushing syndrome, hyperprolactinemia, opioid use, and iron overload syndromes such as hemochromatosis. Hand arthralgias, chondrocalcinosis, hyperpigmentation, and secondary hypogonadism are the earliest manifestations of iron overload syndromes. In men, hereditary hemochromatosis (Answer B) often causes these sequelae in the third and fourth decades. Later in the disease course, patients may experience heart failure, cirrhosis, and diabetes mellitus. Acquired forms of iron overload syndromes (eg, due to multiple transfusions) may also cause disease earlier. Hemochromatosis is inherited in an autosomal recessive manner and has a prevalence of about 0.4% in populations of northern European descent, but it has much lower clinical penetrance. Disease severity is highly variable. Pathogenic variants in the *HFE* gene are responsible, and the most common genotype is homozygosity for the Cys282Tyr (C282Y) variant. Assessment of transferrin saturation is the most useful initial test for hemochromatosis; a transferrin saturation less than 45% is enough to exclude the diagnosis. In the appropriate clinical setting, C282Y homozygosity suffices to diagnose hemochromatosis, but liver biopsy with iron staining remains the criterion standard for diagnosis.

Opioid abuse (Answer C) can cause hypogonadotropic hypogonadism, but it would not cause arthralgias.

Given that this patient has no clinical features of glucocorticoid excess on history and physical examination, screening for Cushing disease (Answer D) is not indicated.

While the patient has a 5-mm pituitary lesion, incidentally discovered microadenomas are seen in 10% to 38% of patients on MRI. In patients with marked hyperprolactinemia due to a large macroadenoma (Answer A), serum prolactin levels can be read as normal unless serial dilution of serum is done to assess for the "hook effect." However, this phenomenon would not be seen with a 5-mm pituitary adenoma.

Inflammatory arthropathies can suppress testosterone secretion and cause arthralgias. This patient has a family history of psoriatic arthropathy and has nonspecific joint pain. However, he has no objective evidence of joint inflammation or rash, making psoriatic arthropathy (Answer E) a very unlikely cause for his presentation.

EDUCATIONAL OBJECTIVE
Diagnose hemochromatosis as a cause of secondary hypogonadism.

REFERENCE(S)
Bhasin S, Brito JP, Cunningham GR, et al. Testosterone therapy in men with hypogonadism: an Endocrine Society clinical practice guideline. *J Clin Endocrinol Metab.* 2018;103(5):1715-1744. PMID: 29562364

McDermott JH, Walsh CH. Hypogonadism in hereditary hemochromatosis. *J Clin Endocrinol Metab.* 2005;90(4):2451-2455. PMID: 15657376

Moyer TP, Highsmith WE, Smyrk TC, Gross JB Jr. Hereditary hemochromatosis: laboratory evaluation. *Clin Chim Acta.* 2011;412(17-18):1485-1492. PMID: 21510925

van Bokhoven MA, van Deursen CT, Swinkels DW. Diagnosis and management of hereditary haemochromatosis. *BMJ.* 2011;342:c7251. PMID: 21248018

10 ANSWER: B) Perform a postejaculatory urine analysis for semen

Ejaculation is the discharge of semen from the male reproductive tract usually accompanied by orgasm. Retrograde ejaculation occurs when semen, which would normally be ejaculated via the urethra, is instead redirected to the bladder. Normally, the sphincter of the bladder contracts before ejaculation, which acts to both inhibit the release of urine and prevent a reflux of seminal fluids into the bladder during ejaculation. Any condition, medication, or surgical procedure that interferes with central control of ejaculation or the autonomic innervation to the seminal tract can cause ejaculatory dysfunction. This patient has partial retrograde ejaculation due to autonomic neuropathy from poorly controlled type 1 diabetes. The diagnosis, which can be suspected from the history, is confirmed by showing that sperm are present in a urine sample obtained after ejaculation (Answer B). In patients not desiring fertility, no treatment is indicated. In patients wishing to start a family, a trial of pseudoephedrine could be considered, as it improves muscle tone at the bladder neck.

There is no indication to start treatment with hCG (Answer A), given that this patient's testosterone level is just below the lower end of normal and that it is intratesticular testosterone that is most important for spermatogenesis. Initiating testosterone therapy (Answer D) would actually suppress sperm production, so it would not be appropriate for a man trying to conceive. Given that sperm are already present in the ejaculate, there is no need to extract them from the testis (Answer C).

Starting an α-adrenergic blocker (Answer E) would actually make the problem worse given that these drugs relax the bladder sphincter and are a common cause of retrograde ejaculation.

EDUCATIONAL OBJECTIVE
Diagnose retrograde ejaculation, characterized by reduced ejaculate volume and oligospermia, in a patient with diabetes and infertility.

REFERENCE(S)
Mehta A, Sigman M. Management of the dry ejaculate: a systematic review of aspermia and retrograde ejaculation. *Fertil Steril.* 2015;104(5):1074-1081. PMID: 26432530

11 **ANSWER: D) Add FSH, 75 IU daily**
For men whose infertility is due to hypogonadotropic hypogonadism as in this case, spermatogenesis can be induced with hormonal therapy in the form of either exogenous gonadotropins (hCG ± FSH) or GnRH. Gonadotropin therapy to induce spermatogenesis consists of subcutaneous administration of hCG alone or in combination with FSH. hCG bears strong structural homology to LH, and acting through the LH receptor on Leydig cells it increases both intratesticular and systemic testosterone production. In men who become hypogonadal after normal puberty has been completed and thus have normal testicular size, treatment with hCG alone is adequate to stimulate spermatogenesis. In contrast, patients who have congenital hypogonadotropic hypogonadism and prepubertal testes (<4 mL), as in this case, need combination therapy with both hCG and FSH (Answer D) to stimulate growth of the seminiferous tubules.

The calculated half-life of hCG is 2.3 days. Therefore, it would be of no benefit to the patient to shorten the interval between injections to daily (Answer C).

In contrast, recombinant LH (Answer A) has a much shorter half-life, estimated at 1 to 5 hours. When used to trigger ovulation in women, the long serum half-life of hCG can be an undesirable characteristic in clinical practice, as residual hCG may be mistaken for early detection of de novo synthesis of hCG by a newly implanted pregnancy. However, when used to stimulate spermatogenesis, the long half-life of hCG means fewer injections for the patient and is therefore more convenient and cheaper than recombinant LH.

This patient's trough testosterone is in the lower part of the normal range, which is where one wants it to be to avoid high estradiol levels and the development of gynecomastia, a common adverse effect when the hCG dosage is too high. Therefore, there would be no benefit to increasing the hCG dosage to 1500 IU every other day (Answer B).

Treatment with clomiphene (Answer E) requires an intact hypothalamus given that it increases LH by blocking estrogen-mediated negative feedback, so it would not be effective in a patient with congenital GnRH deficiency due to Kallmann syndrome.

EDUCATIONAL OBJECTIVE
Recommend the optimal gonadotropin regimen to stimulate spermatogenesis in Kallmann syndrome.

REFERENCE(S)
Burris AS, Rodbard HW, Winters SJ, Sherins RJ. Gonadotropin therapy in men with isolated hypogonadotropic hypogonadism: the response to human chorionic gonadotropin is predicted by initial testicular size. *J Clin Endocrinal Metab.* 1988;66(6):1144-1151. PMID: 3372679

King TFJ, Hayes FJ. Long-term outcome of idiopathic hypogonadotropic hypogonadism. *Curr Opin Endocrinol Diabetes Obes.* 2012;19(3):204-210. PMID: 22499222

Young J, Xu C, Papadakis GE, et al. Clinical management of congenital hypogonadotropic hypogonadism. *Endocr Rev.* 2019;40(2):669-710. PMID: 30698671

12 **ANSWER: A) Y-Chromosome microdeletion**
This couple's infertility is due to azoospermia. Absence of sperm in the ejaculate may occur because of an obstruction in the reproductive tract (obstructive azoospermia) or inadequate production of spermatozoa (nonobstructive azoospermia). The volume and pH of the seminal fluid can be used to determine in which category a patient's azoospermia falls.

This patient has nonobstructive azoospermia based on a normal semen volume and pH. He has normal LH and testosterone levels indicating normal Leydig-cell function, but he has an elevated FSH level due to lack of negative feedback from undetectable inhibin B, which suggests a selective defect in the seminiferous tubule compartment of the testis. This presentation is most likely due to a microdeletion in the Y-chromosome (Answer A), the second most common genetic cause of male infertility after Klinefelter syndrome. The male-specific region on the long arm of the Y chromosome has a locus known as the azoospermia factor (AZF) that contains genes needed for spermatogenesis. This AZF locus contains 3 regions: AZFa, AZFb, and AZFc. Deletions of the entire AZFa region result in complete atrophy of the tubular compartment, with only Sertoli cells seen on testicular biopsy, making sperm retrieval for intracytoplasmic sperm injection virtually impossible. Large deletions in the AZFb region also result in Sertoli-cell–only syndrome. Pathogenic variants in the AZFc region are the most common and account for 80% of Y-chromosome microdeletions. AZFc deletions are compatible with residual spermatogenesis, with oligospermia being a common presentation. These men may be candidates for intracytoplasmic sperm injection. Infertile men who do not have obstructive azoospermia, hypogonadotropic hypogonadism, or a karyotype abnormality should be tested for Y-chromosome microdeletions.

Retrograde ejaculation (Answer B) and congenital bilateral absence of the vas deferens (Answer E) are both causes of obstructive azoospermia, so they would not be consistent with this patient's semen analysis.

Retrograde ejaculation occurs when semen, which would normally be ejaculated via the urethra, is instead redirected to the bladder. Normally, the sphincter of the bladder contracts before ejaculation, which acts to both inhibit the release of urine and prevent a reflux of seminal fluids into the bladder during ejaculation. Any condition, medication or surgical procedure that interferes with central control of ejaculation or the autonomic innervation to the seminal tract, can cause ejaculatory dysfunction.

Congenital bilateral absence of the vas deferens due to a pathogenic variant in the cystic fibrosis transmembrane conductance regulator gene (CFTR) is a relatively frequent cause of infertility in men with obstructive azoospermia. However, given that this patient has a normal semen volume and pH, congenital absence of the vas deferens would not explain his presentation.

Kallmann syndrome (Answer C) is a condition characterized by congenital hypogonadotropic hypogonadism in association with anosmia or hyposmia. This patient's history of normal puberty,

normal testes size, and elevated FSH levels are not consistent with this condition.

This patient does not have mosaic Klinefelter syndrome (Answer D) given his normal testicular size and karyotype.

EDUCATIONAL OBJECTIVE
Describe the presentation of Y-chromosome microdeletions and outline the differential diagnosis of nonobstructive azoospermia.

REFERENCE(S)

Vogt PH, Edelmann A, Kirsch S, et al. Human Y chromosome azoospermia factors (AZF) mapped to different subregions in Yq11. *Hum Mol Genet.* 1996;5(7):933-943. PMID: 8817327

Pryor JL, Kent-First M, Muallem A, et al. Microdeletions in the Y chromosome of infertile men. *N Engl J Med.* 1997;336(8):534-539. PMID: 9023089

Stahl PJ, Schlegel PN. Genetic evaluation of the azoospermic or severely oligozoospermic male. *Curr Opin Obstet Gynecol.* 2012;24(4):221-228. PMID: 22729088

13 ANSWER: B) Normal testosterone, normal/high LH, high FSH

One of the most common long-term adverse effects of chemotherapy in men is gonadal dysfunction. After 1 year of follow-up, azoospermia is seen in 90% of men with Hodgkin lymphoma who have received more than 3 courses of an alkylating agent such as cyclophosphamide. Therefore, all men about to undergo gonadotoxic chemotherapy should be offered the option of sperm cryopreservation.

In the testis, the cells within the seminiferous tubules of the germinal epithelium have the highest mitotic and meiotic indices and are thus most susceptible to the toxic effects of chemotherapy. Damage to the seminiferous tubules decreases secretion of inhibin B from Sertoli cells. This drop in inhibin B, which is the major nonsteroidal regulator of FSH, leads to a 5- to 10-fold increase in FSH levels. By contrast, Leydig cells are less sensitive to the gonadal toxicity of chemotherapeutic agents than the germinal epithelium, which is why LH and testosterone levels are typically maintained within the normal range. In some situations, there may be evidence of subclinical Leydig-cell dysfunction, characterized by testosterone levels that are at the lower end of the normal range in association with elevated LH levels.

Based on this differential sensitivity of the cells of the testes to chemotherapy, the typical hormone profile of a patient with azoospermia following cyclophosphamide is that of normal testosterone, normal LH, and high FSH, which makes Answer B correct. Answer A is incorrect because in the setting of azoospermia, testosterone and LH levels are typically normal, but the FSH level would be elevated. Answer C depicts the hormone milieu of hypogonadotropic hypogonadism, which is what one would see following toxicity to the hypothalamus or pituitary rather than the testis. Answer C reflects a combination of both central (low LH, low testosterone) and peripheral defects in the hypothalamic-pituitary-gonadal axis and is incorrect, as the reproductive effects of cyclophosphamide are confined to the testis.

EDUCATIONAL OBJECTIVE
Explain the impact of cytotoxic chemotherapy on gonadal function and fertility in men.

REFERENCE(S)

Jahnukainen K, Ehmcke J, Hou M, Schlatt S. Testicular function and fertility preservation in male cancer patients. *Best Pract Res Clin Endocrinol Metab.* 2011;25(2):287-302. PMID: 21397199

Hayes FJ, Pitteloud N, DeCruz S, Crowley WF Jr, Boepple PA. Importance of inhibin B in the regulation of FSH secretion in the human male. *J Clin Endocrinol Metab.* 2001;86(11):5541-5546. PMID: 11701733

14 ANSWER: C) Continue current regimen

The goal of gender-affirming hormone therapy in transgender women is to promote a physical appearance that is more congruent with their gender identity. This is achieved by suppressing endogenous hormones of the biologic sex (ie, testosterone) and replacing them with those of the desired gender (ie, estradiol) and maintaining these levels in the physiologic range. For many patients, the physical change that is most desired is breast development. The regimen that the patient is currently using has resulted in the desired hormone milieu. Therefore, continuing this regimen (Answer C) and explaining to the patient that it can take 2 to 3 years for hormone therapy to have the maximum effect on breast development is the best management strategy.

Patients undergoing feminizing hormone therapy should wait a minimum of 12 months to maximize breast growth before breast augmentation surgery. Given that this patient has only been on hormone therapy for 6 months, referral for breast augmentation (Answer E) would be premature at this time.

Doubling the dosage of estrogen replacement (Answer A) when the estradiol level is already in the target range of 100 to 200 pg/mL (367-734 pmol/L) is unnecessary and places the patient at increased risk of adverse effects such as venous thromboembolism and hypertriglyceridemia. Similarly, switching her estrogen from 17β-estradiol to ethinyl estradiol (Answer B), which is the most thrombogenic estrogen, would have a negative effect on the risk-benefit ratio, especially in a patient with obesity.

Her testosterone level is already maximally suppressed, so adding the antiandrogen spironolactone (Answer D) would not provide any additional benefit.

EDUCATIONAL OBJECTIVE
Guide the hormonal care of a transgender patient to optimize breast development.

REFERENCE(S)

Hembree WC, Cohen-Kettenis PT, Gooren L, et al. Endocrine treatment of gender dysphoric/gender incongruent persons: an Endocrine Society clinical practice guideline. *J Clin Endocrinol Metab.* 2017;102(11):1-35. PMID: 28945902

T'Sjoen G, Arcelus J, Gooren L, Klink DT, Tangpricha V. Endocrinology of transgender medicine. *Endocr Rev.* 2019;40(1):97-117. PMID: 30307546

Safer JD, Tangpricha V. Care of transgender persons. *N Engl J Med.* 2019;381(25);2451-2460. PMID: 31851801

15 ANSWER: B) Switch her regimen to a GnRH agonist with a 0.05-mg estradiol patch

In male-to-female transgender patients, estrogen therapy is needed to develop female sexual characteristics. In patients with an intact hypothalamic-pituitary-gonadal axis, the estrogen dosage needed is supraphysiologic given the need to suppress testosterone secretion. However, combined use of a GnRH agonist with estrogen allows physiologic dosages of estrogen to be used, as testosterone secretion is already suppressed. Estrogen therapy can result in marked hypertriglyceridemia. However, the lipid effects of estrogen depend on the route of administration, with the transdermal route having less effect on HDL cholesterol and triglycerides than the oral route. Given this patient's history of hypertriglyceridemia, she is not a suitable candidate for oral estrogen and the most appropriate hormone regimen would be a GnRH agonist and a low-dosage estrogen patch (Answer B), which can be titrated based on clinical response and triglyceride levels. Ethinyl estradiol (Answer D) would not be a good choice because of its negative effects on triglycerides, as well as the fact that it increases the risk of venous thromboembolism significantly more so than 17β-estradiol.

Using spironolactone alone without an estrogen (Answer A) would not provide adequate suppression and blockade of androgen action for the desired physical effects. Based on the laboratory data provided, her testosterone level was not adequately suppressed on this dosage of spironolactone even when previously combined with conjugated equine estrogen. Adding a 5α-reductase inhibitor such as finasteride (Answer E) would neither lower testosterone nor increase estradiol levels. Finasteride can be considered in situations where spironolactone is contraindicated such as hyperkalemia or to alleviate male-pattern balding.

Given that the patient has been living as a woman for more than 2 decades, and considering the increased risk of depression and suicide in the transgender population, withholding further hormone therapy (Answer C) would most likely negatively affect her mental health. In addition, estrogen therapy was not her only risk factor for hypertriglyceridemia.

EDUCATIONAL OBJECTIVE
Guide the hormonal care of a transgender patient with hypertriglyceridemia.

REFERENCE(S)
Hembree WC, Cohen-Kettenis PT, Gooren L, et al. Endocrine treatment of gender-dysphoric/gender-incongruent persons: an Endocrine Society clinical practice guideline. *J Clin Endocrinol Metab.* 2017;102(11):3869-3903. PMID: 28945902

Aljenedil S, Hegele RA, Genest J, Awan Z. Estrogen-associated severe hypertriglyceridemia with pancreatitis. *J Clin Lipidol.* 2017;11(1):297-300. PMID: 28391900

Lufkin EG, Ory SJ. Relative value of transdermal and oral estrogen therapy in various clinical situations. *Mayo Clin Proc.* 1994;69(2):131-135. PMID: 8309263

16 ANSWER: E) Partial androgen insensitivity syndrome

This patient's presentation with hypospadias, cryptorchidism, small testes, gynecomastia, high-normal testosterone level, and elevated gonadotropin concentrations is consistent with partial androgen insensitivity (Answer E). The phenotypic spectrum of androgen insensitivity ranges from that of a phenotypic female at the most severe end of the spectrum (complete androgen resistance) to that of a virilized male with oligospermia at the mildest end of the spectrum. Partial androgen insensitivity is due to a pathogenic variant in the androgen receptor gene located on the X chromosome. In some cases, there may be a history of a family member presenting with primary amenorrhea or an inguinal hernia as a neonate.

Congenital adrenal hyperplasia due to 21 hydroxylase deficiency (Answer A) is the most common form, and it results in impaired conversion of 17-hydroxyprogesterone to 11-deoxycortisol. Males with this form of congenital adrenal hyperplasia have impaired cortisol production but normal testosterone production. Therefore, 21-hydroxylase deficiency would not explain this patient's clinical presentation.

One of the key clinical features that helps to refine the differential diagnosis in this case is the presence of hypospadias. In patients with hypospadias, the urethral opening occurs on the underside of the penis rather than the tip due to insufficient testosterone production in the first trimester of pregnancy when sexual differentiation is occurring. Thus, while a patient with Klinefelter syndrome could present with cryptorchidism, gynecomastia, small testes, and a high-normal testosterone level if he is being treated with testosterone (Answer B), it would not explain his decreased body hair or hypospadias, as testosterone production is normal in utero in a patient with Klinefelter syndrome.

5α-Reductase deficiency (Answer C) is a rare autosomal recessive disorder in which patients with a 46,XY karyotype have impaired virilization during embryogenesis due to defective conversion of testosterone to dihydrotestosterone. These patients often present with ambiguous genitalia and may be reared as girls in childhood. However, patients with a milder phenotype may present with hypospadias. Two of the features that help to distinguish this condition from partial androgen insensitivity are the absence of gynecomastia and gonadotropins in the low-normal range. Thus, 5α-reductase deficiency would not explain this patient's presentation.

Polyglandular autoimmune syndrome type 2 (Answer D) is an autoimmune disorder that affects multiple endocrine organs and most commonly results in type 1 diabetes, Addison disease, and hypothyroidism. While primary hypogonadism can be part of the presentation of polyglandular autoimmune syndrome type 2 and this patient indeed has a diagnosis of hypothyroidism, he does not have any of the other manifestations and it would not explain his cryptorchidism or hypospadias.

EDUCATIONAL OBJECTIVE
Diagnose partial androgen insensitivity and construct a differential diagnosis for hypospadias.

REFERENCE(S)

Mongan NP, Tadokoro-Cuccaro R, Bunch T, Hughes IA. Androgen insensitivity syndrome. *Best Pract Res Clin Endocrinol Metab.* 2015;29(4):569-580. PMID: 26303084

Okeigwe I, Kuohung W. 5-Alpha reductase deficiency: a 40-year retrospective review. *Curr Opin Endocrinol Diabetes Obes.* 2014;21(6):483-487. PMID: 25321150

Merke DP, Auchus RJ. Congenital adrenal hyperplasia due to 21-hydroxylase deficiency. *N Engl J Med.* 2020;383(13):1248-1261. PMID: 32966723

17 ANSWER: C) Estrogen-secreting testicular tumor

Gynecomastia is a benign enlargement of the male breast due mainly to the proliferation of ductal tissue. Gynecomastia develops when there is an increase in the ratio of estrogen to androgens, with the former having a stimulatory effect on breast tissue, while the latter antagonize this effect. A small degree of breast enlargement is a relatively common finding, especially in older men, and it generally does not require any workup when asymptomatic. However, breast enlargement that is prominent, painful, progressive, or of recent onset, as in this case, requires thorough evaluation.

The presence of breast tenderness suggests benign breast growth of recent onset. He has a low testosterone concentration and low gonadotropin concentrations, but the most striking abnormality is a greater than 3-fold increase in estradiol levels. Increased estradiol levels may reflect increased testicular secretion of estradiol, increased extraglandular aromatization of estrogen precursors secreted by the adrenal glands, increased extraglandular aromatase activity, or exposure to exogenous estrogens. Testicular tumors can cause gynecomastia by a number of mechanisms. The production of hCG by germ-cell tumors can stimulate the production of testosterone and estradiol by normal testicular tissue. Unlike germ-cell tumors, Leydig-cell tumors can secrete estradiol directly and in as many as 50% of cases, gynecomastia precedes the development of a palpable testicular mass, but the tumor is usually detectable by ultrasonography. In this patient, the elevated estradiol level, suppressed gonadotropins due to estrogen-mediated negative feedback, and low testosterone levels are best explained by an estrogen-secreting testicular tumor (Answer C).

Hyperprolactinemia (Answer A) can suppress GnRH secretion, resulting in low testosterone levels and gynecomastia. However, the modestly elevated prolactin level in this vignette would not be sufficient to lower testosterone and would also not explain the high estradiol level. In this case, the elevated prolactin is most likely the result of stimulation of the lactotrophs by the estrogen-secreting tumor.

Finasteride (Answer B) modestly raises serum testosterone concentrations by blocking the conversion of testosterone to dihydrotestosterone, so it would not explain this patient's gynecomastia or hormone profile.

The patient's TSH level is not provided. However, his presentation is not consistent with hyperthyroidism (Answer D) given his normal thyroid examination, absence of clinical features of hyperthyroidism, and the fact that his testosterone level is low rather than high-normal, as would be expected in the hyperthyroid state due to high SHBG levels.

EDUCATIONAL OBJECTIVE
Identify the clinical and biochemical features of an estrogen-secreting Leydig-cell tumor.

REFERENCE(S)

Case Records of the Massachusetts General Hospital. Weekly clinicopathological conferences. Case 12-2000. A 60-year-old man with persistent gynecomastia after excision of a pituitary adenoma [published correction appears in *N Engl J Med*. 2000;343(1):76]. *N Engl J Med*. 2000;342(16);1196-1204. PMID: 10770986

Amory JK, Wang C, Swerdloff RS, et al. The effect of 5alpha-reductase inhibition with dutasteride and finasteride on semen parameters and serum hormones in healthy men [published correction appears in *J Clin Endocrinol Metab*. 2007;92(11):4379]. *J Clin Endocrinol Metab*. 2007;92(5):1659-1665. PMID: 17299062

Braunstein GD. Clinical practice. Gynecomastia. *N Engl J Med*. 2007;357(12):1229-1237. PMID: 17881754

18 **ANSWER: D) Testosterone abuse**
This patient has tender gynecomastia. Breast tenderness suggests benign breast growth of recent onset (<6 months). He also has elevated total and free testosterone concentrations, a high estradiol concentration, and low gonadotropin concentrations. This combination can be due to exogenous testosterone abuse (Answer D), endogenous or exogenous testosterone precursors (eg, dehydroepiandrosterone from an adrenal tumor), and endogenous or exogenous hCG (eg, hCG from a germ-cell tumor).

Although chronic hepatitis (Answer A) is commonly associated with elevated SHBG concentrations, the hormone profile in such cases would be a high-normal or elevated total testosterone but a normal free fraction, so it would not explain this patient's hormone profile. An estrogen-secreting testicular tumor (Answer B) would cause elevated estradiol concentrations and suppressed gonadotropins but testosterone levels would not be high. Finasteride (Answer C) modestly raises serum testosterone concentrations by blocking the conversion of testosterone to dihydrotestosterone, but it would not cause suppressed gonadotropin concentrations. In men with hyperthyroidism (Answer E), there is increased hepatic production of SHBG, which results in high levels of total but low or low-normal levels of free testosterone, high estradiol levels, and normal LH levels. Thus, hyperthyroidism would not explain this patient's hormone profile.

EDUCATIONAL OBJECTIVE

Identify the clinical and biochemical features of exogenous testosterone abuse.

REFERENCE(S)

Amory JK, Wang C, Swerdloff RS, et al. The effect of 5alpha-reductase inhibition with dutasteride and finasteride on semen parameters and serum hormones in healthy men [published correction appears in *J Clin Endocrinol Metab.* 2007;92(11):4379]. *J Clin Endocrinol Metab.* 2007;92(5):1659-1665. PMID: 17299062

Braunstein GD. Clinical practice. Gynecomastia. *N Engl J Med.* 2007;357(12):1229-1237. PMID: 17881754

Anawalt BD. Gynecomastia. In: Jameson JL, De Groot LJ, eds. *Endocrinology: Adult and Pediatric.* 7th ed. Philadelphia, PA: Saunders Elsevier; 2015.

Obesity and Lipids Board Review

Sangeeta R. Kashyap, MD

1 **ANSWER: D) Perform a mixed-meal tolerance test to diagnose hyperinsulinemic hypoglycemia after gastric bypass**

Nonspecific postprandial symptoms are common in patients who have had gastric bypass surgery. This patient presents with neuroglycopenia and a home glucose reading of 47 mg/dL (2.6 mmol/L), which resolved with treatment. She requires further evaluation with a mixed-meal tolerance test (Answer D).

Indeed, many hypoglycemia symptoms are common and not specific to hypoglycemia (eg, tremor, tachycardia, and diaphoresis). However, the diagnosis of a true hypoglycemic disorder as presented in this case requires documentation of a low plasma glucose concentration (<50-55 mg/dL [<2.8-3.1 mmol/L]) in the presence of symptoms compatible with neuroglycopenia that are ameliorated by correction of low glucose (Whipple triad). In contrast to dumping syndrome (Answer A), which is noted soon after gastric bypass surgery and improves with time, hyperinsulinemic hypoglycemia presents several months to years (usually >1 year) after surgery. The hallmark of this rare syndrome is severe postprandial neuroglycopenia, which is characteristically absent in dumping.

Hyperinsulinemic hypoglycemia after gastric bypass is characterized by increased prandial GLP-1 levels and would not be treated with a GLP-1 receptor agonist (Answer C). In contrast, a GLP-1 antagonist has been used experimentally to correct this response. Malabsorption after gastric bypass usually presents with steatorrhea and does not lead to low postprandial blood glucose levels. Supplementing with pancreatic enzymes (Answer B) is incorrect.

EDUCATIONAL OBJECTIVE

Diagnose and manage post–gastric bypass hypoglycemia related to hyperinsulinemic hypoglycemia.

REFERENCE(S)

Patti ME, Li P, Goldfine AB. Insulin response to oral stimuli and glucose effectiveness increased in neuroglycopenia following gastric bypass. *Obesity.* 2015;23(4):798-807. PMID: 25755084

Goldfine AB, Mun EC, Devine E, et al. Patients with neuroglycopenia after gastric bypass surgery have exaggerated incretin and insulin secretory responses to a mixed meal. *J Clin Endocrinol Metab.* 2007;92(12):4678-4685. PMID: 17895322

2 **ANSWER: B) 48-year-old patient; hemoglobin A$_{1c}$ of 7.0%; 4-year duration of diabetes; metformin; Roux-en-Y gastric bypass**

Gastric bypass and sleeve gastrectomy result in remission of type 2 diabetes for up to 5 years in randomized controlled trials of metabolic surgery vs medical treatment. The preoperative predictors of diabetes remission include shorter duration of diabetes, younger age, lower hemoglobin A$_{1c}$ level, oral agent vs insulin use, and type of surgery (Roux-en-Y gastric bypass is the most effective). Compared with sleeve gastrectomy, Roux-en-Y gastric bypass results in higher rates of biochemical remission. Laparoscopic gastric banding results in a similar rate of remission to that of metformin when used in patients with new-onset type 2 diabetes. The patient described in Answer B depicts the optimal clinical characteristics: younger age, shorter duration of diabetes, well-controlled diabetes on an oral agent, and Roux-en-Y gastric bypass.

EDUCATIONAL OBJECTIVE
Identify predictors of diabetes remission following bariatric surgery.

REFERENCE(S)

Still CD, Wood GC, Benotti P, et al. Preoperative prediction of type 2 diabetes remission after Roux-en-Y gastric bypass surgery: a retrospective cohort study. *Lancet Diabetes Endocrinol.* 2013;2(1):38-45. PMID: 24579062

Schauer PR, Burguera B, Ikramuddin S, et al. Effect of laparoscopic Roux-en Y gastric bypass on type 2 diabetes mellitus. *Ann Surg.* 2003;238(4):467-484. PMID: 14530719

Brethauer SA, Aminian A, Romero-Talamás H, et al. Can diabetes be surgically cured? Long-term metabolic effects of bariatric surgery in obese patients with type 2 diabetes mellitus. *Ann Surg.* 2013;258(4):628-637. PMID: 24018646

Xiang AH, Trigo E, Martinez M, et al; RISE Consortium; RISE Collaborators. Impact of gastric banding versus metformin on beta-cell function in adults with impaired glucose tolerance or mild type 2 diabetes. *Diabetes Care.* PMID: 30282699

3 ANSWER: A) Reduced total daily energy expenditure; reduced resting metabolic rate; reduced exercise energy expenditure

Weight loss from diet and exercise often leads to weight regain. In response to a hypocaloric diet, an energy deficit occurs, which results in increased hunger and reduced energy expenditure. The difference between energy desired and energy required is termed the energy gap. With weight loss that results in lower body mass index and body surface area, there is a reduction in energy expenditure, resting metabolic rate, and total daily expenditure. On the expenditure side, diet-induced weight loss reduces total daily energy expenditure because of a lower resting metabolic rate and the thermic effect of food, and it often decreases exercise energy expenditure and nonexercise activity thermogenesis. Increased hunger and decreased energy expenditure can readily promote weight regain.

Thus, Answer A correctly identifies the features of metabolic adaptation following weight loss.

EDUCATIONAL OBJECTIVE
Identify metabolic adaptation to weight loss and factors that promote weight gain following caloric restriction.

REFERENCE(S)

Melby CL, Paris HL, Foright RM, Peth J. Attenuating the biologic drive for weight regain following weight loss: must what goes down always go back up? *Nutrients.* 2017;9(5):468. PMID: 28481261

4 ANSWER: B) Worsened dietary adherence; no difference in weight loss; no difference in triglycerides; no difference in blood pressure

Short-term uncontrolled studies have shown that alternate-day fasting results in improved weight loss, increased insulin sensitivity, and improved lipid profiles. However, a recent randomized controlled trial that compared alternate-day fasting with restricted daily caloric intake in adults with obesity (average BMI = 34 kg/m²) did not show any difference in weight loss or lipid profiles. Dietary adherence was, in fact, worse in the alternate-day fasting group vs the restricted daily caloric intake group. Thus, the expected pattern of alternate-day fasting is best depicted in Answer B.

EDUCATIONAL OBJECTIVE
List the clinical outcomes of intermittent fasting for weight loss.

REFERENCE(S)

Trepanowski JF, Kroeger CM, Barnosky A, et al. Effect of alternate-day fasting on weight loss, weight maintenance, and cardioprotection among metabolically healthy obese adults: a randomized clinical trial. *JAMA Intern Med.* 2017;177(7):930-938. PMID: 28459931

Sutton EF, Beyl R, Early KS, Cefalu WT, Ravussin E, Peterson CM. Early time-restricted feeding improves insulin sensitivity, blood pressure, and oxidative stress even without weight loss in men with prediabetes. *Cell Metab.* 2018;27(6):1212-1221. PMID: 29754952

5 ANSWER: A) Start pravastatin, 10 mg daily, and reevaluate in 3 months

The incidence of statin-induced new-onset diabetes is higher in patients with impaired fasting glucose and elevated BMI and usually occurs with more potent statins (eg, rosuvastatin vs pravastatin). Thus, the best course of action is to start with pravastatin and reevaluate this patient for hyperglycemia in 3 months (Answer A). There is no evidence to suggest that metformin treatment prior to initiation of a statin (Answer C) or concomitant use of metformin and pravastatin (Answer D) lowers the risk of statin-induced new-onset diabetes. Post hoc evaluation of previously reported statin trials showed a small increase in the risk of developing new-onset diabetes, which is associated with all statins. Potential mechanisms include reduced insulin secretion and reduced insulin sensitivity.

The JUPITER trial (Justification for Use of Statins in Prevention: An Intervention Trial Evaluating Rosuvastatin), a primary prevention trial in which 17,802 patients were randomly assigned to receive rosuvastatin, 20 mg daily, or placebo over a 1.9-year period showed an overall 27% increase in investigator-reported diabetes mellitus in patients treated with rosuvastatin compared with placebo and a moderate but significant increase of median hemoglobin A_{1c} levels in the rosuvastatin arm. Almost all of the excess risk occurred in participants with baseline evidence of impaired fasting glucose. There were 134 vascular events or deaths avoided for every 54 new cases of diabetes. The statin benefit was as good in those who developed diabetes as in the trial as a whole.

Further studies have identified additional risk factors in statin-treated patients at risk for developing diabetes, including elevated plasma glucose, triglycerides, BMI higher than 30 kg/m², and presence of hypertension.

EDUCATIONAL OBJECTIVE
Identify the adverse effect of new-onset diabetes mellitus in patients treated with statins.

REFERENCE(S)
Ruscica M, Macchi C, Morlotti B, Sirtori CR, Magni P. Statin therapy and related risk of new-onset type 2 diabetes mellitus. *Eur J Intern Med.* 2014;25(5):401-406. PMID: 24685426

Ridker PM, Pradhan A, MacFadyen JG, Libby P, Glynn RJ. Cardiovascular benefits and diabetes risks of statin therapy in primary prevention: an analysis from the JUPITER trial. *Lancet.* 2012;380(9841):565-571. PMID: 22883507

6 ANSWER: C) Significant improvement in quality of life, depression, and sleep apnea

The Look AHEAD trial compared the effect of intensive lifestyle intervention with a control standard regimen of diabetes support and education among patients with type 2 diabetes and a BMI greater than 25 kg/m². At a median follow-up of almost 10 years, there was no significant difference between the 2 groups in cardiovascular morbidity and mortality (thus, Answer A is incorrect). Initial mean weight loss in the intervention group was 8.6% at 12 months. This was followed by weight regain through year 5 and then a subsequent gradual decrease in weight, resulting in an average weight loss of 6.0% at the end of the trial. The weight loss is not expected to be durable (thus, Answer D is incorrect). The control group had gradual but consistent weight loss throughout the study, resulting in an average weight loss of 3.5% at the end of the trial. The intervention group also had greater improvements in fitness, particularly at 1 year, along with improved obesity-related comorbidities such as reduced depression, decreased medication use, and improved quality of life (thus, Answer C is correct and Answer B is incorrect). Even minor weight loss is associated with improved hemoglobin A_{1c} levels (thus, Answer E is incorrect).

EDUCATIONAL OBJECTIVE
Describe the clinical effect of weight loss induced by intensive diet and exercise on mortality from cardiovascular disease and cardiovascular risk factors in patients with type 2 diabetes and overweight or obesity.

REFERENCE(S)

Look AHEAD Research Group, Wing RR, Bolin P, et al. Cardiovascular effects of intensive lifestyle intervention in type 2 diabetes [published correction appears in *N Engl J Med.* 2014;370(19):1866]. *N Engl J Med.* 2013;369(2):145-154. PMID: 23796131

7 ANSWER: E) Antioxidant supplements (ie, vitamins C and E) and folic acid

Antioxidant supplements (ie, vitamins C and E) and folic acid (Answer E) have not been demonstrated to have a protective cardiovascular effect in large observational studies. However, multiple observational studies have consistently documented the association between fish intake and reduced cardiovascular risk. The American Heart Association recommends that individuals without coronary heart disease consume fish at least twice a week, specifically oily fish such as tuna, mackerel, trout, or salmon. Thus, omega-3 fatty acids (Answer A) have a protective, not neutral, effect on cardiovascular risk.

Increased total dietary fiber consumption (Answer B) is associated with reduced risk of cardiovascular disease and coronary health in observational studies. Currently, more than 25 g of total fiber daily is recommended for possibly improving cardiovascular disease outcomes, and 10 to 25 g of soluble fiber daily is recommended for lipid-lowering therapy.

Plant sterols (Answer C) are chemically similar to animal cholesterol, and they can lower LDL cholesterol up to 15% with a maximally effective intake of about 2 g daily. This is primarily achieved by reducing cholesterol absorption in the intestines, but also through downstream biochemical effects of receptor binding.

While alcohol use is not encouraged, for those currently consuming alcohol, the American Heart Association recommends limiting intake to 2 servings per day in men and 1 serving per day in women. Epidemiologic data suggest that this quantity of alcohol (Answer D) may be associated with a decreased risk of cardiovascular disease, but whether initiating consumption of alcohol in those who have abstained lowers cardiovascular disease events is unknown.

EDUCATIONAL OBJECTIVE
Identify dietary factors potentially affecting risk of cardiovascular disease.

REFERENCE(S)

Van Horn L, McCoin M, Kris-Etherton PM, et al. The evidence for dietary prevention and treatment of cardiovascular disease. *J Am Diet Assoc.* 2008;108(2):287-331. PMID: 18237578

Heart Protection Study Collaborative Group. MRC/BHF Heart Protection Study of antioxidant vitamin supplementation in 20,536 high-risk individuals: a randomised placebo-controlled trial. *Lancet.* 2002;360(9326):23-33. PMID: 12114037

American Heart Association Nutrition Committee; Lichtenstein AH, Appel LJ, et al. Diet and lifestyle recommendations revisions 2006: a scientific statement from the American Heart Association Nutrition Committee. *Circulation.* 2006:114(1):82-96. PMID: 16785338

8 ANSWER: B) Vitamin E, 800 IU daily

Nonalcoholic fatty liver disease (NAFLD), the most common cause of chronic liver disease in the western world, encompasses a histologic spectrum of liver disease ranging from simple steatosis to nonalcoholic steatohepatitis (NASH), which can progress to cirrhosis and liver cancer. In the United States, the prevalence of NAFLD and NASH is estimated to be 17% to 33% and 5.7% to 17%, respectively. The disease is closely associated with obesity and diabetes and, due to their ongoing epidemics, the prevalence of NAFLD both in adults and children is likely to increase over time and continue to be a serious public health burden. Currently, there is no definitive treatment for this disease. NASH is characterized histologically by the presence of hepatic steatosis, lobular inflammation, and hepatocyte ballooning. Although the precise mechanism underlying disease progression from steatosis alone to NASH remains poorly understood, it is believed that oxidative stress has a central role contributing to hepatocellular injury. Thus, an effective therapeutic strategy is to target reduction in oxidative stress in patients with this disease.

In the PIVENS trial (Pioglitazone versus Vitamin E versus Placebo for the Treatment of Nondiabetic Patients with Nonalcoholic Steatohepatitis), vitamin E therapy (Answer B) demonstrated significant improvement in steatosis, inflammation, ballooning, and resolution of steatohepatitis in adult patients with aggressive NASH who did not have diabetes or cirrhosis.

Pioglitazone (Answer C) has some benefits for NAFLD and NASH in patients with type 2 diabetes, but the patient in this vignette does not have diabetes.

Vitamin D (Answer A) has no established role in the treatment of NASH. Statin agents are important for reducing cardiovascular disease risk in patients with NAFLD, but they do not treat liver disease itself.

Metformin use (Answer E) is not associated with improvement in nonalcoholic steatohepatitis.

Although atorvastatin (Answer D) is indicated for lowering cardiovascular disease risk, it does not improve nonalcoholic steatohepatitis.

EDUCATIONAL OBJECTIVE
Recommend vitamin E in the management of nonalcoholic steatohepatitis in patients with obesity who do not have diabetes mellitus.

REFERENCE(S)
Sanyal AJ, Chalasani N, Kowdley KV, et al; NASH CRN. Pioglitazone, vitamin E, or placebo for nonalcoholic steatohepatitis. *N Engl J Med.* 2010;362(18):1675-1685. PMID: 20427778

McCullough AJ. Pathophysiology of nonalcoholic steatohepatitis. *J Clin Gastroenterol.* 2006;40(Suppl 1):S17-S29. PMID: 16540762

9 **ANSWER: B) Add alirocumab**
PCSK9 inhibitors (evolocumab and alirocumab [Answer B]) are a new class of medications used to significantly lower LDL cholesterol and reduce cardiovascular disease. They are monoclonal antibodies that target and degrade the PCSK9 protein. PCSK9 circulates in the blood and alters the liver's handling of LDL cholesterol.

Both evolocumab and alirocumab are US FDA approved for clinical atherosclerotic cardiovascular disease and heterozygous familial hyperlipidemia. PCSK9 inhibitors have been studied in statin-intolerant patients (GAUSS-1 and GAUSS-2 studies), but statin intolerance alone is not currently an approved indication in the absence of clinical atherosclerotic cardiovascular disease or familial hyperlipidemia. Clinical trials have shown that LDL cholesterol is lowered approximately 60% by evolocumab and 55% to 60% by alirocumab, which would most likely reduce this patient's LDL-cholesterol concentration below 100 mg/dL (<2.59 mmol/L). The FOURIER trial showed that evolocumab reduced LDL cholesterol 59% in patients with known coronary disease and a baseline LDL-cholesterol level of 70 mg/dL or greater (≥1.81 mmol/L) who were taking a statin compared with placebo and lowered cardiovascular event rates by 15% over 3 years (hazard ratio, 0.85; 95% CI, 0.79-0.92). Additionally, the study indicated there was added benefit at lower LDL-cholesterol levels than previously targeted.

In the ODYSSEY trial of alirocumab vs placebo after acute coronary syndrome, LDL cholesterol was lowered in the alirocumab group by 54.7% compared with LDL cholesterol in the placebo group at 48 months (mean LDL-cholesterol concentration of 53.3 mg/dL vs 101.4 mg/dL, respectively). Risk of a major cardiovascular event was lowered by 15% (hazard ratio, 0.85; 95% CI, 0.78-0.93; P = .0003) (preliminary results released at the American College of Cardiology – 67th Scientific Sessions, March 2010).

The newer data regarding LDL-cholesterol lowering and associated decreased cardiovascular disease risk will most likely shift the focus back to absolute LDL-cholesterol levels from the general group targets recommended in the 2013 American College of Cardiology/American Heart Association Cholesterol-Lowering Guidelines.

Niacin has been shown to lower LDL cholesterol in some trials in men, but it may also worsen this patient's glycemic control. Thus, increasing the dosage (Answer A) is incorrect. Fenofibrate (Answer C) has not been shown to decrease cardiovascular disease event rates.

Lipopheresis (Answer D) has been used to clear LDL particles and reduce cardiovascular disease risk in some patients with heterozygous and homozygous familial hyperlipidemia, but it is invasive, not widely available, and would be an option only if all medications failed. Increasing the pravastatin dosage to 80 mg daily (Answer E) would not effectively lower the LDL cholesterol to target in this case.

EDUCATIONAL OBJECTIVE
Explain the indications for using PCSK9 inhibitors to treat patients with hyperlipidemia.

REFERENCE(S)

Schwartz GG, Steg PG, Szarek M, et al; ODYSSEY OUTCOMES Committees and Investigators. Alirocumab and cardiovascular outcomes after acute coronary syndrome. *N Engl J Med.* 2018;379(22):2097-2107. PMID: 30403574

Sabatine MS, Giugliano RP, Keech AC, et al; FOURIER Steering Committee and Investigators. Evolocumab and clinical outcomes in patients with cardiovascular disease. *N Engl J Med.* 2017; 376(18):1713-1722. PMID: 28304224

Sabatine MS, Giugliano RP, Wiviott SD, et al; Open-Label Study of Long-Term Evaluation against LDL Cholesterol (OSLER) Investigators. Efficacy and safety of evolocumab in reducing lipids and cardiovascular events. *N Engl J Med.* 2015;372(16):1500-1509. PMID: 25773607

Ajufo E, Rader DJ. Recent advances in the pharmacological management of hypercholesterolemia. *Lancet Diabetes Endocrinol.* 2016;4(5):436-446. PMID: 27012540

Steg PG, et al. Joint ACC/JACC Late-Breaking Clinical Trials. Presented at: American College of Cardiology Scientific Session; March 10-12, 2018; Orlando, FL.

10 ANSWER: B) Myositis

A number of medications increase risk of myositis (Answer B) with statins. This is thought to be due to reduced statin clearance by the liver. In this situation, the concern is that interaction with the protease inhibitor will increase the risk of myositis, which might lead to statin discontinuation. Reintroduction of the statin at a lower dosage or after a change in HIV therapy is, however, a possibility. The best-studied drug interaction is that with gemfibrozil, which markedly increases circulating statin levels. Cyclosporine, which is often used as a long-term treatment in transplant recipients, also increases myositis risk. Greater LDL-cholesterol reduction in patients such as this one may be achieved with the use of low statin dosages supplemented with other LDL-cholesterol reduction therapies such as ezetimibe. Resins are likely to increase the patient's triglyceride levels. Other drugs that increase myositis risk include ketoconazole and erythromycin. Patients taking a short-term course of these drugs are advised to stop their statins.

Patients such as the one in this vignette often develop diabetes mellitus (Answer A). High-dosage statin therapy will probably increase this risk, but it would not be a reason to avoid lowering LDL cholesterol in a patient at high risk of cardiovascular disease. Statins do not inhibit antiviral agents (Answer C). Increased transaminase levels occur in 1% to 2% of patients taking statins. However, liver disease (Answer E) caused by statins is rare, and provided the increases in transaminase levels are less than 3 times the upper normal limit, it is acceptable to continue lipid-lowering therapy. For this reason, the US FDA has recently changed its guidelines on monitoring liver function in statin-treated patients—it now recommends checking liver enzymes "as clinically indicated." Worsening of lipoatrophy (Answer D) is not expected with the use of statins.

EDUCATIONAL OBJECTIVE
Identify the potential interaction of statins with protease inhibitors, which may lead to an increased risk of myositis.

REFERENCE(S)

Venero CV, Thompson PD. Managing statin myopathy. *Endocrinol Metab Clin North Am.* 2009;38(1):121-136. PMID: 19217515

Thompson PD, Clarkson P, Karas RH. Statin-associated myopathy. *JAMA*. 2003;289(13):1681-1690. PMID: 12672737

Kirchner JT. Clinical management considerations for dyslipidemia in HIV-infected individuals. *Postgrad Med*. 2012;124(1):31-40. PMID: 22314112

11 ANSWER: D) Switch metoprolol to amlodipine

Patients with collagen-vascular disease can develop severe hyperlipidemia. Occasionally, this is due to the production of antibodies that can inhibit lipoprotein lipase or heparin (and lipase binding to endothelium). Antibodies can also be directed to apolipoproteins: antibodies to apolipoprotein B lead to hypobetalipoproteinemia, and antibodies to apolipoprotein AI lead to low HDL-cholesterol levels. Several medications in this setting, as well as in patients without collagen-vascular disease, can exacerbate hypertriglyceridemia. One such class of medications is β-adrenergic blockers. Thus, substituting a calcium-channel blocker for metoprolol (Answer D) is correct.

Changing from one steroid to another (Answer A) should not affect hypertriglyceridemia. Although thiazide diuretics increase triglycerides, so do loop diuretics (Answer C). Lisinopril (Answer B) does not affect triglyceride levels.

EDUCATIONAL OBJECTIVE
Advise patients on medications, such as β-adrenergic blockers, that increase triglyceride levels.

REFERENCE(S)
Stone NJ. Secondary causes of hyperlipidemia. *Med Clin North Am*. 1994;78(1):117-141. PMID: 8283927

Dinu AR, Merrill JT, Shen C, Antonov IV, Myones BL, Lahita RG. Frequency of antibodies to the cholesterol transport protein apolipoprotein A1 in patients with SLE. *Lupus*. 1998;7(5):355-360. PMID: 9696140

12 ANSWER: D) Skin irritation/rash

The adverse event profile of PCSK9 inhibitor medications is favorable. In the FOURIER trial of evolocumab vs placebo, all adverse events were similar between evolocumab and placebo with the exception of injection site reactions that were uncommon but were slightly higher in the evolocumab group (2.1% vs 1.6%; $P < .001$), although allergic reactions were similar (3.1% vs 2.9%). Neurocognitive dysfunction (Answer A) was rare and similar between groups (1.6% vs 1.5%). Although there has been no evidence of cognitive dysfunction to date in clinical trials, there remains concern for patients who achieve very low levels of LDL cholesterol (eg, <30 mg/dL [<0.78 mmol/L]) on therapy. The incidence of liver enzyme elevation (Answer B) 3 or more times the upper normal limit was similar between groups (1.8% vs 1.8%). Myalgias (Answer C) (5.0 vs 4.8%), elevated creatine kinase (0.7% vs 0.7%), and rhabdomyolysis (0.1% vs 0.1%) were similar in treatment vs placebo groups, respectively.

In the ODYSSEY trial of alirocumab vs placebo after acute coronary syndrome, the only adverse event more common in the alirocumab group was injection site reaction on the skin (Answer D) (3.8% vs 2.1%, respectively; hazard ratio, 1.82; 95% CI, 1.54-2.17) (preliminary results released at the American College of Cardiology – 67th Scientific Sessions, March 2010).

There is also concern for the development of new-onset diabetes with use of PCSK9 inhibitor therapy similar to what has been observed with statins. This is based on genetic epidemiology studies showing that loss-of-function pathogenic variants in the gene encoding PCSK9 are associated with lower LDL cholesterol and lower risk of cardiovascular disease but increased risk of type 2 diabetes. Increased risk of type 2 diabetes has not been demonstrated in clinical trials so far, but longer-term studies are needed to fully elucidate this risk.

EDUCATIONAL OBJECTIVE
Describe the adverse effect profile of the new class of cholesterol-lowering medications, PCSK9 inhibitors.

REFERENCE(S)

Sabatine MS, Giugliano RP, Keech AC, et al; FOURIER Steering Committee and Investigators. Evolocumab and clinical outcomes in patients with cardiovascular disease. *N Engl J Med.* 2017;376(18):1713-1722. PMID: 28304224

Sabatine MS, Giugliano RP, Wiviott SD, et al; Open-Label Study of Long-Term Evaluation against LDL Cholesterol (OSLER) Investigators. Efficacy and safety of evolocumab in reducing lipids and cardiovascular events. *N Engl J Med.* 2015;372(16):1500-1509. PMID: 25773607

Steg PG, et al. Joint ACC/JACC Late-Breaking Clinical Trials. Presented at: American College of Cardiology Scientific Session; March 10-12, 2018; Orlando, FL.

Schwartz GG, Steg PG, Szarek M, et al; ODYSSEY OUTCOMES Committees and Investigators. Alirocumab and cardiovascular outcomes after acute coronary syndrome. *N Engl J Med.* 2018;379(22):2097-2107. PMID: 30403574

13 ANSWER: A) Vitamin B_{12}

Roux-en-Y gastric bypass is associated with thiamine deficiency, B_{12} deficiency, and, less commonly, zinc deficiency that typically causes a rash and diarrhea. Laparoscopic gastric banding procedures do not bypass any intestinal segment and therefore do not cause malabsorption. Laparoscopic gastric banding is not associated with vitamin or mineral deficiencies. Biliopancreatic diversion (duodenal switch) can cause significant malabsorption and vitamin and mineral deficiencies as late complications due to depleted body stores.

Vitamin B_{12} deficiency (Answer A) can cause the neurologic symptoms and signs observed in this patient, as well as megaloblastic anemia, but the body stores a sizeable amount of B_{12} in the liver. Vitamin B_{12} deficiency does not usually occur until 6 to 24 months after bariatric surgery. Sleeve gastrectomy can be associated with B_{12} deficiency, but it is not as common after this procedure as it is with gastric bypass. Vitamin B_{12} is an essential micronutrient that the body cannot produce; it must be ingested. Vitamin B_{12} is found in animal-based foods including dairy, eggs, fish, meat, poultry. Persons following a vegan diet may not get vitamin B_{12} unless they take a supplement or eat a fortified food such as cereal. Vitamin B_{12} deficiency can occur in other gastrointestinal disorders, including pernicious anemia, malabsorption from inflammatory bowel disease, gastrectomy, small-bowel bypass, or bowel resection. Vitamin B_{12} deficiency presents with glossitis, angular stomatitis, and neurologic changes with paresthesias in a stocking and glove distribution, loss of vibratory sense, progressive weakness, ataxia, and ultimately dementia if untreated.

Thiamine deficiency (Answer C) causes neuronal death due to metabolic dysfunction of astrocytes within the central nervous system. The classic triad of this condition is confusion, ataxia, and nystagmus. A wide range of other abnormalities can be seen, including cranial nerve dysfunction, peripheral neuropathies, seizures, and psychosis. Because thiamine is a water-soluble vitamin, body stores can be depleted within days to weeks of inadequate intake. The condition typically presents 4 to 12 weeks after bariatric surgery but can occur as early as 2 weeks. Although most commonly reported following Roux-en-Y gastric bypass, Wernicke encephalopathy can occur after any type of bariatric surgery. The most common antecedent is persistent vomiting, which then severely limits thiamine intake. Other less common precipitating factors are intravenous glucose or parenteral nutrition administration without thiamine supplementation. The condition is important to recognize, as treatment with parenteral thiamine (100 mg daily for 7 to 14 days, or 500 mg 3 times daily for 3 days) must be administered to prevent serious persistent morbidity.

Folate deficiency (Answer B) is uncommon and typically presents as anemia. Zinc deficiency (Answer D) is rare. It is associated with skin and hair findings and is primarily seen as a late complication after biliary pancreatic diversion. Copper deficiency (Answer E) can be present following gastric bypass and is often unrecognized but may present with neuromuscular symptoms different from those described in this vignette.

EDUCATIONAL OBJECTIVE
Differentiate among the vitamin deficiencies that can occur after gastric bypass surgery.

REFERENCE(S)
Aasheim ET. Wernicke encephalopathy after bariatric surgery, a systematic review. *Ann Surg.* 2008;248(5): 714-720. PMID: 18948797

Serra A, Sechi G, Singh S, Kumar A. Wernicke encephalopathy after obesity surgery: a systematic review. *Neurology.* 2007;69(6):615. PMID: 17679686

Mechanick JI, Kushner RF, Sugerman HJ, et al; American Association of Clinical Endocrinologists; Obesity Society; American Society for Metabolic & Bariatric Surgery. American Association of Clinical Endocrinologists, The Obesity Society, and American Society for Metabolic & Bariatric Surgery medical guidelines for clinical practice for the perioperative nutritional, metabolic, and nonsurgical support of the bariatric surgery patient [published correction appears in *Obesity (Silver Spring).* 2010;18(3):649]. *Obesity (Silver Spring).* 2009;17(Suppl 1):S1-S70. PMID: 19319140

14 ANSWER: B) Melanocortin 4 receptor (*MC4R*) pathogenic variant

Although knowledge of the monogenic forms of severe childhood obesity is most relevant for pediatric endocrinologists, adult endocrinologists will on occasion encounter a patient with one of these syndromes, and genetic forms of obesity provide insights into important pathways that regulate body weight. The most common monogenic form of early-onset obesity involves pathogenic variants in the gene than encodes the melanocortin 4 receptor (*MC4R*) (Answer B). *MC4R* pathogenic variants are thought to occur in as many as 1 in 1000 individuals. The melanocortin 4 receptor is involved in hypothalamic signaling along the neural pathway that responds to leptin.

Individuals who have pathogenic variants in the genes encoding leptin (Answer C) or the leptin receptor (Answer D) have hypothalamic hypogonadism and subtle impairments in GH and immune function. In contrast, individuals with *MC4R* pathogenic variants present with severe obesity but normal reproductive function. They also have normal growth and "big bones" that are thought to be due to increased insulin levels during development. Prader-Willi syndrome (Answer A) is a multisystem disorder that is caused by the lack of expression of paternally inherited imprinted genes on chromosome 15q11-q13. The typical features of Prader-Willi syndrome include hypotonia, poor feeding after birth, learning disabilities, growth retardation, behavioral problems, hypothalamic hypogonadism, and cryptorchidism. The initial screening genetic test, DNA methylation analysis, is important in making a definitive diagnosis.

EDUCATIONAL OBJECTIVE
Differentiate among the common monogenic forms of severe childhood obesity.

REFERENCE(S)
Farooqi S, O'Rahilly S. Genetics of obesity in humans. *Endocr Rev.* 2006;27(7):710-718. PMID: 17122358

Ranadive SA, Vaisse C. Lessons from extreme human obesity: monogenic disorders. *Endocrinol Metab Clin North Am.* 2008;37(3):733-751. PMID: 18775361

Farooqi S. Insights from the genetics of severe childhood obesity. *Horm Res.* 2007;68(Suppl 5):5-7. PMID: 18174694

15 ANSWER: B) Liraglutide

Liraglutide, 3.0 mg daily, (Answer B) is approved for patients with a BMI of 27 kg/m² or greater with an obesity-related comorbidity (of which this patient has multiple). The most common adverse effects of liraglutide are gastrointestinal in nature and include nausea in about 30% to 40% of patients, vomiting, abdominal pain, and diarrhea or constipation. Gastrointestinal adverse effects are significant enough in approximately 6% of patients in clinical trials to prompt them to withdraw and stop the medication. Gallbladder disease occurs in about 5% of patients on liraglutide compared with placebo and should be used with caution in someone who has had known gallstones. However, this patient already had a cholecystectomy, so this is not a risk for her.

Topiramate (Answer D) is FDA approved for epilepsy and migraine headaches, which makes it a potentially attractive choice for this patient given her history of migraines. Although there are a number of studies in which it was used specifically for weight loss, it is not FDA approved for this purpose. However, there is strong evidence that it produces a 6% to 8% weight loss that is sustained at 1 year. However, topiramate is associated with the formation of kidney stones due to its acid-base effects and urine metabolite excretion. Topiramate is contraindicated in patients with kidney stones. The combination of phentermine and topiramate (Answer C) is also contraindicated for this patient because of her history of kidney stones.

Naltrexone/bupropion (Answer E) is contraindicated in patients with uncontrolled hypertension, which makes it a suboptimal choice for this patient.

Orlistat (Answer A) is an over-the-counter lipase inhibitor that aids in weight loss, but it is far less effective than liraglutide in clinical trials.

EDUCATIONAL OBJECTIVE
Appropriately select weight-loss medications on the basis of a patient's clinical circumstances and current medications.

REFERENCE(S)

Rosenstock J, Hollander P, Gadde KM, Sun X, Strauss R, Leung A; OBD-202 Study Group. A randomized, double-blind, placebo-controlled, multicenter study to assess the efficacy and safety of topiramate controlled release in the treatment of obese type 2 diabetic patients. *Diabetes Care.* 2007;30(6):1480-1486. PMID: 17363756

Eliasson B, Gudbjörnsdottir S, Cederholm J, Liang Y, Vercruysse F, Smith U. Weight loss and metabolic effects of topiramate in overweight and obese type 2 diabetic patients: randomized double-blind placebo-controlled trial. *Int J Obes (London).* 2007;31(7):1140-1147. PMID: 17264849

Apovian CM, Aronne LJ, Bessesen DH, et al; Endocrine Society. Pharmacological management of obesity: an Endocrine Society clinical practice guideline. *J Clin Endocrinol Metab.* 2015;100(2):342-362. PMID: 25590212

16 ANSWER: C) Apolipoprotein E2/E2

The apolipoprotein (apo) E2/E2 phenotype (Answer C) is present in patients with dysbetalipoproteinemia, which is also referred to as type III hyperlipidemia, or broad-beta disease. Classic skin manifestations include tuberoeruptive lesions at the elbows and palmar xanthomas as observed in this patient. The apo E2/E2 phenotype occurs in about 1 per 100 persons, but the development of characteristic dyslipidemia is infrequent and usually appears later in life due to acquired medical conditions such as hypothyroidism, obesity, diabetes mellitus, or estrogen replacement therapy. The lipoprotein that accumulates is a remnant of triglyceride metabolism (beta VLDL) and is associated with an increased risk of atherosclerotic vascular disease. Although the calculated LDL-cholesterol level is increased in this patient, it is spurious due to accumulation of beta VLDL. This remnant is cholesterol ester–enriched and has "balanced" concentrations of cholesterol and triglyceride, which accounts for the nearly equal serum cholesterol and triglyceride levels.

ABCA1 is a protein involved in moving cholesterol from peripheral tissues onto HDL particles. Deficiency of this protein (Answer A) results in the condition known as Tangier disease, characterized by very low HDL-cholesterol levels and the classic physical examination finding of orange tonsils, which this patient does not have. LDL-receptor deficiency (Answer B) results in the condition known as familial hypercholesterolemia. Patients with familial hypercholesterolemia have very high LDL-cholesterol levels, tendinous xanthomas, and premature coronary artery disease. Apolipoprotein C2 is a cofactor for lipoprotein lipase. Deficiency of apolipoprotein C2 (Answer D) therefore results in marked hypertriglyceridemia such as that seen in lipoprotein lipase deficiency. Overproduction of apolipoprotein B (Answer E) is the underlying problem in patients with familial combined hyperlipidemia. These individuals can have elevations in both triglycerides and LDL cholesterol such as that described in this patient, but this condition is not associated with the classic skin lesions (tuberoeruptive and palmar xanthomas) that are characteristic of dysbetalipoproteinemia.

Identify the clinical features of dysbetalipoproteinemia.

REFERENCE(S)
Garg A, Simha V. Update of dyslipidemia. *J Clin Endocrinol Metab.* 2007;92(5):1581-1589. PMID: 17483372

Walden CC, Hegele RA. Apolipoprotein E in hyperlipidemia. *Ann Intern Med.* 1994;120(12):1026-1036. PMID: 8185134

Marais AD, Solomon GA, Blom DJ. Dysbetalipoproteinaemia: a mixed hyperlipidaemia of remnant lipoproteins due to mutations in apolipoprotein E. *Crit Rev Clin Lab Sci.* 2014;51(1):46-62. PMID: 24405372

17 **ANSWER: A) Coronary calcium score**

Of these options, the test with the best predictive value for cardiovascular disease events in middle-aged men is the coronary artery calcium score (Answer A) obtained using CT imaging. Coronary calcium is thought to indicate response to inflammation in the artery. Although no screening test is perfect, this test is meant to detect early disease and the 5-year risk of coronary events. Moreover, a positive score is associated with better adherence to lifestyle modification. However, in younger patients (eg, those with familial hypercholesterolemia), this imaging fails to detect disease because atherosclerotic plaques in these patients are often not calcified. Coronary calcium has also been used to indicate subclinical cardiovascular disease in younger patients with type 1 diabetes.

Although LDL particle size has been promoted as an independent risk factor, small, dense LDL is highly correlated with hypertriglyceridemia, low HDL cholesterol, and metabolic syndrome. Moreover, there are no guidelines for use of LDL particle size distribution (Answer B) to alter therapy. Measurement of apolipoprotein B (Answer C) provides similar data to that from assessment of non-HDL cholesterol. Apolipoprotein A1 measurement (Answer D) would not add more information than what is obtained with measuring HDL cholesterol.

HOMA-IR (Answer E) is a measure of insulin sensitivity and has no clinical role in cardiovascular risk assessment. Additional blood tests that might be performed with some justification include measurement of lipoprotein (a), C-reactive protein, and hemoglobin A_{1c}. White blood cell counts are a well-established indicator of cardiac risk, but variability precludes their use as a screening test.

This man does not require therapy for LDL-cholesterol reduction. Additional lipid-lowering therapies are not indicated unless there is concern for or evidence of vascular disease. With a family history of premature disease, one could argue that knowing whether he is at higher than expected risk would change this calculation.

Recommend coronary artery calcium scoring as a possible tool to assess cardiovascular disease risk.

REFERENCE(S)
Guerci AD, Arad Y, Agatston A. Predictive value of EBCT scanning. *Circulation.* 1998;97(25):2583-2584. PMID: 9657482

Orakzai RH, Nasir K, Orakzai SH, et al. Effect of patient visualization of coronary calcium by electron beam computed tomography on changes in beneficial lifestyle behaviors. *Am J Cardiol.* 2008;101(7):999-1002. PMID: 18359321

18 **ANSWER: B) Start rosuvastatin once weekly**

Statin intolerance is a common clinical problem, and it is especially an issue in patients with underlying conditions that may predispose to muscular-skeletal adverse effects. Aside from reviewing other medications that might interfere with statin metabolism (eg, gemfibrozil, cyclosporine, amiodarone), screening for hypothyroidism is also important, as it is in all patients with hypercholesterolemia. The only reasonable management option listed is to treat the patient with a once-weekly (or alternate-day) statin (Answer B). This strategy might result in fewer muscle symptoms.

Coenzyme Q10 (Answer A) circulates in the blood associated with LDL cholesterol, and statin treatment reduces coenzyme Q10. Although coenzyme Q10 has been used for statin-induced myalgia, no data confirm that this supplement is beneficial. However, it also does not appear to have any downside risk, so it is often used. Red yeast rice extract (Answer C) has been used in several supplement formulations to lower cholesterol. One meta-analysis published in 2006 showed some moderate lipid-lowering effects with red yeast rice extracts, but there are no rigorous trials, cardiovascular outcome trials, or long-term safety data available to support its recommendation for patients with hyperlipidemia. Fish oil (Answer D) is used for hypertriglyceridemia, but it has no significant LDL-cholesterol–lowering effects. Although omega-3 fatty acids have been touted as antiinflammatory agents, they also have no known benefit in this condition. Creatine phosphokinase levels are usually in the normal range in patients with myalgias, so its measurement (Answer E) is not indicated.

EDUCATIONAL OBJECTIVE
Develop a management strategy for statin-induced myalgia.

REFERENCE(S)
Backes JM, Gibson CA, Ruisinger JF, Moriarty PM. The high-dose rosuvastatin once weekly study (The HD-ROWS). *J Clin Lipidol.* 2012;6(4):362-367. PMID: 22836073

Marcoff L, Thompson PD. The role of coenzyme Q10 in statin-associated myopathy: a systematic review. *J Am Coll Cardiol.* 2007;49(23):2231-2237. PMID: 17560286

19 ANSWER: D) Kidney stones
Many different diets result in weight loss. Varying the macronutrient content has less effect on long-term weight loss than adherence to a reduced-calorie diet that allows weight loss of approximately 1 lb per week. Reducing caloric intake by 500 calories a day should result in meaningful weight loss over time. The low-carbohydrate, moderate-protein, high-fat ketogenic diet is based on restricting carbohydrates to 20 to 60 g daily while maintaining adequate protein intake and replacing carbohydrate calories with fat calories. This approach forces the body to switch from burning carbohydrates to breaking down fat (lipolysis) into fatty acids for fuel and generating ketone bodies causing ketosis. Both low-fat and low-carbohydrate dietary approaches with the same total daily caloric intake have been shown to result in a similar amount of weight loss at 1 year (11-13 lb [5-6 kg]).

The ketogenic diet is associated with typical adverse effects, including severe fatigue and headaches in the first few weeks, as well as constipation, potentially significant increases in LDL cholesterol from the high-fat content, and bad breath from ketosis. Drinking plenty of fluids is important, as dehydration is also common with ketogenic diets and this can contribute to kidney stone formation (Answer D). Kidney stone formation can occur due to the increased production and build-up of uric acid. Also, the accompanying mild acidemia has been theorized to increase bone turnover, causing increased calcium excretion and potentially contributing to stone formation.

Cataract formation (Answer A) due to increased fat intake has not been reported in patients following a ketogenic diet. Eruptive xanthoma (Answer C) can occur with extremely high triglycerides (>1000 mg/dL [>11.30 mmol/L]), which is not likely on a ketogenic diet in the absence of an underlying genetic disorder causing hypertriglyceridemia. Low-carbohydrate ketogenic diets improve glycemic control, so glucosuria (Answer B) is not a common finding in the absence of diabetes.

EDUCATION OBJECTIVE
List the risks and benefits of common diet plans for weight loss, including ketogenic diets.

REFERENCE(S)
Gardner CD, Trepanowski JF, Del Gobbo LC, et al. Effect of low-fat vs low-carbohydrate diet on 12-month weight loss in overweight adults and the association with genotype pattern or insulin secretion: the DIETFITS randomized clinical trial. *JAMA.* 2018;319(7):667-679. PMID: 29466592

20

ANSWER: A) Ezetimibe

This patient's clinical picture is consistent with familial hypercholesterolemia, which is associated with very high risk of cardiovascular disease. Fenofibrate (Answer B) and niacin (Answer D) have not been shown to reduce cardiovascular event rates when added to statin therapy. However, data from the IMPROVE-IT trial recently demonstrated that ezetimibe (Answer A) added to a regimen of simvastatin, 40 mg daily, resulted in a modest but significant 6.4% reduction in a composite cardiovascular endpoint.

Evolocumab (Answer C) is a monoclonal antibody that targets and degrades the protein PCSK9. It was approved by the US FDA in 2015. PCSK9 circulates in the blood and alters the liver's handling of LDL cholesterol by stimulating degradation of LDL receptors, which allows less LDL to be cleared from the circulation. Inhibition of PCSK9 with evolocumab lowers circulating LDL by 50% to 60% and significantly lowers the risk of cardiovascular disease. It is specifically approved for use in addition to diet and maximally tolerated statin therapy in adult patients with heterozygous or homozygous familial hypercholesterolemia. The other US FDA–approved medication in this class is alirocumab. Although a PCSK9 inhibitor will lower LDL cholesterol more than ezetimibe, the recently updated 2018 American Heart Association/American College of Cardiology cholesterol management guidelines state that ezetimibe should be added before a PCSK9 inhibitor. This recommendation is due in part to a cost-effectiveness analysis that showed that PSCK9 inhibitors cost approximately $150,000 per QUALY (quality-adjusted life year—the general threshold for value is ≤~$50,000 per QUALY). The best next step would be to add ezetimibe, although this patient will most likely benefit from the subsequent addition of a PCSK9 inhibitor. An additional treatment option for patients with familial hypercholesterolemia is lipopheresis, although this is not widely available.

EDUCATIONAL OBJECTIVE

Explain current recommendations for the addition of lipid-lowering pharmacologic agents to statin therapy for LDL-cholesterol lowering and cardiovascular risk reduction.

REFERENCE(S)

Cannon CP, Blazing MA, Giugliano RP, et al; IMPROVE-IT Investigators. Ezetimibe added to statin therapy after acute coronary syndromes. *N Engl J Med.* 2015;372(25):2387-2397. PMID: 26039521

Sabatine MS, Giugliano RP, Wiviott SD, et al; Open-Label Study of Long-Term Evaluation against LDL Cholesterol (OSLER) Investigators. Efficacy and safety of evolocumab in reducing lipids and cardiovascular events. *N Engl J Med.* 2015;372(16):1500-1509. PMID: 25773607

Ajufo E, Rader DJ. Recent advances in the pharmacological management of hypercholesterolaemia. *Lancet Diabetes Endocrinol.* 2016;4(5):436-446. PMID: 27012540

Grundy SM, Stone NJ, Bailey AL, et al. 2018 AHA/ACC/AACVPR/AAPA/ABC/ACPM/ADA/AGS/APhA/ASPC/NLA/PCNA guideline on the management of blood cholesterol. *Circulation.* 2019;139(25):e1082-e1143. PMID: 30586774

Grundy SM, Stone NJ, Bailey AL, et al. 2018 AHA/ACC/AACVPR/AAPA/ABC/ACPM/ADA/AGS/APhA/ASPC/NLA/PCNA guideline on the management of blood cholesterol: executive summary. *Circulation.* 2019;139(25):e1046-e1081. PMID: 30565953

21

ANSWER: D) Elevated lipoprotein (a)

Additional biomarkers of increased cardiovascular risk beyond LDL cholesterol have been used to further quantify cardiovascular risk in patients who have persistent disease despite good response to lipid-lowering therapy, including non-HDL cholesterol, apolipoprotein B, and lipoprotein (a).

Lipoprotein (a) (Answer D) is highly atherogenic and is associated with increased risk of cardiovascular disease, particularly premature cardiovascular disease. Lipoprotein (a) is an LDL particle with a large protein, apo (a), attached covalently to apolipoprotein B that can incorporate into the arterial wall and contribute to atherosclerosis. Lipoprotein (a) may be modestly elevated in familial hyperlipidemia, but very high levels are associated with a significant increase in atherosclerotic disease. Persons with a lipoprotein (a) level in the upper tertile have an increased risk of cardiovascular disease (odds ratio, 1.7; 95% CI, 1.4-1.9) compared with persons whose level is in the lowest tertile.

Apolipoprotein B (Answer B) is a lipoprotein found on all atherogenic lipid particles, including LDL and triglyceride-rich particles. Non-HDL cholesterol has been suggested as a marker of cardiovascular risk because it also includes non-LDL (triglyceride risk) atherogenic particles. Apolipoprotein B and non-HDL cholesterol predict risk along with LDL cholesterol in patients with primarily elevated LDL cholesterol and elevated triglycerides as found in patients with type 2 diabetes. This patient does not have diabetes or elevated triglycerides, which suggest apolipoprotein B and non-HDL cholesterol are not likely to be additionally informative beyond his LDL-cholesterol level. Apolipoprotein B elevation can support a diagnosis of familial hyperlipidemia and is associated with high risk of cardiovascular disease, but this patient's baseline LDL-cholesterol level was not typical of a patient with familial hyperlipidemia.

The 2013 American College of Cardiology/American Heart Association cholesterol-lowering guidelines do not currently recommend measurement of biomarkers such as apolipoprotein B, lipoprotein (a), and high-sensitivity C-reactive protein for the purpose of primary risk stratification in addition to the lipid profile, but these measures may be used in select cases. Newer guidelines suggest additional markers may be used in select cases to further risk stratify patients, although clear pharmacologic strategies to lower cardiovascular disease risk by targeting lipoprotein (a) reduction are still lacking. However, the particle is effectively removed by apheresis.

Apolipoprotein A1 (Answer A) is an important structural lipoprotein in HDL particles. Genetic variants leading to the deficiency of apolipoprotein A1 result in very low HDL-cholesterol levels, generally less than 20 mg/dL (<0.52 mmol/L), and high risk of heart disease. This man's HDL-cholesterol level is greater than 40 mg/dL (>1.04 mmol/L), which is not consistent with apolipoprotein A1 deficiency.

ATP-binding cassette A1 (ABCA1) deficiency (Answer C), or Tangier disease, is a cause of very low HDL cholesterol and is associated with very early-onset cardiovascular disease, frequently when individuals are in their 20s and 30s. Tangier disease is associated with accumulation of cholesterol in lymphoid tissue giving a classic physical finding: orange tonsils. However, patients with ABCA1 deficiency typically have HDL-cholesterol levels less than 20 mg/dL (<0.52 mmol/L).

EDUCATIONAL OBJECTIVE
Explain the cardiovascular risk associated with elevated lipoprotein (a).

REFERENCE(S)
Stone NJ, Robinson JG, Lichtenstein AH, et al; American College of Cardiology/American Heart Association Task Force on Practice Guidelines. 2013 ACC/AHA guideline on the treatment of blood cholesterol to reduce atherosclerotic cardiovascular risk in adults: a report of the American College of Cardiology/American Heart Association Task Force on Practice Guidelines [published correction appears in *Circulation.* 2014;129(25 Suppl 2):S46-S48]. *Circulation.* 2014;129(25 Suppl 2):S1-S45. PMID: 24222016

Danesh J, Collins R, Peto R. Lipoprotein(a) and coronary heart disease. Meta-analysis of prospective studies. *Circulation.* 2000;102(10):1082-1085. PMID: 10973834

Kamstrup PR, Benn M, Tybjaerg-Hansen A, Nordestgaard BG. Extreme lipoprotein(a) levels and risk of myocardial infarction in the general population: The Copenhagen City Heart Study. *Circulation.* 2008;117(2):176-184. PMID: 18086931

Nordestagarrd BG, Chapman MJ, Ray K, et al; European Atherosclerosis Society Consensus Panel. Lipoprotein(a) as a cardiovascular risk factor: current status. *Eur Heart J.* 2010;31(23):2844-2853. PMID: 20965889

Chalasani N, Younossi Z, Lavine JE, et al. The diagnosis and management of nonalcoholic fatty liver disease: practice guidance from the American Association for the Study of Liver Diseases. *Hepatology.* 2018;67(1):328-357. PMID: 28714183

22 ANSWER: C) Icosapent ethyl, 2 g twice daily

Many patients who are high risk for cardiovascular disease, including those with diabetes, have residual cardiovascular disease risk even after receiving appropriate therapy with statins and ezetimibe. Elevated triglycerides are atherogenic and represent residual cardiovascular disease risk beyond LDL cholesterol. Thus, making no changes in this patient's current therapy (Answer A) is not the best option.

Icosapent ethyl (Answer C) is a purified eicosapentaenoic acid ethyl ester (an omega-3 fatty acid). Although omega-3 fatty acids have been shown to lower triglycerides, in aggregate they have not been shown to lower the risk of cardiovascular disease. Over-the-counter omega-3 fatty acid preparations are not regulated and may contain a variety of fatty acids and other components. In January 2019, the REDUCE-IT trial published in the *New England Journal of Medicine* showed that adding icosapent ethyl, 2 g twice daily, vs placebo to a statin in patients with persistent mildly elevated fasting triglycerides (135 to 500 mg/dL [1.52-5.65 mmol/L]) and an LDL-cholesterol concentration between 41 and 100 mg/dL (1.06-2.59 mmol/L) for a median of 4.9 years (n = 8179) lowered the risk of major cardiovascular events (cardiovascular death, or nonfatal myocardial infarction, stroke, coronary revascularization, or unstable angina) by 25% (17.2% vs 22%; hazard ratio, 0.75; 95% CI, 0.68-0.83). Cardiovascular death was 4.3% in the icosapent ethyl group and 5.2% in the placebo group (hazard ratio, 0.80; 95% CI, 0.66-0.98). There have been concerns about omega-3 fatty acids promoting arrhythmia and possibly increasing bleeding risk. Hospitalization for atrial fibrillation was higher in the icosapent ethyl treatment group than in the placebo group (3.1% vs 2.1%; *P* = .004), and there was a trend toward more

serious bleeding in the icosapent ethyl treatment group compared with placebo (2.7% vs 2.1%; *P* = .06). More work is needed to fully characterize the risk of these potential adverse events in the context of potential benefits for cardiovascular disease risk reduction.

While fenofibrate (Answer D) and niacin ER (Answer E) lower triglycerides, they have not been shown to lower cardiovascular disease risk when added to appropriate medical therapy, including statins. Similarly, in aggregate, omega-3 fatty acids have not been shown to lower cardiovascular disease risk. Fibrate treatment in patients with diabetes failed to reduce primary cardiovascular endpoints in the Bezafibrate Infarction Prevention (BIP) trial and more recently in the Action to Control Cardiovascular Risk in Diabetes (ACCORD) trial. The ACCORD trial specifically assessed whether adding a fibrate to a statin conferred any additional cardiovascular benefits. The results were negative. These studies have been criticized for not selecting individuals with elevated triglycerides at baseline, and post hoc analyses suggest a benefit among those with high baseline triglyceride levels. The Fenofibrate Intervention and Event Lowering in Diabetes (FIELD) study enrolled nearly 10,000 patients with type 2 diabetes, of which about 3650 were women. This study also failed to demonstrate that fenofibrate reduced cardiovascular events. The AIM-HIGH study included a large number of patients with diabetes and examined the effectiveness of adding niacin to aggressive statin therapy. Despite the fact that niacin reduced triglyceride levels and increased HDL-cholesterol levels, the trial was stopped early because of a failure of niacin treatment to reduce cardiovascular endpoints, as well as an unexpected increase in stroke rates.

Gemfibrozil (Answer B) should not be used in combination with a statin.

EDUCATIONAL OBJECTIVE

Describe the benefits of the omega-3 fatty acid, icosapent ethyl, for both triglyceride lowering and cardiovascular risk reduction for patients with triglyceride levels above target and residual risk of cardiovascular disease despite good response to statin treatment.

REFERENCE(S)

Bhatt DL, Steg PG, Miller M, et al; REDUCE-IT Investigators. Cardiovascular risk reduction with icosapent ethyl for hypertriglyceridemia. *N Engl J Med*. 2019;380(1):1-22. PMID: 30415628

23 ANSWER: A) Atorvastatin

An estimated 25% of persons globally have nonalcoholic fatty liver disease (NAFLD), with the highest rates in the Middle East (32%) and the lowest rates in Africa (13%). Both obesity and type 2 diabetes are strong predictors of NAFLD. A subset of individuals with NAFLD progress to nonalcoholic steatohepatitis (NASH) and ultimately cirrhosis. By 2020, NASH is expected to be the leading cause of liver transplant. Persons with NAFLD are also at increased risk for cardiovascular disease. Cardiovascular disease is the leading cause of death in individuals with NAFLD, not death due to liver-related causes. The American Association for the Study of Liver Disease recommends aggressive risk factor modification in patients with NAFLD to lower their cardiovascular disease risk, including treatment of dyslipidemia. Patients with NAFLD typically have dyslipidemia with high triglycerides, low HDL cholesterol, and increased small, dense LDL cholesterol.

The American Heart Association/American College of Cardiology 2013 guidelines state that this patient's clinical profile and 10-year cardiovascular disease risk score (diabetes, aged 40-75 years, LDL cholesterol 70-189 mg/dL, >7.5% risk of cardiovascular disease event in the next 10 years) suggest that he would benefit from a high-intensity statin. Furthermore, the presence of NAFLD puts him at even greater risk of a cardiovascular event than someone with a similar profile without NAFLD. The American Association for the Study of Liver Disease recommends the use of statins in the presence of fatty liver disease for the reduction of cardiovascular risk, as patients with NAFLD are not at increased risk of liver toxicity from statin use. Furthermore, secondary analysis from the IMPROVE-IT trial shows that patients with NAFLD may have greater cardiovascular disease risk reduction with dual therapy given that the study showed greater benefit in the subset with NAFLD with the addition of ezetimibe to simvastatin than with simvastatin alone. Data from at least one clinical trial (secondary endpoint) showed that ALT decreased in patients with NAFLD who were placed on a statin vs placebo.

While there has been concern for some time about the potential risk of treating individuals who have abnormal liver function tests with lipid-lowering drugs, there is no evidence that these drugs cause severe or progressive hepatic damage or that they cannot be safely used in patients with chronic liver disease. The GREACE study (Greek Atorvastatin and Coronary Heart Disease Evaluation) demonstrated that in individuals with liver transaminase values less than 3 times the upper normal limit, there are no adverse effects of lipid-lowering drugs on liver function over time and there are significant benefits to lipid-lowering therapy in cardiovascular disease risk reduction.

In the absence of serious or progressive liver disease, this patient first requires therapy with a statin (Answer A). Omega-3 fatty acids (Answer B), fenofibrate (Answer C), ezetimibe (Answer D), and niacin (Answer E) would not provide the cardiovascular disease risk reduction comparable to that of a statin. Since a statin is safe to use in this patient and it has the greatest benefits, it is the treatment of choice. He may gain additional benefit from the addition of ezetimibe to a statin, but a statin is the best first choice.

EDUCATIONAL OBJECTIVE

Assess the benefits and risks of statin use in patients with fatty liver disease.

REFERENCE(S)

Younossi ZM, Koenig AB, Abdelatif D, Fazel Y, Henry L, Wymer M. Global epidemiology of nonalcoholic fatty liver disease-meta-analytic assessment of prevalence, incidence, and outcomes. *Hepatology*. 2016;64:73-84. PMID: 26707365

Chalasani N, Younossi Z, Lavine JE, et al. The diagnosis and management of nonalcoholic fatty liver disease: practice guidance from the American Association for the Study of Liver Diseases. *Hepatology.* 2018;67(1):328-357. PMID: 28714183

Motamed N, Rabiee B, Poustchi H, et al. Non-alcoholic fatty liver disease (NAFLD) and 10-year risk of cardiovascular diseases. *Clin Res Hepatol Gastroenterol.* 2017;41(1):31-38. PMID: 27597641

Bril F, PoNrtillo Sanchez P, Lomonaco R, et al. Liver safety of statins in prediabetes or T2DM and nonalcoholic steatohepatitis: post hoc analysis of a randomized trial. *J Clin Endocrinol Metab.* 2017;102(8):2950-2961. PMID: 28575232

Athyros VG, Tziomalos K, Gossios TD, et al; GREACE Study Collaborative Group. Safety and efficacy of long-term statin treatment for cardiovascular events in patients with coronary heart disease and abnormal liver tests in the Greek Atorvastatin and Coronary Heart Disease Evaluation (GREACE) Study: a post-hoc analysis. *Lancet.* 2010;376(9756):1916-1922. PMID: 21109302

Demyen M, Alkhalloufi K, Pyrsopoulos NT. Lipid-lowering agents and hepatotoxicity. *Clin Liver Dis.* 2013;17(4):699-714. PMID: 24099026

24 ANSWER: C) Stop gemfibrozil

Serum total cholesterol, HDL-cholesterol, LDL-cholesterol, and triglyceride levels increase during pregnancy (typically the increases are by 75%, 40%, 70%, and 300%, respectively). The mean values for total cholesterol and triglycerides during pregnancy are 317 mg/dL (8.21 mmol/L) and 300 mg/dL (3.39 mmol/L), respectively. After delivery, lipids slowly return to prepregnancy levels. In women with underlying disorders of triglyceride metabolism, levels may rise during pregnancy to a degree that puts the mother at risk for pancreatitis, which could have serious implications for both the mother and the fetus. In addition, the development of gestational diabetes could increase the risk of marked hypertriglyceridemia.

Drugs used for the treatment of lipid disorders should generally be stopped before conception, including gemfibrozil (thus, Answer C is correct and Answer A is incorrect) and fenofibrate (thus, Answer B is incorrect). Statins are teratogenic and contraindicated in pregnancy (thus, Answer D is incorrect). Ideally, all medications should be avoided during pregnancy, particularly during the first trimester when embryogenesis and tissue differentiation occur. Omega-3 fatty acids have been used to treat hypertriglyceridemia during pregnancy, but the available data suggest that they are not very effective. However, omega-3 fatty acids may be the treatment of choice in the first trimester.

Observational studies and case reports suggest that fibrates may be used safely and effectively during pregnancy after the first trimester. Fenofibrate is more potent than omega-3 fatty acids, so it is the best choice in the second and third trimesters.

When pancreatitis due to hypertriglyceridemia develops during pregnancy, a number of treatment approaches have been used. The standard approach of fasting, fluid administration, and pain control is the best first step. If hyperglycemia is present, then intravenous insulin can be administered. Other treatments that have been tried include intravenous heparin, plasma exchange, lipoprotein apheresis, and cesarean delivery if the pregnancy is far enough along.

EDUCATIONAL OBJECTIVE
Develop an approach to treating hypertriglyceridemia during pregnancy.

REFERENCE(S)
Amin T, Poon LC, Teoh TG, et al. Management of hypertriglyceridaemia-induced acute pancreatitis in pregnancy. *J Matern Fetal Neonatal Med.* 2015;28(8):954-958. PMID: 25072837

Crisan LS, Steidl ET, Rivera-Alsina ME. Acute hyperlipidemic pancreatitis in pregnancy. *Am J Obstet Gynecol.* 2008;198(5):e57-e59. PMID: 18359475

Whitten AE, Lorenz RP, Smith JM. Hyperlipidemia-associated pancreatitis in pregnancy managed with fenofibrate. Obstet Gynecol. 2011;117(2 Pt 2):517-519. PMID: 21252809

Nakao J, Ohba T, Takaishi K, Katabuchi H. Omega-3 fatty acids for the treatment of hypertriglyceridemia during the second trimester. *Nutrition.* 2015;31(2):409-412. PMID: 25592021

25
ANSWER: C) Metoprolol

Drug-induced weight gain is a common clinical problem. A number of drug classes can have this effect, including antidiabetes medications, β-adrenergic blockers, antipsychotic agents, antidepressant agents, mood stabilizers, glucocorticoids, and progestational agents. Several management options are available for patients who have drug-induced weight gain. One strategy is to reduce the dosage of the offending medication or to reconsider the value of that medication and potentially to stop it. Alternatively, a behavioral weight-management program can be instituted. Finally, the problematic medication can be stopped and an alternative medication can be prescribed. For example, a GLP-1 agonist or an SGLT-2 inhibitor can be used in place of, or in addition to, a sulfonylurea.

Of the available antihypertensive medications, β-adrenergic blockers such as metoprolol (Answer C) are associated with weight gain, while ACE inhibitors (Answer A), angiotensin-receptor blockers, calcium-channel blockers, and diuretics are not.

Many diabetes medications are associated with weight gain (up to 10-20 lb [4.5-9.1 kg] in the first 6 to 12 months), including the anabolic hormone insulin, insulin secretagogues such as the sulfonylurea glipizide, meglitinides, and thiazolidinediones such as pioglitazone. Metformin (Answer B) is weight neutral in general, although it is associated with mild weight loss in some patients. DPP-4 inhibitors and α-glucosidase inhibitors are weight neutral, and GLP-1 receptor agonists promote weight loss in addition to improving blood glucose control. SGLT-2 inhibitors are associated with mild weight loss in the context of glucosuria and water loss.

More recently, antihistamines have been recognized as weight promoting. The more potent the antihistamine, the more likely the patient is to gain weight with long-term use. H1-antihistamines such as cetirizine are the most likely to be associated with weight gain.

Statins (Answer D) are not associated with significant weight gain.

Other medication classes that can lead to weight gain include glucocorticoids, antidepressants, antipsychotic agents, and hormonal contraceptives. Of the antidepressants, the selective serotonin reuptake inhibitors sertraline, citalopram, and escitalopram (Answer E) are weight neutral. Fluoxetine and bupropion are associated with weight loss.

EDUCATIONAL OBJECTIVE
Identify weight-promoting and weight-neutral medications among commonly prescribed medications for adults.

REFERENCE(S)
Apovian CM, Aronne LJ, Bessesen DH, et al; Endocrine Society. Pharmacological management of obesity: an Endocrine Society clinical practice guideline. *J Clin Endocrinol Metab.* 2015;100(2):342-362. PMID: 25590212

26
ANSWER: B) Travoprost ophthalmic solution

Topiramate is FDA-approved for the reduction of migraine headaches and seizures. Although a number of studies have been conducted in which it was used specifically for weight loss, it is not FDA-approved for weight loss, but it is commonly used off-label for this purpose. There is strong evidence that it produces a 6% to 8% weight loss that is sustained at 1 year. Topiramate is FDA-approved for weight loss in combination with phentermine (phentermine/topiramate, 15/92 mg extended release formulation), which was approved in 2015. Topiramate is contraindicated in pregnancy due to the risk of birth defects, including cleft lip and cleft palate. It is also contraindicated in patients with glaucoma or hyperthyroidism or in patients who have used monoamine oxidase inhibitors antidepressants within the last 2 weeks. Therefore, topiramate would be contraindicated in this patient taking travoprost ophthalmic solution (Answer B) for glaucoma.

Common adverse effects of topiramate include paresthesias in the fingers and toes, dysgeusia (altered taste including metallic taste, particularly when drinking carbonated drinks), difficulty concentrating ("brain fog"), mood disturbances (depressed mood in some, rarely suicidal thoughts), trouble sleeping, and constipation. Topiramate shifts the acid-base status to become more acidic, resulting in metabolic acidosis in some individuals. Due to the shift toward acidemia, topiramate increases the risk of kidney stones and possibly osteoporosis through increased bone turnover. For this reason, topiramate should not be used in patients with kidney stones. There is a small risk of lactic acidosis with topiramate, so it should be used with caution with metformin, which is also associated with a small risk of lactic acidosis. However, prediabetes and metformin use (Answer D) are not contraindications to combination therapy with topiramate.

Topiramate is used to treat migraines and could be a preferable choice in someone who has chronic headaches. Neither metoprolol (Answer A) nor pioglitazone (Answer C) is a contraindication for use of topiramate.

EDUCATIONAL OBJECTIVE
List potential adverse effects of weight-loss medications and select medications appropriately in the context of other medical conditions.

REFERENCE(S)
Apovian CM, Aronne LJ, Bessesen DH, et al; Endocrine Society. Pharmacological management of obesity: an Endocrine Society clinical practice guideline. *J Clin Endocrinol Metab.* 2015;100(2):342-362. PMID: 25590212

Yanovski SZ, Yanovski JA. Long-term drug treatment for obesity: a systematic and clinical review. *JAMA.* 2014;311(1):74-86. PMID: 24231879

Rosenstock J, Hollander P, Gadde KM, Sun X, Strauss R, Leung A; OBD-202 Study Group. A randomized, double-blind, placebo-controlled, multicenter study to assess the efficacy and safety of topiramate controlled release in the treatment of obese type 2 diabetic patients. *Diabetes Care.* 2007;30(6):1480-1486. PMID: 17363756

Eliasson B, Gudbjörnsdottir S, Cederholm J, Liang Y, Vercruysse F, Smith U. Weight loss and metabolic effects of topiramate in overweight and obese type 2 diabetic patients: randomized double-blind placebo-controlled trial. *Int J Obes (London).* 2007;31(7):1140-1147. PMID: 17264849

27 ANSWER: A) Lifestyle modification to achieve 10% weight loss

The overall prevalence of nonalcoholic fatty liver disease (NAFLD) and nonalcoholic steatohepatitis (NASH) is estimated to be 24% in North America with a projected global cost of $50 trillion by 2025. NAFLD/NASH are examples of obesity-associated organ damage; detailed in the Edmonton Obesity Staging System (EOSS). Patients with NASH are at increased risk for progression of cirrhosis with increasing fibrosis determined by liver biopsy (fibrosis stage 1 to 4). In 2016, NASH replaced hepatitis C infection as the main cause of liver transplant. NASH, even with fibrosis, is a dynamic condition with opportunities for both progression and remission. However, the natural course of NASH with stage 3 fibrosis is to progress to cirrhosis rather than regress. Currently, there are no FDA-approved medications to treat NAFLD/NASH, although there are many compounds in development. Pioglitazone has been shown to improve liver fibrosis based on liver biopsy and is commonly used in the setting of diabetes and NAFLD/NASH, although it is weight-promoting, which dampens enthusiasm for its long-term use.

The mainstay of therapy is lifestyle modification (Answer A) with changes in diet and increases in physical activity. Exercise independent of weight loss has been shown to result in regression of NASH. Weight loss of 5% to 10% results in significant regression in NASH as demonstrated by liver biopsy. Weight loss of 5% to 7% has been associated with regression by at least one stage of fibrosis in 50% of patients depending on BMI. Weight loss of 10% or more results in NASH regression in 97% of patients. No medication has been associated with this degree of NAFLD/NASH regression without weight loss.

Some GLP-1 receptor agonists have been associated with improvement of NASH. A small randomized, placebo-controlled trial of liraglutide, 1.8 mg daily (dosing targeted to improved glycemic control), has been shown to result in NASH regression. Liraglutide, 1.8 mg daily, vs placebo for 48 weeks in patients with biopsy-proven NASH resulted in resolution of steatohepatitis as determined by liver biopsy in 9 of 23 patients (39%)

in the liraglutide group vs 2 of 23 patients (9%) in the placebo group (LEAN trial, 2016). Moderate weight loss and improved glycemic control with liraglutide, 1.8 mg daily, resulted in less regression than did weight loss of 5% to 10% through lifestyle modification. Moreover, there is evidence that exenatide (Answer B), which belongs to the same drug class as liraglutide, would result in improvement of NASH.

Improved glycemic control is associated with lowered triglycerides and is beneficial for fatty liver, but the effects of NASH regression with fibrosis have not been demonstrated with other diabetes medications. Canagliflozin (Answer C), an SGLT-2 inhibitor that promotes glucosuria, is associated with mild weight loss, improved glycemic control, and improved circulating markers of liver function, including ALT, AST, and g-glutamyl transferase, but it has not been shown to lead to regression of NASH as determined by liver biopsy. Current research is focusing on SGLT inhibition to treat NAFLD and NASH, and it may become an important treatment modality for NAFLD/NASH in the future.

Metformin (Answer D) improves glycemic control and was shown to decrease progression from prediabetes to type 2 diabetes in the Diabetes Prevention Trial in conjunction with weight loss, but metformin alone has not been associated with improvement of NASH.

EDUCATIONAL OBJECTIVE
Recommend an approach to weight management for obesity complicated by nonalcoholic liver disease and nonalcoholic steatohepatitis.

REFERENCE(S)
Younossi Z, Tacke F, Arrese M, et al. Global perspectives on non-alcoholic fatty liver disease and non-alcoholic steatohepatitis. *Hepatology.* 2019;69(6):2672-2682. PMID: 30179269

Wong VW, Chan RS, Wong GL, et al. Community-based lifestyle modification programme for non-alcoholic fatty liver disease: a randomized controlled trial. *J Hepatol.* 2013;59(3):536-542. PMID: 23623998

Cusi K. Pioglitazone for the treatment of NASH in patients with prediabetes or type 2 diabetes mellitus. *Gut.* 2018;67(7):1371. PMID: 28408383

Boettcher E, Csako G, Pucino F, Wesley R, Loomba R. Meta-analysis: pioglitazone improves liver histology and fibrosis in patients with non-alcoholic steatohepatitis. *Aliment Pharmacol Ther.* 2012;35(1):66-75. PMID: 22050199

Armstrong MJ, Gaunt P, Aithal GP, et al. Liraglutide safety and efficacy in patients with non-alcoholic steatohepatitis (LEAN): a multicentre, double-blind, randomized, placebo-controlled trial phase 2 study. *Lancet.* 2016;387(10019):679-690. PMID: 26608256

Inoue M, Hayashi A, Taguchi T, et al. Effects of canagliflozin on body composition and hepatic fat content in type 2 diabetes patients with non-alcoholic fatty liver disease. *J Diabetes Investig.* 2019;10(4):1004-1011. PMID: 30461221

Leiter LA, Forst T, Polidori D, Balis DA, Xie J, Sha S. Effect of canagliflozin on liver function tests in patients with type 2 diabetes. *Diabetes Metab.* 2016;42(1):25-32. PMID: 26575250

Li B, Wang Y, Ye Z, et al. Effects of canagliflozin on fatty liver indexes in patients with type 2 diabetes: a meta-analysis of randomized controlled trials. *J Pharm Pharm Sci.* 2018;21(1):222-235. PMID: 29935547

28 ANSWER: B) Mediterranean diet
Over the last 10 years, many randomized controlled trials have examined the efficacy of diets that differ in macronutrient composition for weight loss. Study findings have led to the general conclusion that diet composition is not that important for weight loss. Low-carbohydrate, low-fat, and high-protein diets all can produce weight loss if patients adhere to the diet. Which diet is best for weight loss? The answer appears to be: whichever diet to which one can adhere. Another important question, however, is which diet is best for cardiovascular health? As far back as 1999, the Lyon Heart Study demonstrated that a Mediterranean-style diet (Answer B) was associated with a reduction in cardiovascular events in individuals who had known cardiovascular disease. More recently, a

multicenter randomized controlled primary prevention trial done in Spain demonstrated a reduction in major cardiovascular events. The epidemiologic data suggesting cardiovascular benefits of a Mediterranean diet also continue to accumulate. It may be that other dietary approaches, such as a vegetarian diet, an Asian-style diet, or others, might have similar benefits; they simply have not been well studied yet.

EDUCATIONAL OBJECTIVE
Review the data from randomized controlled trials on the effects of different dietary strategies on cardiovascular disease.

REFERENCE(S)
de Lorgeril M, Salen P, Martin JL, Monjaud I, Delaye J, Mamelle N. Mediterranean diet, traditional risk factors, and the rate of cardiovascular complications after myocardial infarction: final report of the Lyon Diet Heart Study. *Circulation.* 1999;99(6):779-785. PMID: 9989963

Shai I, Schwarzfuchs D, Henkin Y, et al; Dietary Intervention Randomized Controlled Trial (DIRECT) Group. Weight loss with a low-carbohydrate, Mediterranean, or low-fat diet. *N Engl J Med.* 2008;359(3):229-241. PMID: 18635428

Estruch R, Ros E, Salas-Salvadó J, et al; PREDIMED Study Investigators. Primary prevention of cardiovascular disease with a Mediterranean diet [published correction appears in *N Engl J Med.* 2014;370(9):886]. *N Engl J Med.* 2013;368(14):1279-1290. PMID: 23432189

Sofi F, Abbate R, Gensini GF, Casini A. Accruing evidence on benefits of adherence to the Mediterranean diet on health: an updated systematic review and meta-analysis. *Am J Clin Nutr.* 2010;92(5):1189-1196. PMID: 20810976

Pituitary Board Review

Laurence Katznelson, MD

1 ANSWER: D) Osilodrostat

This patient has Cushing disease, with residual disease despite 2 attempts at transsphenoidal resection. Medical therapy is indicated. Osilodrostat (Answer D) is a potent oral 11β-hydroxylase inhibitor that was recently approved for adults with Cushing disease who either cannot undergo pituitary gland surgery or have undergone surgery but still have the disease. Osilodrostat effectively reduces cortisol levels. It is well tolerated overall, but in some women, it has been associated with hirsutism (noted in this patient), acne, and elevated serum testosterone levels.

Mifepristone (Answer A) is a glucocorticoid-receptor blocker that is effective in the treatment of patients with all forms of Cushing syndrome. Because it blocks the glucocorticoid receptor, cortisol and ACTH levels may actually rise during treatment (the cortisol level fell in this vignette). Mifepristone effectively improves the clinical manifestations of Cushing syndrome, as well as improves glucose control. Ketoconazole (Answer B) is a steroidogenesis blocker, and it is useful for lowering cortisol. Patients with Cushing syndrome are at risk for liver dysfunction that may be associated with a rise in ACTH levels. However, ketoconazole is not associated with an increase in androgen levels, as noted in this vignette. Pasireotide (Answer C) is a somatostatin analogue that can reduce ACTH secretion and lead to cortisol control in approximately 20% to 25% of patients, and it is frequently associated with hyperglycemia (not noted in this patient). Mitotane (Answer E) is an adrenolytic drug used for both Cushing syndrome and adrenocortical carcinoma. Mitotane can normalize hypercortisolism in up to 60% of patients, but adverse effects such as nausea and anorexia limit its use, and it was therefore not recommended for this patient.

EDUCATIONAL OBJECTIVE

Describe the effects of medical therapy in the treatment of Cushing disease.

REFERENCE(S)

Fleseriu M, Pivonello R, Young J, et al. Osilodrostat, a potent oral 11β-hydroxylase inhibitor: 22-week, prospective, Phase II study in Cushing's disease. *Pituitary.* 2016;19(2):138-148. PMID: 26542280

Hinojosa-Amaya JM, Cuevas-Ramos D, Fleseriu M. Medical management of Cushing's syndrome: current and emerging treatments. *Drugs.* 2019;79(9):935-956. PMID: 31098899

2 ANSWER: D) Maintenance of normal IGF-1 levels (in most patients)

An oral octreotide capsule was recently approved to treat acromegaly in patients who previously responded to and tolerated treatment with octreotide or lanreotide. In a recent phase 3 randomized, double-blind, placebo-controlled trial, IGF-1 levels were maintained in 78% of patients on the study drug vs in 19% of patients taking placebo. IGF-1 levels are thus expected to be maintained in most patients (Answer D). IGF-1 levels are not expected to increase (Answer E) in most patients taking the oral octreotide capsule. Gastrointestinal adverse effects (Answer A) and occurrence of hyperglycemia (Answer C) are similar between the oral octreotide capsule and injectable analogues. As the oral octreotide capsule is a somatostatin analogue, GH levels decrease, not increase (Answer B), on the medication.

EDUCATIONAL OBJECTIVE

Describe the use of the oral octreotide capsule in the treatment of acromegaly.

REFERENCE(S)

Melmed S, Popovic V, Bidlingmaier M, et al. Safety and efficacy of oral octreotide in acromegaly: results of a multicenter phase III trial. *J Clin Endocrinol Metab.* 2015;100(4):1699-1708. PMID: 25664604

Samson SL, Nachtigall LB, Fleseriu M, et al. Maintenance of acromegaly control in patients switching from injectable somatostatin receptor ligands to oral octreotide. *J Clin Endocrinol Metab.* 2020;105(10):e3785-e3797. PMID: 32882036

3 ANSWER: A) Serum α-subunit measurement

This patient has hyperthyroidism, increased thyroid gland iodine uptake, and the unexpected finding of a TSH value that is not suppressed—an indication that a TSH-secreting tumor is the cause of her hyperthyroidism. Surgery would be the best option, with use of a somatostatin analogue as adjuvant therapy. Elevation of α-subunit is present in up to 85% of patients with a TSH-secreting pituitary adenoma, and its measurement (Answer A) would be an appropriate next test in this patient's evaluation. The relative increase in serum α-subunit is greater than that of serum TSH, resulting in a high molar ratio of α-subunit to TSH.

Somatostatin inhibits both GH and TSH, and somatostatin analogues can inhibit TSH secretion from the tumor, as well as decrease tumor size. However, scintography for presence of somatostatin receptors (Answer B) is not necessary, as these patients are usually sensitive to somatostatin analogues. The differential diagnosis of high TSH and T_4 levels includes thyroid hormone resistance. Assessment for a pathogenic variant in the gene encoding the thyroid hormone receptor (Answer C) may be diagnostic in a patient with presumed resistance to thyroid hormone, but this patient does not have evidence of thyroid hormone resistance despite the elevated free T_4. The presence of heterophile antibodies (Answer D) may result in a higher than expected TSH value. However, given the presence of a sellar mass, increased thyroid gland iodine uptake, and clinical hyperthyroidism, an artifactually elevated TSH value is inconsistent with the present diagnosis.

Measurement of thyroid-stimulating immunoglobulin (Answer E) is important for the assessment of Graves disease, but it is not necessary for this patient given the presence of a TSH-secreting adenoma.

EDUCATIONAL OBJECTIVE

Confirm the diagnosis of a TSH-secreting tumor.

REFERENCE(S)

Beck-Peccoz P, Giavoli C, Lania A. A 2019 update on TSH-secreting pituitary adenomas. *J Endocrinol Invest.* 2019;42(12):1401-1406. PMID: 31175617

Beck-Peccoz P, Persani L, Mannavola D, Campi I. Pituitary tumours: TSH-secreting adenomas. *Best Pract Res Clin Endocrinol Metab.* 2009;23(5):597-606. PMID: 19945025

4 ANSWER: A) Start hCG injections, 3 times weekly

This male patient has infertility based on azoospermia on semen analysis. In his case, infertility is most likely the result of hypogonadotropic hypogonadism. He had preexisting fertility, as he fathered a child before diagnosis and treatment of his pituitary tumor. The goal now would be to reestablish fertility through gonadotropin therapy. In up to 90% of men with hypogonadotropic hypogonadism, gonadotropin treatment results in the appearance of sperm in the ejaculate, although the achieved sperm is often not normal. Even if pregnancy does not occur spontaneously, the number of sperm is often sufficient for pregnancy to be achieved by insemination with the patient's semen (intrauterine insemination) or with the help of assisted reproductive technology, such as in vitro fertilization with or without intracytoplasmic sperm injection. LH, through its substitute hormone hCG, is always replaced first before FSH because hCG alone may be sufficient for stimulation of spermatogenesis (thus, Answer A is correct and Answer B is incorrect). Men treated with both hCG and hMG (human menopausal gonadotropin) achieve sperm in approximately 6 to 10 months, but the time to pregnancy is longer.

A blockage in the patient's duct system is unlikely in this setting of secondary hypogonadism, and testicular sperm extraction (Answer C) would not be a technique used initially. Because clomiphene citrate (Answer D) requires an intact pituitary gland for efficacy, this medication would not be useful in the setting of hypopituitarism. The chances for fertility in a patient such as this are well over 50%, and suggesting adoption at this point (Answer E) would be premature.

EDUCATIONAL OBJECTIVE
Manage infertility in men with hypopituitarism.

REFERENCE(S)
Shiraishi K, Matsuyama H. Gonadotropin actions on spermatogenesis and hormonal therapies for spermatogenic disorders [Review]. *Endocr J.* 2017;64(2):123-131. PMID: 28100869

Farhat R, Al-zidjali F, Alzahrani AS. Outcome of gonadotropin therapy for male infertility due to hypogonadotrophic hypogonadism. *Pituitary.* 2010;13(2):105-110. PMID: 19838805

5 ANSWER: C) Craniopharyngioma

The key feature in this vignette is that the patient has diabetes insipidus, which indicates a primarily hypothalamic origin of his tumor. Craniopharyngiomas may occur in children and teenagers, and there is a distinct second peak in older adults (age 50-74 years). The presence of a cystic tumor in this man, as well as diabetes insipidus, points to a craniopharyngioma (Answer C). Diabetes insipidus is very uncommon in patients with pituitary adenomas (gonadotroph adenomas [Answer A], prolactinoma [Answer B], and silent corticotroph adenoma [Answer D]). Craniopharyngiomas are typically described on MRI as calcified, solid, and/or cystic lesions, usually with a lobular shape and diameter of 20 to 40 mm. The solid elements are often isointense or hypointense on T1-weighted images, exhibit inhomogeneous high intensity on T2-weighted images, and heterogeneously enhance after gadolinium administration.

The very mild prolactin elevation in this case is from hypothalamic damage rather than from a prolactinoma and could accompany any of these other tumors/lesions. Langerhans cell histiocytosis (Answer E) usually presents as an infiltrative disease of the hypothalamus and stalk with stalk thickening on MRI rather than as a mass lesion.

EDUCATIONAL OBJECTIVE
Differentiate among hypothalamic and pituitary mass lesions.

REFERENCE(S)
Bogusz A, Müller HL. Childhood-onset craniopharyngioma: latest insights into pathology, diagnostics, treatment, and follow-up. *Expert Rev Neurother.* 2018;18(10):793-806. PMID: 30257123

Müller HL. Craniopharyngioma. *Endocr Rev.* 2014;35(3):513-543. PMID: 24467716

Zada G, Lin N, Ojerholm E, Ramkissoon S, Laws ER. Craniopharyngioma and other cystic epithelial lesions of the sellar region: a review of clinical, imaging, and histopathological relationships. *Neurosurg Focus.* 2010;28(4):E4. PMID: 20367361

Erfurth EM, Holmer H, Fjalldal SB. Mortality and morbidity in adult craniopharyngioma. *Pituitary.* 2013;16(1):46-55. PMID: 22961634

6 ANSWER: D) Referral for psychiatric evaluation

The results of the patient's fluid-deprivation test indicate that he is able to concentrate urine. The failure to completely concentrate urine results from impaired renal concentrating mechanisms that occur with prolonged washout of the renal medullary gradient because of his constant excessive water intake and excretion. The treatment of choice, then, is referral for psychiatric evaluation (Answer D) rather than prescribing DDAVP (Answer E), as he is able to concentrate urine appropriately with water deprivation, which rules out diabetes insipidus.

The remaining options (amiloride [Answer A], thiazide diuretic [Answer B], or indomethacin [Answer C]) would be appropriate to ameliorate polyuria resulting from nephrogenic diabetes insipidus. In a recent study, measurement of copeptin, the C-terminal segment of the arginine vasopressin prohormone, following an infusion of hypertonic saline had greater diagnostic accuracy than the fluid-deprivation test in patients with hypotonic polyuria.

EDUCATIONAL OBJECTIVE
Interpret results from a fluid-deprivation test in the evaluation of diabetes insipidus.

REFERENCE(S)
Fenske W, Allolio B. Clinical review: current state and future perspectives in the diagnosis of diabetes insipidus: a clinical review. *J Clin Endocrinol Metab.* 2012;97(10):3426-3437. PMID: 22855338

de Fost M, Oussaada SM, Endert E, et al. The water deprivation test and a potential role for the arginine vasopressin precursor copeptin to differentiate diabetes insipidus from primary polydipsia. *Endocr Connect.* 2015;4(2):86-91. PMID: 25712898

Fenske W, Refardt J, Chifu I, et al. A copeptin-based approach in the diagnosis of diabetes insipidus. *N Engl J Med.* 2018;379(5):428-439. PMID: 30067922

7   ANSWER: A) Late-night salivary cortisol measurement
Following transsphenoidal surgery for Cushing disease, the recurrence rate is approximately 25% at 5 years. The degree of the cortisol decrease after surgery correlates with long-term remission. Therefore, it is important to perform serial evaluation for possible recurrence. Patients are often perceptive as to whether they have had recurrence, and this information is useful in planning testing. The most accurate test for recurrence is late-night salivary cortisol measurement (Answer A). In recent studies, late-night salivary cortisol measurement had the highest predictive value compared with overnight dexamethasone testing and 24-hour urinary free cortisol excretion (Answer D).

Repeating an ACTH measurement (Answer E) is not useful for determining recurrence. Once recurrence has been confirmed, pituitary MRI (Answer B) should be performed to evaluate for a visible adenoma. A plan to perform serial monitoring with serum cortisol measurement in 6 months (Answer C) is not an ideal option for this patient,

as she does have some signs consistent with Cushing disease recurrence, so further testing should be performed now. In addition, an isolated serum cortisol measurement is not useful for determining recurrence.

EDUCATIONAL OBJECTIVE
Assess patients with Cushing disease for recurrence following successful surgery.

REFERENCE(S)
Amlashi FG, Swearingen B, Faje AT, et al. Accuracy of late-night salivary cortisol in evaluating postoperative remission and recurrence in Cushing's disease. *J Clin Endocrinol Metab.* 2015;100(10), 3770-3777. PMID: 26196950

Braun LT, Rubinstein G, Zopp S, et al. Recurrence after pituitary surgery in adult Cushing's disease: a systematic review on diagnosis and treatment. *Endocrine.* 2020;70(2):218-231. PMID: 32743767

Danet-Lamasou M, Asselineau J, Perez P, et al. Accuracy of repeated measurements of late-night salivary cortisol to screen for early-stage recurrence of Cushing's disease following pituitary surgery. *Clin Endocrinol (Oxf).* 2015;82(2):260-266. PMID: 24975391

8   ANSWER: C) Chest CT
Pituitary hormone excess syndromes are usually due to overproduction of these hormones in an unregulated fashion from pituitary adenomas. However, rare neuroendocrine tumors can produce ACTH, resulting in ectopic ACTH Cushing syndrome. In this circumstance, the pituitary gland may appear normal in size. For interpretation of the inferior petrosal sinus catheterization, corticotropin-releasing hormone–stimulated central ACTH values should be at least 3-fold higher than peripheral values. This patient had a 1.5-fold increase only, so this situation does not meet criteria for diagnosing Cushing disease. Thus, in this patient without a significant central-to-peripheral ACTH gradient and with lack of lateralization on inferior petrosal catheterization, the possibility of a neuroendocrine tumor producing ectopic ACTH, such as a bronchial carcinoid, should be considered. As bronchial

carcinoid is the most common source of ectopic ACTH secretion, CT of the chest (Answer C) should be the first imaging performed to identify the source. Other forms of imaging such as MRI and ^{68}Ga DOTATATE PET/CT could also be performed to investigate the possibility of a bronchial carcinoid or pancreatic neuroendocrine tumor. Additionally, corticotropin-releasing hormone levels could be measured. If an ectopic tumor is not detected, then exploratory transsphenoidal surgery could be considered.

Performing a corticotropin-releasing hormone test (Answer A), a dexamethasone corticotropin-releasing hormone test (Answer B), or another inferior petrosal sinus sampling (Answer D) would not aid in diagnosis. A high-dose dexamethasone-suppression test (Answer E) may be useful for evaluating causes of ACTH-dependent Cushing syndrome, but it does not reliably distinguish between pituitary and ectopic disease. Of note, transsphenoidal surgical exploration is a reasonable alternative, as there are cases of false-negative petrosal catheterizations, but it is very reasonable to search for ectopic disease first with imaging.

EDUCATIONAL OBJECTIVE
Differentiate among the different causes of ACTH-dependent Cushing syndrome.

REFERENCE(S)
Young J, Haissaguerre M, Viera-Pinto O, Chabre O, Baudin E, Tabarin A. Management of endocrine disease: Cushing's syndrome due to ectopic ACTH secretion: an expert operational opinion. *Eur J Endocrinol.* 2020;182(4):R29-R58. 31999619

Sathyakumar S, Paul TV, Asha HS, et al. Ectopic Cushing syndrome: a 10-year experience from a tertiary care center in southern India. *Endocr Pract.* 2017;23(8):907-914. PMID: 28614007

Frete C, Corcuff JB, Kuhn E, et al. Non-invasive diagnostic strategy in ACTH-dependent Cushing's syndrome. *J Clin Endocrinol Metab.* 2020;105(10): dgaa409. PMID: 32594169

9 ANSWER: A) Mifepristone
All of these treatment modalities can improve Cushing disease, and treatment during pregnancy is advocated because it results in better fetal outcomes. Transsphenoidal surgery (Answer C) has a cure rate of 80% to 90% in expert neurosurgical hands with very low complication and fetal loss rates when done in the second trimester. Metyrapone (Answer B) has been used safely in pregnancy in a few cases, but there is limited clinical experience. There is experience with only about 50 cases in which somatostatin analogues have been used to treat acromegaly during pregnancy, with relatively minor adverse effects. However, somatostatin analogues cross the placenta and have unknown effects on the fetus. There is no experience with pasireotide (Answer D) during pregnancy, and it would be expected to worsen glucose tolerance in this population susceptible to gestational diabetes. Although cabergoline (Answer E) is safe when stopped after conception, there is little experience when used throughout pregnancy, and its ability to normalize cortisol levels in Cushing disease is only modest. Neither pasireotide nor cabergoline is absolutely contraindicated during pregnancy.

Mifepristone (Answer A) was originally developed as a progesterone receptor blocker and is a potent abortifacient (RU486); therefore, its use in pregnancy is absolutely contraindicated.

EDUCATIONAL OBJECTIVE
Identify which options are contraindicated in the treatment of Cushing disease during pregnancy.

REFERENCE(S)
Machado MC, Fragoso MCBV, Bronstein MD. Pregnancy in patients with Cushing's syndrome. *Endocrinol Metab Clin North Am.* 2018;47(2):441-449. PMID: 29754643

Brue T, Amodru V, Castinetti F. Management of endocrine disease: management of Cushing's syndrome during pregnancy: solved and unsolved questions. *Eur J Endocrinol.* 2018;178(6):R259-R266. PMID: 29523633

Caimari F, Valassi E, Garbayo P, et al. Cushing's syndrome and pregnancy outcomes: a systematic review of published cases. *Endocrine.* 2017;55(2): 555-563. PMID: 27704478

10 ANSWER: B) Perform a macimorelin-stimulation test to assess GH levels

This patient is at risk for GH deficiency given his history of craniopharyngioma, sellar radiation therapy, and panhypopituitarism. He has signs and symptoms of GH deficiency, including increased abdominal girth, fatigue, and reduced short-term memory and attention span. In the setting of at least 3 deficient axes, the presence of a serum IGF-1 level less than 85 ng/dL (<15.1 nmol/L) is consistent with GH deficiency. However, IGF-1 can be normal or low normal in persons with GH deficiency. The next step would be to perform a provocative GH test, and of the listed answer choices, a macimorelin-stimulation test (Answer B) would be best. Either an insulin tolerance test (Answer D) or a glucagon-stimulation test would be other potential options. Although an insulin tolerance test is considered the gold standard test for assessment of GH deficiency, this patient's history of seizures precludes its use given the risk of profound hypoglycemia.

Measuring a random GH level (Answer C) is not useful in the diagnosis of GH deficiency. Patients with GH deficiency may have mild depression, and although referral for psychiatry (Answer A) is not incorrect, addressing the underlying cause is a better first step.

EDUCATIONAL OBJECTIVE
Determine the most appropriate approach to diagnose GH deficiency.

REFERENCE(S)
Yuen KCJ, Biller BMK, Radovick S, et al. American Association of Clinical Endocrinologists and American College of Endocrinology guidelines for management of growth hormone deficiency in adults and patients transitioning from pediatric to adult care. *Endocr Pract.* 2019;25(11):1191-1232. PMID: 31760824

Yuen KC, Tritos NA, Samson SL, Hoffman AR, Katznelson L. American Association of Clinical Endocrinologists and American College of Endocrinology disease state clinical review: update on growth hormone stimulation testing and proposed revised cut-point for the glucagon stimulation test in the diagnosis of adult growth hormone deficiency. *Endocr Pract.* 2016;22(10):1235-1244. PMID: 27409821

Ramos-Leví AM, Marazuela M. Treatment of adult growth hormone deficiency with human recombinant growth hormone: an update on current evidence and critical review of advantages and pitfalls. *Endocrine.* 2018;60(2):203-218. PMID: 29417370

Garcia JM, Biller BMK, Korbonits M, et al. Macimorelin as a diagnostic test for adult GH deficiency. *J Clin Endocrinol Metab.* 2018;103(8):3083-3093. PMID: 29860473

11 ANSWER: E) Decreased peak bone mass

The *transition period* refers to the time of life between the end of puberty and full maturation of bone, muscle, and body fat composition. Peak bone mass usually occurs by age 25 years, and GH deficiency during the transition period results in a failure to attain this peak bone mass (Answer E). Once GH is discontinued, there may be a change in body composition with a reduction in lean mass and an increase in fat mass, but overall weight does not increase significantly (Answer A). GH deficiency may be associated with a reduction in lean body mass, not an increase (Answer D). Some studies have suggested that GH deficiency is associated with an increased risk of mortality. No data clearly prove that GH treatment reduces the risk of mortality in patients with hypopituitarism, although findings from some recent studies suggest that this may be true. Thus, a reduced mortality rate (Answer C) is incorrect. GH therapy may result in insulin resistance and glucose intolerance (Answer B), but this is not usually seen when GH is discontinued.

Discuss the effects of GH in the transition period (between the end of puberty and full maturation of bone, muscle, and body fat composition).

REFERENCE(S)

Yuen KCJ, Biller BMK, Radovick S, et al. American Association of Clinical Endocrinologists and American College of Endocrinology guidelines for management of growth hormone deficiency in adults and patients transitioning from pediatric to adult care. *Endocr Pract.* 2019;25(11):1191-1232. PMID: 31760824

Çamtosun E, Şıklar Z, Berberoğlu M. Prospective follow-up of children with idiopathic growth hormone deficiency after termination of growth hormone treatment: is there really need for treatment at transition to adulthood? *J Clin Res Pediatr Endocrinol.* 2018;10(3):247-255. PMID: 29553045

Richmond E, Rogol AD. Treatment of growth hormone deficiency in children, adolescents and at the transitional age. *Best Pract Res Clin Endocrinol Metab.* 2016;30(6):749-755. PMID: 27974188

12 ANSWER: C) Add pegvisomant

Although studies do show that increasing the somatostatin analogue dosage (Answer A) may be beneficial, these regimens are not generally adopted. Cabergoline (Answer B) can be useful in the setting of modest acromegaly, and it may show benefit in combination with octreotide. However, this regimen is effective in less than half of patients and is unlikely to be effective in this patient with more active disease. Radiation therapy (Answer D) often takes a number of years to be effective and it is therefore unlikely to be effective within 6 months. Reoperation (Answer E) is unlikely to be effective in this case, as the tumor is in the cavernous sinus and is difficult to approach surgically.

The addition of pegvisomant (Answer C) would be the most effective regimen in this timeframe. In this setting, pegvisomant is often prescribed weekly or twice weekly, in contrast to use of pegvisomant as monotherapy (prescribed daily). Because this patient has had some response to the somatostatin analogue with a partial reduction in IGF-1, it is reasonable to add pegvisomant as combination therapy instead of switching to pegvisomant as monotherapy.

EDUCATIONAL OBJECTIVE

Recommend the best therapeutic approach in a patient with acromegaly who has had a partial response to adjuvant therapy with somatostatin analogue therapy.

REFERENCE(S)

Katznelson L, Laws ER Jr, Melmed S, et al; Endocrine Society. Acromegaly: an endocrine society clinical practice guideline. *J Clin Endocrinol Metab.* 2014;99(11):3933-3951. PMID: 25356808

Fleseriu M, Biller BMK, Freda PU, et al. A Pituitary Society update to acromegaly management guidelines. *Pituitary.* 2021;24(1):1-13. PMID: 33079318

Giustina A, Mazziotti G, Cannavò S, et al. High-dose and high-frequency lanreotide Autogel in acromegaly: a randomized, multicenter study. *J Clin Endocrinol Metab.* 2017;102(7):2454-2464. PMID: 28419317

Melmed S, Bronstein MD, Chanson P, et al. A consensus statement on acromegaly therapeutic outcomes. *Nat Rev Endocrinol.* 2018;14(9):552-561. PMID: 30050156

13 ANSWER: B) Decrease the GH dosage

Oral estrogens can act on the liver to decrease the responsiveness of the liver to GH with respect to IGF-1 production. Therefore, to maintain a steady level of IGF-1, the GH dosage may actually need to be decreased in this setting (thus, Answer B is correct and Answer C is incorrect). Interestingly, estrogens also stimulate hepatic thyroxine-binding globulin, so increases in levothyroxine dosages are sometimes needed and, presumably, the converse is also true (thus, Answer A is incorrect). Although increasing the hydrocortisone dosage (Answer D) could be considered useful given that GH may metabolize cortisol and lead to relative adrenal insufficiency, the first step for this patient would be to reduce the GH dosage (Answer B). Stopping estrogen has no effect on hydrocortisone dosage requirements, so decreasing the hydrocortisone dosage (Answer E) is incorrect.

EDUCATIONAL OBJECTIVE
Describe interactions among hormonal replacement therapies.

REFERENCE(S)
Glynn N, Kenny H, Quisenberry L, et al. The effect of growth hormone replacement on the thyroid axis in patients with hypopituitarism: in vivo and ex vivo studies. *Clin Endocrinol (Oxf)*. 2017;86(5):747-754. PMID: 27809356

Birzniece V, Ho KKY. Sex steroids and the GH axis: implications for the management of hypopituitarism. *Best Pract Res Clin Endocrinol Metab*. 2017; 31(1):59-69. PMID: 28477733

Fleseriu M, Hashim IA, Karavitaki N, et al. Hormonal replacement in hypopituitarism in adults: an Endocrine Society clinical practice guideline. *J Clin Endocrinol Metab*. 2016;101(11):3888-3921. PMID: 27736313

14 ANSWER: A) Pathogenic variant in the *PROP1* gene

This patient had childhood-onset GH deficiency, as well as hypothyroidism. He also has empty sella on MRI. Pathogenic variants in the genes encoding a number of transcription factors, including *POU1F1* (formerly *PIT1*) and *PROP1*, can cause disruption in the development of many pituitary cell types during embryogenesis, resulting in multiple pituitary hormone deficiencies. Pathogenic variants in *PROP1* (Answer A) result in a decrease in the amount of PROP1 protein, a transcription factor important for the development of the somatotroph, lactotroph, and thyrotroph lineages with deficiencies of their respective hormones. Some affected individuals also have delayed puberty. Combined pituitary hormone deficiency (GH, prolactin, TSH) has an incidence of about 1 in 8000 births, and 10% of patients have an affected family member. Between 25% and 50% of these cases are due to pathogenic variants in *POU1F1* or *PROP1*. In this patient, the history of GH and thyroid hormone treatment starting in childhood suggests congenital combined pituitary hormone deficiency.

In some children with PROP1 deficiency, there is early pituitary enlargement of uncertain cause, which results in sellar enlargement and subsequent loss of pituitary volume, leading to an empty sella. In most series, when patients with empty sellas have evaluations of pituitary function, between one-quarter and one-third have varying degrees of hypopituitarism.

Acute trauma causing pituitary infarction (Answer B) may reveal subsequent empty sella, but this patient does not have a history of significant trauma and his hypopituitarism predated his concussion. The *TBX19* gene encodes a transcription factor necessary for differentiation of the corticotroph cell and production of proopiomelanocortin. Pathogenic variants in *TBX19* (Answer C) lead to central adrenal insufficiency, which is not present in this patient. Langerhans cell histiocytosis (Answer D) is an infiltrative disease of the hypothalamus and pituitary stalk that might present with stalk thickening rather than an empty sella. Langerhans cell histiocytosis usually presents with diabetes insipidus. Hemochromatosis (Answer E) can cause iron deposition in the pituitary and usually affects the gonadotroph cells; it is not associated with empty sella.

EDUCATIONAL OBJECTIVE
Determine the cause of childhood-onset combined hypopituitarism.

REFERENCE(S)
Prince KL, Walvoord EC, Rhodes SJ. The role of homeodomain transcription factors in heritable pituitary disease. *Nat Rev Endocrinol*. 2011;7(12): 727-737. PMID: 21788968

Pavel ME, Hensen J, Pfäffle R, Hahn EG, Dörr HG. Long-term follow-up of childhood-onset hypopituitarism in patients with the PROP-1 gene mutation. *Horm Res*. 2003;60(4):168-173. PMID: 14530604

Mendonca BB, Osorio MG, Latronico AC, Estefan V, Lo LS, Arnhold IJ. Longitudinal hormonal and pituitary imaging changes in two females with combined pituitary hormone deficiency due to deletion of A301,G302 in the PROP1 gene. *J Clin Endocrinol Metab.* 1999;84(3):942-945. PMID: 10084575

Guitelman M, Garcia Basavilbaso N, Vitale M, et al. Primary empty sella (PES): a review of 175 cases. *Pituitary.* 2013;16(2):270-274. PMID: 22875743

15 ANSWER: A) Inability to lactate

This patient has Sheehan syndrome, referring to infarction of the pituitary gland after a complicated delivery with postpartum hemorrhage. The hemorrhage may be of sufficient severity to cause hypotension and require blood transfusion. When the blood loss results in hypotension and the diagnosis of Sheehan syndrome is considered, evaluation and treatment of adrenal insufficiency should be initiated. The serum cortisol level may not be severely low in such patients, as cortisol-binding globulin is elevated with pregnancy, resulting in measurement of a normal or higher total cortisol. When hypopituitarism is mild, there can be a delay in diagnosis for up to many years. When hypopituitarism is more severe, there is a failure to lactate (Answer A), which would be notable in the first days following delivery. Subsequently, menses may fail to resume (Answer D), and there may be loss of sexual hair. Affected patients may also describe fatigue, weight loss, and anorexia, possibly from adrenal insufficiency. Hypothyroidism can occur as well, although measurement of free T_4 (Answer B) and TSH may not reveal evidence of central hypothyroidism for several weeks. With hypopituitarism, she may gain weight (Answer C), but the inability to lactate would occur first.

EDUCATIONAL OBJECTIVE
Identify the endocrine sequelae of Sheehan syndrome.

REFERENCE(S)

Diri H, Tanriverdi F, Karaca Z, et al. Extensive investigation of 114 patients with Sheehan's syndrome: a continuing disorder. *Eur J Endocrinol.* 2014;171(3):311-318. PMID: 24917653

Dökmetaş HS, Kilicli F, Korkmaz S, Yonem O. Characteristic features of 20 patients with Sheehan's syndrome. *Gynecol Endocrinol.* 2006; 22(5):279-283. PMID: 16785150

Diri H, Karaca Z, Tanriverdi F, Unluhizarci K, Kelestimur F. Sheehan's syndrome: new insights into an old disease. *Endocrine.* 2016;51(1):22-31. PMID: 26323346

16 ANSWER: C) Start tolvaptan

This patient has undergone 2 of the 3 phases of the triphasic response following pituitary surgery. She had immediate diabetes insipidus, followed by hyponatremia, which is usually due to syndrome of inappropriate antidiuretic hormone secretion. Diabetes insipidus in the subsequent phase would complete the 3 phases. This patient has severe hyponatremia, which occurred rapidly. Tolvaptan (Answer C) is an oral vasopressin receptor antagonist that is administered daily for up to 4 days, and it is very effective in the treatment of moderate to severe hyponatremia following pituitary surgery. A vasopressin receptor antagonist may facilitate recovery from syndrome of inappropriate antidiuretic hormone secretion in this setting. Tolvaptan administration (15 mg) will result in the most rapid normalization of sodium compared with the other listed options. Hypertonic saline can also be used in this setting, usually at a recommended dose and rate of 0.5 to 1.0 mL/kg body weight per hour, which, in this patient, translates to 30 to 60 mL per hour. A rate of 5 mL/h (Answer E) is too low.

If fluid restriction is to be successful, it should be to less than 500 to 1000 mL/24 h. A 1500-mL limit (Answer A) is too high. Demeclocycline (Answer B) causes partial nephrogenic diabetes insipidus and can be useful for patients with chronic, symptomatic hyponatremia, such as that associated with malignancy; it is generally not used when hyponatremia develops acutely. Saline infusion with intermittent furosemide (Answer D) combines salt infusion with an increase in urinary excretion of water in excess of sodium. However, this form of sodium correction is slow and is minimally useful.

EDUCATIONAL OBJECTIVE

Manage moderate to severe hyponatremia in the postoperative setting following transsphenoidal surgery.

REFERENCE(S)

Verbalis JG, Goldsmith SR, Greenberg A, et al. Diagnosis, evaluation, and treatment of hyponatremia: expert panel recommendations. *Am J Med.* 2013;126(10 Suppl 1):S1-S42. PMID: 24074529

Jahangiri A, Wagner J, Tran MT, et al. Factors predicting postoperative hyponatremia and efficacy of hyponatremia management strategies after more than 1000 pituitary operations. *J Neurosurg.* 2013;119(6):1478-1483. PMID: 23971964

Woodmansee WW, Carmichael J, Kelly D, Katznelson L; AACE Neuroendocrine and Pituitary Scientific Committee. American Association of Clinical Endocrinologists and American College of Endocrinology disease state clinical review: postoperative management following pituitary surgery. *Endocr Pract.* 2015;21(7):832-838. PMID: 26172128

17 ANSWER: D) Lymphocytic hypophysitis

The most likely lesion in this patient is lymphocytic hypophysitis (Answer D). The key historical point is that these lesions usually develop in the intrapartum or postpartum period and present as mass lesions towards the latter part of pregnancy. A symmetrically enlarged pituitary on MRI is characteristic of hypophysitis, often with extension up the stalk as in this case. Gadolinium was not administered, as the patient is pregnant. ACTH insufficiency occurs in two-thirds of patients with these lesions and should be investigated and treated if found, as adrenal insufficiency is a major cause of death in this setting. In this patient, the progressive, severe fatigue and weight loss point to the possibility of ACTH deficiency. Expectant management will usually suffice for lymphocytic hypophysitis, as the size of most lesions decreases after delivery.

Nonsecreting and prolactin-secreting pituitary adenomas are far more common sellar lesions in women in this age group, but nonsecreting pituitary adenomas (Answer B) generally do not enlarge and cause symptoms during pregnancy. Prolactinomas (Answer A) can, of course, enlarge during pregnancy. However, this patient was previously well, had regular menses before pregnancy, and had no difficulty getting pregnant, implying that she had not been having difficulty with fertility as might be expected with a prolactinoma. The prolactin levels in this case are also helpful in that a patient with a macroprolactinoma should have prolactin levels exceeding 500 ng/mL (>21.7 nmol/L), but a patient with lymphocytic hypophysitis usually has prolactin levels less than 200 ng/mL (<8.7 nmol/L). Although craniopharyngiomas (Answer C) do occur in this age group, they are much less common, and there have been only 3 reports of a change in size during pregnancy. Pituitary apoplexy (Answer E) is usually due to hemorrhage into a preexisting tumor and has a dramatic presentation with sudden onset of severe headache, stiff neck, and often a decreased level of consciousness. Her presentation of gradually worsening headaches with lack of other central nervous system findings does not suggest a hemorrhage. The MRI findings are also not compatible with hemorrhage.

EDUCATIONAL OBJECTIVE

Construct the differential diagnosis of mass lesions in pregnancy.

REFERENCE(S)

Carmichael JD. Update on the diagnosis and management of hypophysitis. *Curr Opin Endocrinol Diabetes Obes.* 2012;19(4):314-321. PMID: 22543347

Joshi MN, Whitelaw BC, Carroll PV. Mechanisms in endocrinology: hypophysitis: diagnosis and treatment. *Eur J Endocrinol.* 2018;179(3):R151-R163. PMID: 29880706

Allix I, Rohmer V. Hypophysitis in 2014. *Ann Endocrinol (Paris)*. 2015;76(5):585-594. PMID: 26514950

18 ANSWER: D) Metastasis

The key features in this patient are the rapid growth of the mass and the presence of diabetes insipidus. This is most consistent with a metastasis (Answer D). Metastasis to the sella is most commonly seen in patients with a known primary and is uncommonly the first manifestation of a metastatic neoplasm. Diabetes insipidus occurs because the metastasis involves the posterior pituitary. The most common cancers causing such metastases are breast cancer in women and lung cancer in men. This patient's history of breast cancer makes this the most likely diagnosis.

Clinically nonfunctioning pituitary adenomas (Answer A) are usually slow growing and are rarely associated with diabetes insipidus. Prolactinoma (Answer B) is unlikely given the modestly elevated serum prolactin, the rapid increase in tumor size, and the presence of diabetes insipidus (rarely associated). Craniopharyngioma (Answer C) can also be associated with diabetes insipidus, but lesions are cystic and patients usually present at a younger age. There is no clinical evidence of sarcoidosis (Answer E) based on history or chest imaging.

EDUCATIONAL OBJECTIVE
Differentiate metastases from other pituitary mass lesions.

REFERENCE(S)
Al-Aridi R, El Sibai K, Fu P, Khan M, Selman WR, Arafah BM. Clinical and biochemical characteristic features of metastatic cancer to the sella turcica: an analytical review. *Pituitary*. 2014;17(6):575-587. PMID: 24337713

Ariel D, Sung H, Coghlan N, Dodd R, Gibbs IC, Katznelson L. Clinical characteristics and pituitary dysfunction in patients with metastatic cancer to the sella. *Endocr Pract*. 2013;19(6):914-919. PMID: 23757610

Cai H, Liu W, Feng T, Li Z, Liu Y. Clinical presentation and pathologic characteristics of pituitary metastasis from breast carcinoma: cases and a systematic review of the literature. *World Neurosurg*. 2019;S1878-S8750(18)32949-8. PMID: 30630045

19 ANSWER: C) An adverse effect of cabergoline

Several studies have shown that dopamine agonists, both cabergoline and bromocriptine, can cause impulse control disorders, including hypersexuality compulsive behavior, in 15% to 20% of treated patients (Answer C). The effect appears to be somewhat dosage dependent, so lowering the dosage, if not discontinuing the dopamine agonist, may be helpful.

This patient's tumor is probably not large enough to cause substantial hypothalamic damage (Answer B). Increasing the serum testosterone to the normal range (Answer A) should not lead to impulse control behavior. While a behavior change unrelated to this tumor or treatment (Answer D) is possible, an adverse effect of cabergoline is the most likely explanation.

EDUCATIONAL OBJECTIVE
Describe potential adverse effects of dopamine agonist treatment in patients with prolactinomas.

REFERENCE(S)
Ioachimescu AG, Fleseriu M, Hoffman AR, Vaughan TB, Katznelson L. Psychological effects of dopamine agonist treatment in patients with hyperprolactinemia and prolactin-secreting adenomas. *Eur J Endocrinol*. 2019;180(1):31-40. PMID: 30400048

Bancos I, Nannenga MR, Bostwick JM, Silber MH, Erickson D, Nippoldt TB. Impulse control disorders in patients with dopamine agonist-treated prolactinomas and nonfunctioning pituitary adenomas: a case-control study. *Clin Endocrinol (Oxf)*. 2014;80(6):863-868. PMID: 24274365

De Sousa SMC, Baranoff J, Rushworth RL, et al. Impulse control disorders in dopamine agonist-treated hyperprolactinemia: prevalence and risk factors. *J Clin Endocrinol Metab*. 2020;105(3):dgz076. PMID: 31580439

20 ANSWER: C) Perform transsphenoidal surgery

This patient presents with a large sellar mass, with suprasellar extension and mild chiasmal compression. The relatively low serum prolactin concentration (<150 to 200 ng/mL [<6.5-8.7 nmol/L]) in this case is not consistent with a macroprolactinoma and is more likely due to stalk effect. Therefore, the lesion is probably a nonfunctioning pituitary macroadenoma, and transsphenoidal surgery (Answer C) is indicated.

Given that the patient probably does not have a prolactinoma, neither higher-dosage bromocriptine (Answer A) nor cabergoline (Answer D) is indicated to reduce tumor size. Stereotactic radiosurgery (Answer E) is not indicated, as surgical resection with chiasmal decompression is necessary. Radiosurgery is unlikely to reduce tumor size and improve optic chiasmal function in a short timeframe. Further, radiosurgery is contraindicated when the tumor touches the chiasm, given risk of optic chiasmal injury. Somatostatin analogue therapy (Answer B) is generally not useful for these tumors, as there have been inconsistent results.

EDUCATIONAL OBJECTIVE
Distinguish between hyperprolactinemia resulting from hypothalamic/stalk dysfunction and tumor production.

REFERENCE(S)
Freda PU, Post KD. Differential diagnosis of sellar masses. *Endocrinol Metab Clin North Am.* 1999;28(1):81-117. PMID: 10207686

Lucas JW, Zada G. Imaging of the pituitary and parasellar region. *Semin Neurol.* 2012;32(4):320-331. PMID: 23361479

Huang W, Molitch ME. Management of nonfunctioning pituitary adenomas (NFAs): observation. *Pituitary.* 2018;21(2):162-116. PMID: 29280025

Samperi I, Lithgow K, Karavitaki N. Hyperprolactinaemia. *J Clin Med.* 2019;8(12):2203. PMID: 31847209

21 ANSWER: C) Another MRI in 12 months

This 48-year-old patient has been found incidentally to have a microlesion of the pituitary gland. Because this is a microlesion without associated symptoms (eg, no diabetes insipidus), there is no indication for surgery (Answer B) or irradiation (Answer D). Appropriate management would simply be to perform serial monitoring and assess for a change in tumor size in 12 months with another MRI (Answer C). Tumors such as this one grow quite slowly (0.6 mm/y on average), so he is in no imminent danger from tumor growth. If the MRI had shown significant suprasellar extension with abutment of the optic chiasm, then visual field testing (Answer A) should have been performed; otherwise, it should not.

EDUCATIONAL OBJECTIVE
Manage a pituitary incidentaloma.

REFERENCE(S)
Molitch ME. Pituitary tumours: pituitary incidentalomas. *Best Pract Res Clin Endocrinol Metab.* 2009;23(5): 667-675. PMID: 19945030

Freda PU, Beckers AM, Katznelson L, et al; Endocrine Society. Pituitary incidentalomas: an Endocrine Society clinical practice guideline. *J Clin Endocrinol Metab.* 2011;96(4):894-904. PMID: 21474686

Scangas GA, Laws ER Jr. Pituitary incidentalomas. *Pituitary.* 2014;17(5):486-491. PMID: 24052242

22 ANSWER: E) Repeat the MRI in 6 months

This 75-year-old man with known coronary artery disease, hypertension, and mild renal insufficiency was found to have an incidental macroadenoma. He has adequate pituitary function. He has hyperprolactinemia, but the prolactin value is in the range consistent with stalk effect and would be expected to be higher in the presence of a macroprolactinoma. Thus, this patient most likely has a clinically nonfunctioning adenoma. Given the lack of local mass effects and the presence of adequate pituitary function, there is no indication for surgery (Answer B) or irradiation (Answer C), and he should be assessed for change in tumor size in 6 months with a repeated MRI (Answer E). Such tumors grow quite slowly (0.6 mm/y on average), so he is in no imminent danger from tumor growth. If the MRI showed clinically significant suprasellar extension with abutment of the optic chiasm, then visual field testing (Answer A) should be performed; otherwise, it should not. Although there are reports of tumor shrinkage with dopamine agonists (Answer D), these agents are not consistently found to be useful in reducing the size of nonfunctioning pituitary macroadenomas. Also, there is no indication to try to shrink the tumor at this time.

EDUCATIONAL OBJECTIVE
Manage pituitary incidentalomas.

REFERENCE(S)

Freda PU, Beckers AM, Katznelson L, et al; Endocrine Society. Pituitary Incidentaloma: an Endocrine Society clinical practice guideline. *J Clin Endocrinol Metab*. 2011;96(4):894-904. PMID: 21474686

Molitch ME. Nonfunctioning pituitary tumors. *Handb Clin Neurol*. 2014;124:167-184. PMID: 25248587

Thyroid Board Review

Jacqueline Jonklaas, MD, PhD, MPH

1 ANSWER: E) Administer ^{131}I activity that is 50% of standard activity

Following radioactive iodine administration, iodine that is not taken up into the thyroid remnant or thyroid cancer tissue is cleared from the body primarily via the kidneys and excreted in the urine. This can be illustrated during posttherapy scanning when iodine accumulation in the bladder can be visualized. In a biokinetic model developed using in vivo gamma camera scanning, the metabolism and clearance of iodine were demonstrated in 6 patients with thyroid cancer and normal kidney function, as activity was demonstrated successively in the stomach, body fluid, whole body, bladder, and thyroid remnant. In an anuric patient with end-stage kidney disease, iodine cannot be cleared by the usual routes and there is potential for excessive exposure of the whole body and bone marrow.

In this particular patient, administration of radioactive iodine is indicated because of her multifocal tumor with extrathyroidal extension and significant lymph node involvement (thus, Answer A is incorrect). If radioactive iodine ablation is intended, administering radioactive iodine as the ^{123}I isotope (Answer B) will not suffice, as this isotope can only be used be used for imaging and not for ablation because it emits only gamma particles that can be imaged with a gamma camera (not destructive beta particles). The ^{131}I isotope, however, emits both gamma and beta particles. Regarding the need for an extended duration of a low-iodine diet, this has not been well studied, but use of an empiric activity of radioactive iodine (Answer C) will most likely lead to excessive bone marrow exposure.

Case examples of patients with end-stage kidney disease who were treated with radioactive iodine for thyroid cancer are shown (see table).

Table. Examples of Radioactive Iodine Administered for Ablation Under Hypothyroid Conditions in Patients With End-Stage Kidney Disease

Author, year (number of cases reported)	Hemodialysis or peritoneal dialysis	Activity selected (mCi)	How determined
Willegaignon 2010 (1 case)	Peritoneal	100	Dosimetry
Holst 2005 (1 case)	Hemodialysis	98	60% reduction
Bhat 2017 (1 case)	Hemodialysis	50	Based on AUC for ^{131}I excretion
Jiminez 2001 (3 cases)	Hemodialysis	75 87 120	Dosimetry
Yeyin 2015 (3 cases)	Hemodialysis	50 50 75	50% reduction
Alevizaki 2006 (5 cases)	Hemodialysis	30 35 35 40 70	40%-50%
Murcutt 2008 (1 case)	Hemodialysis	81	No reduction

Although approaches varied in these case reports, in general, patients were treated with reduced activities, compared with the anticipated empiric activity. However, there are other case reports in which patients were treated with higher than standard activities. The activity chosen depends strongly on the dialysis schedule, generally with hemodialysis being pursued 24 to 48 hours after radioisotope administration to reduce whole-body and bone marrow exposure. The administration of radioactive iodine to a patient receiving dialysis requires careful planning and precautions to avoid exposure of the staff caring for the patient and performing the dialysis, as well as appropriate measures to avoid contamination of dialysis equipment. Based on the mathematical modeling and dosimetric calculations that have been reported, a reasonable approach is to administer 50% of standard activity (Answer E), or, if available, to determine the activity based on dosimetric calculations. Giving 10% of standard activity (Answer D) would most likely not be sufficient to provide effective ablation.

EDUCATIONAL OBJECTIVE

Explain that radioactive iodine is excreted via the kidneys and that reduction of radioactive iodine activity is required for a patient with thyroid cancer and end-stage kidney disease.

REFERENCE(S)

Huang CC, Lin YH, Kittipayak S, Hwua YS, Wang SY, Pan LK. Biokinetic model of radioiodine I-131 in nine thyroid cancer patients subjected to in-vivo gamma camera scanning: a simplified five-compartmental model. *PLoS One.* 2020;15(5):e0232480. PMID: 32365074

Holst JP, Burman KD, Atkins F, Umans JG, Jonklaas J. Radioiodine therapy for thyroid cancer and hyperthyroidism in patients with end-stage renal disease on hemodialysis. *Thyroid.* 2005;15(12):1321-1331. PMID: 16405403

Jiménez RG, Moreno AS, Gonzalez EN, et al. Iodine-131 treatment of thyroid papillary carcinoma in patients undergoing dialysis for chronic renal failure: a dosimetric method. *Thyroid.* 2001;11(11):1031-1034. PMID: 11762712

Alevizaki C, Molfetas M, Samartzis A, et al. Iodine 131 treatment for differentiated thyroid carcinoma in patients with end stage renal failure: dosimetric, radiation safety, and practical considerations. *Hormones (Athens).* 2006;5(4):276-287. PMID: 17178703

Willegaignon J, Ribeiro VPB, Sapienza M, Ono C, Watanabe CB. Is it necessary to reduce the radioiodine dose in patients with thyroid cancer and renal failure? *Arq Bras Endocrinol Metabol.* 2010;54(4):413-418. PMID: 20625654

Bhat M, Mozzor M, Chugh S. Dosing of radioactive iodine in end-stage renal disease patient with thyroid cancer. *Endocrinol Diabetes Metab Case Rep.* 2017;2017:17-0111. PMID: 29158901

Yeyin N, Cavdar I, Uslu L, Abuqbeitah M, Demir M. Effects of hemodialysis on iodine-131 biokinetics in thyroid carcinoma patients with end-stage chronic renal failure. *Nucl Med Commun.* 2016;37(3):283-287. PMID: 26619394

Murcutt G, Edwards J, Boakye J, Davenport A. Hemodialysis of chronic kidney failure patients requiring ablative radioiodine therapy. *Kidney Int.* 2008;73(11):1316-1319. PMID: 18354377

2 ANSWER: D) Defer radioactive iodine for at least 3 months

The cornerstones of preparation for radioactive iodine ablation are generally considered to include serum TSH elevation using recombinant human TSH and iodine depletion by following a low-iodine diet. If a spot urine iodine is checked to verify that iodine levels have been sufficiently lowered, urinary iodine excretion less that 50 µg/g creat is considered to be evidence of success. The problem that may be encountered in this patient is that the iodine load that he was exposed to as a result of the iodinated contrast media could contain 15 to 37 g of iodine. Some studies suggest that urinary iodine may return to baseline 4 to 6 weeks after iodinated contrast exposure. The time approximates 4 weeks in athyreotic individuals and 6 weeks or even longer in those with intact thyroid glands in whom the thyroid concentrates iodine and thus allows whole-body iodine retention. In those with renal insufficiency, the clearance of iodine may be slower.

If the goal is to achieve a low urinary iodine concentration, rather than simply a normal one, maintaining the same instructions and schedule for the patient (Answer C) may be inadvisable. Hydration and diuretic regimens (Answer A) have been used to potentially prevent radiocontrast-induced nephropathy and have also been used to clear iodine as a result of a contrast load. However, this has not been evaluated as a strategy and theoretically could increase the risk of hyponatremia during the low-iodine diet.

It is possible that a longer duration of a low-iodine diet for 3 weeks (Answer B), rather than 1 to 2 weeks (which is followed in most institutions), may help lower the iodine load caused by the iodinated contrast media. However, the success of this approach has not been documented.

Based on studies suggesting that urinary iodine levels may have normalized by 4 weeks after exposure to iodinated contrast media in athyreotic patients, it may at first seem that delaying his schedule by 1 week (Answer E) could be correct, as this would allow a full 6 weeks to elapse, and a return of urinary iodine levels to baseline might be anticipated. However, this may not be the best answer, as urinary iodine levels that are lower than normal are the goal. Moreover, there are also data suggesting that despite the return to "baseline" urinary iodine concentration, delay after contrast exposure for at least 3 to 4 months (Answer D) may be associated with better response rates to radioactive iodine in patients with intermediate-risk thyroid cancer. It has been suggested based on animal models that iodinated contrast media may reduce iodine uptake in the thyroid even after iodine has cleared, perhaps through an effect to decrease sodium-iodide symporter expression. Proteomic studies in mice show that many cellular pathways are modulated by contrast exposure, perhaps providing a mechanism for reduction of iodine uptake in thyroid tissue.

EDUCATIONAL OBJECTIVE
Explain how exposure to iodinated contrast media provides a significant iodine load and may necessitate a delay of radioactive iodine administration.

REFERENCE(S)

Lan W, Renjie W, Qichang W, Feiyue T, Qingjie M, Bin J. Preoperative use of intravenous contrast media is associated with decreased excellent response rates in intermediate-risk DTC patients who subsequently receive total thyroidectomy and low-dose RAI therapy. *Front Oncol.* 2020;10:1297. PMID: 33042786

Padovani RP, Kasamatsu TS, Nakabashi CC, et al. One month is sufficient for urinary iodine to return to its baseline value after the use of water-soluble iodinated contrast agents in post-thyroidectomy patients requiring radioiodine therapy. *Thyroid.* 2012;22(9):926-930. PMID: 22827435

Sohn SY, Choi JH, Kim NK, et al. The impact of iodinated contrast agent administered during preoperative computed tomography scan on body iodine pool in patients with differentiated thyroid cancer preparing for radioactive iodine treatment. *Thyroid.* 2014;24(5):872-877. PMID: 24295076

Hichri M, Vassaux G, Guigonis JM, et al. Proteomic analysis of iodinated contrast agent-induced perturbation of thyroid iodide uptake. *J Clin Med.* 2020;9(2):329. PMID: 31979418

Sawka AM, Ibrahim-Zada I, Galacgac P, et al. Dietary iodine restriction in preparation for radioactive iodine treatment or scanning in well-differentiated thyroid cancer: a systematic review. *Thyroid.* 2010;20(10):1129-1138. PMID: 20860420

3 **ANSWER: D) Minimal uptake throughout both lobes of the thyroid**
This patient has developed subacute thyroiditis following coronavirus infection. This type of thyroiditis is well documented to follow infections with various types of viruses such as coxsackievirus and adenovirus. There are at least a dozen reports of subacute thyroiditis following COVID-19, with more reports continuing to accumulate. The characteristics of the thyroiditis and the pattern of thyroid function appear to be similar with all the aforementioned viruses, with younger women mostly being affected and the symptoms developing in the 2 to 4 weeks after resolution of the viral symptoms. Neck pain and fever accompany the symptoms of thyrotoxicosis, and thyroid function tests and imaging are suggestive of destructive thyroiditis. Thyroid function subsequently normalizes, with some cases of temporary hypothyroidism.

As is the case with other instances of viral thyroiditis, radionuclide scans with either technetium or ^{123}I show absent or minimal uptake (Answer D). Elevated or normal uptake (Answers A, B, C, and E) would not be expected. If performed, thyroid ultrasonography might show diffuse areas of hypoechogenicity and color Doppler ultrasonography usually shows mild to absent vascularity.

The angiotensin-converting enzyme 2 degrades angiotensin II to angiotensin as part of its regulation of the renin-angiotensin-aldosterone system in the kidney. The angiotensin-converting enzyme 2 receptor is present in many tissues in addition to the kidney. Expression studies have shown that the highest levels occur in the small intestine, testis, kidney, heart, and thyroid. Severe acute respiratory syndrome coronavirus 2 (SARS-CoV-2), the virus causing coronavirus disease (COVID-19), has been shown to bind to the angiotensin-converting enzyme 2 receptor. Endocytosis of this virus-receptor complex allows entry of SARS-CoV-2 into affected cell. This internalization of the virus into thyrocytes may underlie the thyroiditis symptoms that occur following COVID-19, reflecting injury of the thyroid gland.

Some of the injury seen in various tissues may be due to the host immune responses to the virus, which, if excessive, could add to tissue injury in the form of "cytokine storm." With respect to the subacute thyroiditis associated with COVID-19, it is not known whether the cytokine storm explanation must be invoked or whether the virus itself causes injury as presumably occurs in subacute thyroiditis caused by other viruses.

EDUCATIONAL OBJECTIVE
Describe how SARS-CoV-2 has been associated with subacute thyroiditis.

REFERENCE(S)

Li MY, Li L, Zhang Y, Wang XS. Expression of the SARS-CoV-2 cell receptor gene ACE2 in a wide variety of human tissues. *Infect Dis Poverty.* 2020;9(1):45. PMID: 32345362

Campos-Barrera E, Alvarez-Cisneros T, Davalos-Fuentes M. Subacute thyroiditis associated with COVID-19. *Case Rep Endocrinol.* 2020;2020: 8891539. PMID: 33005461

Chakraborty U, Ghosh S, Chandra A, Ray AK. Subacute thyroiditis as a presenting manifestation of COVID-19: a report of an exceedingly rare clinical entity. *BMJ Case Rep.* 2020;13(12):e239953. PMID: 33370933

Rotondi M, Coperchini F, Ricci G, et al. Detection of SARS-COV-2 receptor ACE-2 mRNA in thyroid cells: a clue for COVID-19-related subacute thyroiditis. *J Endocrinol Invest.* 2021;44(5):1085-1090. PMID: 33025553

Brancatella A, Ricci D, Cappellani D, et al. Is subacute thyroiditis an underestimated manifestation of SARS-CoV-2 infection? Insights from a case series. *J Clin Endocrinol Metab.* 2020;105(10):dgaa537. PMID: 32780854

4 ANSWER: B) Methimazole was stopped on day 1

When the full medical record became available, it was clear that this patient was initially overtreated for Graves disease and developed iatrogenic hypothyroidism when he continued to take his medication without having follow-up testing. On day 1 (admission to first hospital), he was taking 40 mg methimazole daily. This was stopped (Answer B), and his next laboratory assessment shows the rapid increase in total T_3 as his underlying Graves disease with its predominant T_3 production becomes evident.

Starting levothyroxine on day 1 (Answer C) would be unlikely to provide such a significant increase in total T_3 in such a short period as is seen in the day 5 laboratory results. Liothyronine started on day 5 (Answer D) might account for the increase in total T_3 by day 11 but is unlikely to account for the increase in free T_4. Similarly, levothyroxine started on day 5 (Answer E) would be unlikely to produce a doubling of total T_3 by day 11. Starting amiodarone on day 1 (Answer A) as a sole medication change would be unlikely to cause the rapid increase in total T_3 specifically seen by day 5.

The full course of events for this patient is shown (*see table*).

The full trajectory of the patient's laboratory results indicates several important aspects of using thionamides to treat hyperthyroidism. One is initially choosing a methimazole dosage based on

Analyte	5 Months prior	4 Months prior	2 Months prior	Day 1	Day 5	Day 11	Day 18	Day 26	Day 40
TSH	<0.005 mIU/L	<0.008 mIU/L	89 mIU/L	178 mIU/L	155 mIU/L	0.819 mIU/L	0.179 mIU/L	0.102 mIU/L	0.386 mIU/L
Free T$_4$	3.28 ng/dL (SI: 42.2 pmol/L)	1.10 ng/dL (SI: 14.2 pmol/L)	0.9 ng/dL (SI: 11.6 pmol/L)	<0.10 ng/dL (SI: 1.3 pmol/L)	0.13 ng/dL (SI: 1.7 pmol/L)	0.43 ng/dL (SI: 5.5 pmol/L)	0.85 ng/dL (SI: 10.9 pmol/L)	0.66 ng/dL (SI: 8.5 pmol/L)	0.43 ng/dL (SI: 5.5 pmol/L)
Total T$_3$	279 ng/dL (SI: 4.3 nmol/L)	201 ng/dL (SI: 3.1 nmol/L)	65 ng/dL (SI: 1.0 nmol/L)	32 ng/dL (SI: 0.5 nmol/L)	212 ng/dL (SI: 3.3 nmol/L)	574 ng/dL (SI: 8.8 nmol/L)	627 ng/dL (SI: 9.7 nmol/L)	182 ng/dL (SI: 2.8 nmol/L)	134 ng/dL (SI: 2.1 nmol/L)
TRAb	28 IU/L	...	...	...	...	...	...	...	...
Daily methimazole dosage	7.5 mg	30 mg	30 mg (mistaken as 30 mg twice daily)	40 mg	0	0	5 mg	5 mg	5 mg

Reference ranges: TSH, 0.5-5.0 mIU/L; free T$_4$, 0.8-1.8 ng/dL (SI: 10.30-23.17 pmol/L); total T$_3$, 70-200 ng/dL (SI: 1.08-3.08 nmol/L); TRAb, <1.75 IU/L.

the degree of elevation of the thyroid hormones, but then further adjusting the methimazole, usually by dosage reduction as the patient responds to therapy. The American Thyroid Association guidelines, for example, recommend an initial methimazole dosage of 10 to 20 mg daily for free T$_4$ values that are 1.5 to 2 times the upper normal limit. According to these guidelines, once the patient is euthyroid, the methimazole dosage can generally be reduced by 30% to 50%. It appears that iatrogenic hypothyroidism ensued in this patient when it was believed that he was erroneously taking 60 mg methimazole daily and it was determined that a reduction to 40 mg daily was appropriate, even in the face of a TSH value of 89 mIU/L. A quick rebound into T$_3$ thyrotoxicosis occurred when the patient's methimazole was stopped. These data suggest the important of monitoring therapy, clear communications about drug dosages, and ideally continuity of care during supervision of the patient's therapy.

EDUCATIONAL OBJECTIVE

Monitor thyroid function during thionamide therapy to avoid both undertreatment of hyperthyroidism and iatrogenic hypothyroidism.

REFERENCE(S)

Ross DS, Burch HB, Cooper DS, et al. 2016 American Thyroid Association guidelines for diagnosis and management of hyperthyroidism and other causes of thyrotoxicosis. *Thyroid.* 2016;26(10):1343-1421. PMID: 27521067

5 **ANSWER: C) Hyperemesis gravidarum**
Normal pregnancy is characterized by transient gestation thyrotoxicosis as β-hCG levels peak at approximately weeks 10 to 12 towards the end of the first trimester. Due to the TSH-like activity of β-hCG, there is stimulation of the thyroid gland. Typically, free T$_4$ and T$_3$ increase, although the elevation is relatively mild, and TSH levels are correspondingly reduced in a mirror image of the β-hCG changes. In some pregnancies, these changes in thyroid parameters can be of greater magnitude. In a classic 1992 study of 57 patients with hyperemesis gravidarum (Answer C), 30% of patients had undetectable TSH, defined as less than 0.04 mIU/L. The pattern of the hormonal changes is shown (*see figure on the following page*), with the highest hCG and free T$_4$ levels seen in patients with the most severe hyperemesis.

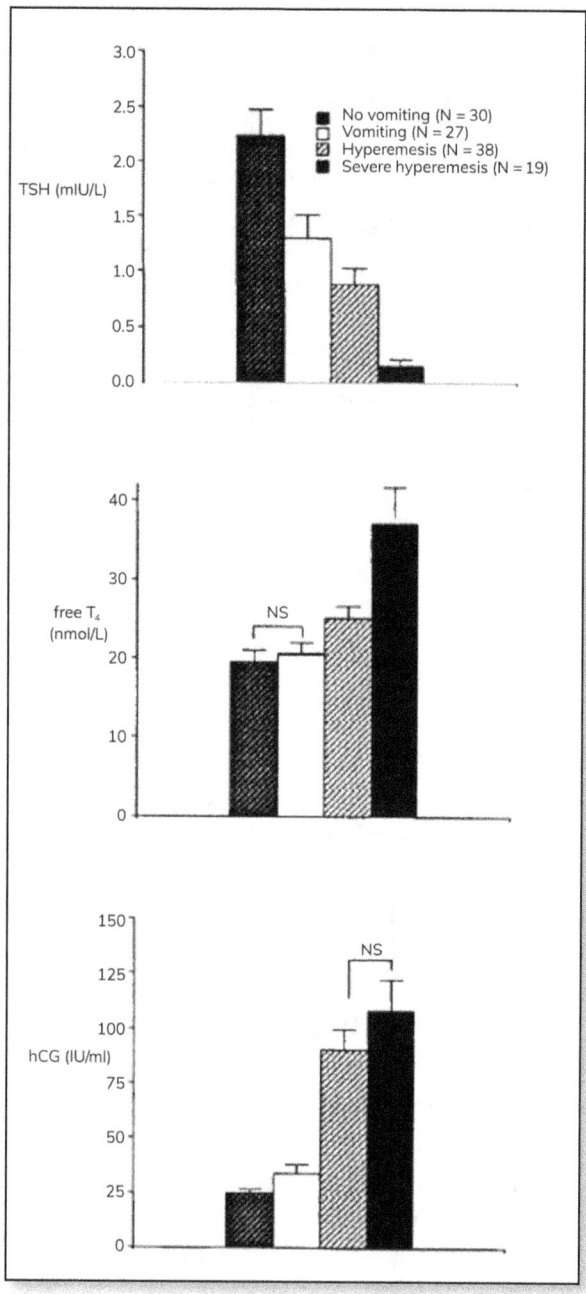

Figure reprinted from Goodwin TM, Montoro M, Mestman JH, Pekary AE, Hershman JM. The role of chorionic gonadotropin in transient hyperthyroidism of hyperemesis gravidarum. *J Clin Endocrinol Metab.* 1992;75(5):1333-1337. © Endocrine Society.

The changes seen in TSH and thyroid hormone levels can overlap with those in Graves disease. Features that may aid in the distinction between gestational thyrotoxicosis and Graves disease are symptoms predating pregnancy, goiter, orbitopathy, and TRAb in Graves disease. In gestational thyrotoxicosis, the symptoms begin during pregnancy with a strong component of nausea and vomiting that is not usually seen in Graves hyperthyroidism. The ratio of T_3 to T_4 is also typically higher in Graves disease than in hyperemesis gravidarum. This patient has hyperemesis gravidarum. As is typically seen in this disorder, the symptoms and thyroid abnormalities resolve as the patient moves into the second trimester. The treatment for hyperemesis gravidarum is supportive with use of antiemetics, fluid replacement, and correction of electrolyte abnormalities. Antithyroidal treatment is not needed, although it was used in this patient because of her extreme presentation with unusual thyroid hormone elevations and tachyarrhythmia. Her course, however, was typical of hyperemesis gravidarum, as her nausea, vomiting, and thyroid abnormalities resolved in the second trimester.

Growth/differentiation factor 15, which is a hormone produced by the placenta, has been postulated to contribute to the nausea and vomiting seen in hyperemesis gravidarum by its stimulation of the area postrema in the brainstem.

The patient's pelvic ultrasonography showed a singleton pregnancy, so a twin pregnancy (Answer E) is incorrect. There is no need to invoke a diagnosis of trophoblastic disease in a patient with a viable pregnancy, so choriocarcinoma (Answer A) and hydatidiform mole (Answer D) are not the best choices. Familial gestational hyperthyroidism (Answer B) is due to pathogenic variants in the TSH receptor gene, which enhance its response to β-hCG stimulation. While the vignette does not provide a family history, this condition is ruled out because the patient did not experience severe nausea and vomiting during her first pregnancy.

EDUCATIONAL OBJECTIVE
Construct the differential diagnosis for hyperthyroidism associated with elevated β-hCG levels.

REFERENCE(S)

Goodwin TM, Montoro M, Mestman JH, Pekary AE, Hershman JM. The role of chorionic gonadotropin in transient hyperthyroidism of hyperemesis gravidarum. *J Clin Endocrinol Metab*. 1992;75(5):1333-1337. PMID: 1430095

Goldman AM, Mestman JH. Transient non-autoimmune hyperthyroidism of early pregnancy. *J Thyroid Res*. 2011;2011:142413. PMID: 21785688

Fejzo MS, Trovik J, Grooten IJ, et al. Nausea and vomiting of pregnancy and hyperemesis gravidarum. *Nat Rev Dis Primers*. 2019;5(1):62. PMID: 31515515

6   ANSWER: C) Benign follicular adenoma

RAS variants are the most frequent genetic alteration found in thyroid nodules with indeterminate cytology. They are also the second most common pathogenic variant found in malignant thyroid nodules. The *BRAF* V600E pathogenic variant (not found in this patient's nodule) is a strong predictor of papillary thyroid cancer. However, *RAS* variants do not have a good predictive value for thyroid cancer and, overall, *RAS*-like variants are generally associated with low-risk thyroid cancer. *RAS* variants can be present in benign nodules; noninvasive follicular thyroid neoplasms with papillary-like nuclear features (NIFTP); and cancers such as follicular variant of papillary thyroid cancer, papillary thyroid cancer, and poorly differentiated thyroid cancer. Benign follicular adenomas develop from a clonal process and can acquire additional variants. In thyroid nodules with a *RAS* variant, NIFTP can be considered a precursor lesion for invasive encapsulated follicular variant of papillary thyroid cancer, and follicular adenoma can be thought of as a precursor of follicular thyroid carcinoma. Of the answer options given, benign follicular adenoma (Answer C) is the answer most congruent with having a *RAS* variant present, but not having a *BRAF* V600E pathogenic variant.

RAS tumors typically have the sonographic features shown in this case: regular margins, mixed echogenicity or isoechoic or hyperechoic appearance, and lack of calcifications. *BRAF* tumors are more likely to have irregular margins, hypoechogenicity, calcifications, and abnormal lymph nodes. In a retrospective study of 78 thyroid nodules with indeterminate cytology that underwent resection, 50 had *RAS*-like variants. Of these, 36% were benign, 32% were NIFTP, and 32% were cancer (6% follicular cancer, 10% follicular variant of papillary thyroid cancer, and 16% classic papillary thyroid cancer). Most had low-risk sonographic features. In the same study, 8 nodules had *BRAF*-like variants, most had a high-risk sonographic appearance, and all were papillary thyroid cancer.

Nodules harboring the tall cell variant of papillary thyroid cancer (Answer A) are often microlobulated, hypoechoic, have microcalcifications, and are frequently associated with lymph node metastases. Most tumors have the *BRAF* V600E pathogenic variant. The sonographic features of the diffuse sclerosing variant of papillary thyroid cancer (Answer B) include an ill-defined hypoechoic nodule and scattered microcalcifications, with the major genetic rearrangement being *RET/PTC*. The hobnail variant of papillary thyroid cancer (Answer D) is rare, but findings reported on ultrasonography include hypoechogenicity, microcalcifications, and metastatic lymph nodes. The *BRAF* V600E pathogenic variant may be present. Columnar cell variants (Answer E) are also rare, and their sonographic features include being hypoechoic, having microcalcifications, and having capsular protrusions representing extrathyroidal extension and nodal metastases. The *BRAF* V600E pathogenic variant may be present. The sonographic findings in this vignette are not consistent with this entity.

Note: Image in vignette stem is reprinted with permission from Shin JH. Ultrasonographic imaging of papillary thyroid carcinoma variants. *Ultrasonography*. 2017;36(2):103-110. © Korean Society of Ultrasound in Medicine.

EDUCATIONAL OBJECTIVE

Predict the type of histology likely to be associated with a thyroid nodule with a *RAS* pathogenic variant and low-risk sonographic appearance.

REFERENCE(S)

Chin PD, Zhu CY, Sajed DP, et al. Correlation of ThyroSeq results with surgical histopathology in cytologically indeterminate thyroid nodules. *Endocr Pathol*. 2020;31(4):377-384. PMID: 32671653

Nikiforov YE. Role of molecular markers in thyroid nodule management: then and now. *Endocr Pract*. 2017;23(8):979-988. PMID: 28534687

Angell TE. RAS-positive thyroid nodules. *Curr Opin Endocrinol Diabetes Obes*. 2017;24(5):372-376. PMID: 28639967

Guan H, Toraldo G, Cerda S, et al. Utilities of *RAS* mutations in preoperative fine needle biopsies for decision making for thyroid nodule management: results from a single-center prospective cohort. *Thyroid*. 2020;30(4):536-547. PMID: 31996097

Shin JH. Ultrasonographic imaging of papillary thyroid carcinoma variants. *Ultrasonography*. 2017;36(2):103-110. PMID: 28222584

7 ANSWER: B

When given orally, estrogen therapy exposes the liver to circulating levels of estrogen delivered via the portal circulation. The effect of estrogen in the liver is to increase the synthesis of a number of binding proteins. The proteins that are known to be increased by estrogen include SHBG, cortisol-binding globulin, and thyroxine-binding globulin. Estrogen delivered by the transdermal route does not appear to increase the levels of any of these binding proteins, presumably because the estrogen does not reach the liver in sufficient quantities. When healthy women who are menopausal, but have no other hormonal deficiencies are provided with oral vs transdermal estrogen, only the oral estrogen causes an increase in SHBG, cortisol-binding globulin, and thyroxine-binding globulin. In these women without hypothyroidism, the increased thyroxine-binding globulin is associated with a corresponding increase in total T_4, modest decrease in free T_4, but no change in serum TSH.

In a classic study of women taking levothyroxine either for replacement therapy or TSH suppression therapy, oral conjugated estrogens were associated with increased thyroxine-binding globulin, increased total T_4, decreased free T_4, and increased serum TSH. In some women, the TSH increase was not clinically significant, but in 40% of women, the degree of TSH elevation was sufficient to prompt an increase in the patient's levothyroxine dosage.

Answers A and C are incorrect, as transdermal estrogen does not increase T_4 and thyroxine-binding globulin. Answer D is incorrect, as oral estrogen is not associated with a decrease in T_4 and thyroxine-binding globulin. Oral androgen given in the past as therapy for breast cancer has been shown to have this effect and to thereby decrease levothyroxine requirement. Answer E is incorrect, as this does not reflect the known stimulation of T_4 and thyroxine-binding globulin by oral estrogen. Answer B correctly portrays the increase in T_4, thyroxine-binding globulin, and TSH seen with oral estrogen, while also incorporating the lack of effect of transdermal estrogen on these parameters.

EDUCATIONAL OBJECTIVE

Explain that estrogen reaching the liver in sufficient quantities increases the synthesis of thyroxine-binding globulin and thereby increases total T_4 levels.

REFERENCE(S)

Shifren JL, Desindes S, McIlwain M, Doros G, Mazer NA. A randomized, open-label, crossover study comparing the effects of oral versus trans-dermal estrogen therapy on serum androgens, thyroid hormones, and adrenal hormones in naturally menopausal women. *Menopause*. 2007;14(6):985-994. PMID: 17507833

Arafah BM. Increased need for thyroxine in women with hypothyroidism during estrogen therapy. *N Engl J Med*. 2001;344(23):1743-1749. PMID: 11396440

Tahboub R, Arafah BM. Sex steroids and the thyroid. *Best Pract Res Clin Endocrinol Metab*. 2009;23(6):769-780. PMID: 19942152

Arafah BM. Decreased levothyroxine requirement in women with hypothyroidism during androgen therapy for breast cancer. *Ann Intern Med*. 1994;121(4):247-251. PMID: 7518657

8 ANSWER: D) Patient error in taking levothyroxine

This patient's levothyroxine dosage is 225 mcg daily, which involves him taking 2 tablets of levothyroxine (one 200-mcg tablet and one 25-mcg tablet). The most likely explanation for his current thyroid function test results is patient error (Answer D). When first questioned about his out-of-range laboratory results, the patient confirmed that he was taking the correct dosage of 225 mcg daily and affirmed his adherence to his treatment regimen. He was prescribed an increased dosage of 300 mcg daily on the basis of this history. However, the patient contacted his physician the next day and explained that he had actually mistakenly filled his pill dispenser with 2 tablets of 25 mcg instead of 1 each of 25 mcg and 200 mcg, and that based on his tablet count he had been doing this for the last 3 weeks. He patient then resumed his correct dosage of 225 mcg daily.

Errors of this nature are not uncommon in patients taking long-term medications, especially if they are taking several medications. Making medication regimens and schedules as simple and convenient as possible is advisable. Taking levothyroxine with food and with interfering medications is commonly reported in patients with elevated TSH values. This patient was using a pill dispenser, which is helpful. Perhaps reminding the patient about the colors of different levothyroxine doses would be a good educational opportunity. However, some studies indicate low rates of adherence to long-term therapies, with one study reporting an adherence rate of 68% for hypothyroidism therapy.

Pharmacy errors can also occur and are more likely to involve issues such as polypharmacy or undesirable medication interaction, rather than providing a patient with an erroneous dose of medication. However, this was not an offered answer option.

Large doses of biotin (Answer C) are not the most likely explanation, as this would be expected to cause false lowering of TSH values and false increases in free T_4 values when measured using sandwich and competitive assays, respectively, that use the streptavidin–biotin interaction. Similarly, storage of levothyroxine at extreme temperatures (Answer E) may result in product deterioration, but this is not the most likely explanation if the patient is storing his levothyroxine in the bedroom.

MacroTSH (Answer B) and heterophilic antibodies (Answer A) are not the best answers, as these would be expected to be associated with a false elevation in TSH but normal free T_4 level. In this case, the patient had a low free T_4 level and some symptoms compatible with hypothyroidism. Thus, it seems most likely that the patient would be biochemically hypothyroid.

EDUCATIONAL OBJECTIVE
Appreciate that errors in taking medications are common and should be considered in a patient who has abnormal thyroid function.

REFERENCE(S)
Briesacher BA, Andrade SE, Fouayzi H, Chan KA. Comparison of drug adherence rates among patients with seven different medical conditions. *Pharmacotherapy.* 2008;28(4):437-443. PMID: 18363527

Kucukler FK, Akbaba G, Arduc A, Simsek Y, Guler S. Evaluation of the common mistakes made by patients in the use of levothyroxine. *Eur J Intern Med.* 2014;25(9):e107-e108. PMID: 25240626

Favresse J, Burlacu MC, Maiter D, Gruson D. Interferences with thyroid function immunoassays: clinical implications and detection algorithm. *Endocr Rev.* 2018;39(5):830-850. PMID: 29982406

Loh TP, Kao SL, Halsall DJ, et al. Macro-thyrotropin: a case report and review of literature. *J Clin Endocrinol Metab.* 2012;97(6):1823-1828. PMID: 22466337

9 ANSWER: D) Decrease levothyroxine dosage, schedule repeated TSH measurement in 6 to 8 weeks

Following surgery and radioactive iodine ablation, this patient's tumor would initially have been staged as intermediate risk. In addition, the tall cell variant of papillary thyroid cancer is known to be an aggressive variant. However, she has had an excellent response to therapy, with no current evidence of disease on the basis of the undetectable unstimulated thyroglobulin level and ultrasound with evidence of only benign-appearing lymph nodes. Current American Thyroid Association guidelines recommend continual modification of risk status based on new information obtained in the course of follow-up. An excellent response to therapy, defined as negative imaging and a suppressed serum thyroglobulin concentration less than 0.2 ng/mL (<0.2 μg/L) or stimulated thyroglobulin concentration less than 1 ng/mL (<1 μg/L) in the absence of thyroglobulin antibodies should lead to both a decrease in the level of TSH suppression and to lessening of the intensity and frequency of follow-up. A TSH target in the low-normal range would be reasonable for this patient, thus maintaining or increasing the TSH-suppressive levothyroxine dosage (Answers A, B, and C) is incorrect. There is no role for another radioactive iodine whole-body scan (Answer E), given evidence of her excellent response to therapy and the previously negative whole-body scan. The best course of action is to decrease her levothyroxine dosage and to measure TSH in 6 to 8 weeks (Answer D).

EDUCATIONAL OBJECTIVE

Explain restaging in the setting of thyroid cancer and guide appropriate surveillance and treatment in a patient with an excellent response to thyroid cancer therapy.

REFERENCE(S)

Haugen BR, Alexander EK, Bible KC, et al. 2015 American Thyroid Association management guidelines for adult patients with thyroid nodules and differentiated thyroid cancer: the American Thyroid Association Guidelines Task Force on Thyroid Nodules and Differentiated Thyroid Cancer. *Thyroid.* 2016;26(1):1-133. PMID: 26462967

Tuttle RM, Tala H, Shah J, et al. Estimating risk of recurrence in differentiated thyroid cancer after total thyroidectomy and radioactive iodine remnant ablation: using response to therapy variables to modify the initial risk estimates predicted by the new American Thyroid Association staging system. *Thyroid.* 2010;20(12): 1341-1349. PMID: 21034228

Tuttle RM, Alzahrani AS. Risk stratification in differentiated thyroid cancer: from detection to final follow-up. *J Clin Endocrinol Metab.* 2019;104(9):4087-4100. PMID: 30874735

10 ANSWER: C) Hook effect

Serum calcitonin levels are generally proportional to the degree of medullary cancer tumor burden. Monitoring calcitonin levels at least every 6 months postoperatively is recommended by current American Thyroid Association guidelines, and the calcitonin doubling time is an independent predictor of survival. However, it is important to be aware of potential pitfalls in calcitonin measurement. The hook effect (Answer C) refers to artificially low calcitonin measurements in the setting of very high serum levels of calcitonin that saturate the binding capacity of the antibody used in the immunoassay. This is more likely to occur with immunoradiometric assays than with immunochemiluminometric or immunofluorometric assays. For example, in one description of an immunofluorometric assay, the hook effect was observed only with calcitonin concentrations greater than 200,000 pg/mL (>58,400 pmol/L). The presence of the hook effect should be suspected in patients with a large tumor burden and surprisingly low serum calcitonin levels, or in the setting of discordance with prior values without intervening therapy. If the hook effect is present, serial dilution of the sample will demonstrate a nonlinear relationship.

Chronic kidney disease (Answer A) lowers the renal calcitonin clearance rate and thus may increase serum calcitonin levels, rather than decrease them. Use of omeprazole (Answer B) and other proton-pump inhibitors may increase gastrin secretion, which will, in turn, increase calcitonin levels, not cause them to be lower than expected. Heterophilic antibodies (Answer D) have been reported to interfere with calcitonin measurements, but heterophilic antibodies typically result in artificially elevated calcitonin values (due to cross-linking of capture and tracer antibodies in the absence of analyte) rather than artificially low values. Cross-reactivity of procalcitonin with calcitonin (Answer E) appears to be minimal. Moreover, if procalcitonin was also being measured by the calcitonin assay, this might be expected to lead to a higher value rather than a lower one.

EDUCATIONAL OBJECTIVE
Describe pitfalls in the use of serum calcitonin to monitor medullary cancer.

REFERENCE(S)

Wells SA Jr, Asa SL, Dralle H, et al; American Thyroid Association Guidelines Task Force on Medullary Thyroid Carcinoma. Revised American Thyroid Association guidelines for the management of medullary thyroid carcinoma. *Thyroid.* 2015;25(6):567-610. PMID: 25810047

Leboeuf R, Langlois MF, Martin M, Ahnadi CE, Fink GD. "Hook effect" in calcitonin immunoradiometric assay in patients with metastatic medullary thyroid carcinoma: case report and review of the literature. *J Clin Endocrinol Metab.* 2006;91(2):361-364. PMID: 16278263

Camacho CP, Lindsey SC, Kasamatsu TS, et al. Development and application of a novel sensitive immunometric assay for calcitonin in a large cohort of patients with medullary and differentiated thyroid cancer, thyroid nodules, and autoimmune thyroid diseases. *Eur Thyroid J.* 2014;3(2):117-124. PMID: 25114875

11 ANSWER: B) Excessive dental caries
Salivary gland dysfunction after treatment with radioactive iodine is quite common. This can take the form of sialadenitis, xerostomia, and taste alterations. The incidence of xerostomia is between 15% and 54%, and it tends to improve over time. Prolonged or persistent xerostomia predisposes patients to excessive caries (Answer B).

Alteration of taste, which occurs commonly after radioiodine therapy, is typically transient rather than permanent (Answer A). Patients may describe a metallic or chemical taste that occasionally persists for months after therapy. Permanent hypoparathyroidism (Answer E) is a very rare consequence of radioiodine therapy, with only 2 cases described in the literature to date. Transient depression of sperm count occurs following radioiodine, and there is a cumulative

effect on the testes, manifested as an elevation in serum FSH and slight decrease in sperm count, but not azoospermia (Answer C). Men desiring future fertility and receiving radioiodine doses greater than 400 mCi should be counseled about sperm cryopreservation. Leukemia (Answer D) is a potential consequence of receiving very high doses of radioiodine, with a frequency of 0.3%, typically occurring in older patients receiving a cumulative dose greater than 800 mCi. Patients who receive the highest doses over the shortest intervals are most likely to develop this rare complication, with a latency period of less than 10 years. Ideally, patients requiring repeated treatments with radioiodine should receive treatment at intervals of at least 1 year, but patients with aggressive radioiodine-avid disease should not be denied therapy at shorter intervals when appropriate.

EDUCATIONAL OBJECTIVE
Anticipate the most likely adverse effects of high-dose radioactive iodine treatment.

REFERENCE(S)

Clement SC, Peeters RP, Ronckers CM, et al. Intermediate and long-term adverse effects of radioiodine therapy for differentiated thyroid carcinoma--a systematic review. *Cancer Treat Rev.* 2015;41(10):925-934. PMID: 26421813

Singer MC, Marchal F, Angelos P, et al. Salivary and lacrimal dysfunction after radioactive iodine for differentiated thyroid cancer: American Head and Neck Society Endocrine Surgery Section and Salivary Gland Section joint multidisciplinary clinical consensus statement of otolaryngology, ophthalmology, nuclear medicine and endocrinology. *Head Neck.* 2020;42(11):3446-3459. PMID: 32812307

12 ANSWER: D) Atenolol
This patient has developed what appears to be painless thyroiditis while taking interferon alfa. β-Adrenergic blockade (Answer D) is indicated to control his rapid pulse, but the other measures listed are unnecessary. Patients with hepatitis C have a higher prevalence of positive TPO antibodies, even before treatment with

interferon alfa, than do patients with other forms of viral hepatitis (11.2% vs 3.6%, respectively). The most common thyroid manifestation of interferon alfa therapy is hypothyroidism, which occurs in approximately 5% of all treated patients but in 36% of patients who have positive TPO antibodies before treatment. Women are twice as likely as men to develop this disorder (8.7% vs 3.4% in one study). A smaller number of patients develop thyrotoxicosis during interferon alfa therapy; this is more often painless thyroiditis rather than Graves disease, although both have been described. The percentage of patients with positive TPO antibodies increases after treatment with interferon alfa (from 3.7% to 9.7% in one study). Most patients (60%) with interferon alfa–associated thyroid dysfunction have improvement in their thyroid symptoms after drug discontinuation.

Methimazole therapy (Answer A) would not be effective for thyroiditis, as thyroid hormone is being released from the damaged thyroid gland rather than reaching the blood stream from ongoing synthesis. Propylthiouracil (Answer E) would also be ineffective in the setting of thyroiditis. Even in hyperthyroidism due to Graves disease or toxic nodular disease, it is not generally a first-line drug. Prednisone therapy (Answer B) is sometimes used to treat painful subacute thyroiditis, but it is not indicated for painless drug-induced thyroiditis. Intravenous immunoglobulin (Answer C) is not indicated for the treatment of thyroiditis.

EDUCATIONAL OBJECTIVE
Diagnose and manage drug-induced thyroiditis.

REFERENCE(S)
Nair Kesavachandran C, Haamann F, Nienhaus A. Frequency of thyroid dysfunctions during interferon alpha treatment of single and combination therapy in hepatitis C virus-infected patients: a systematic review based analysis. *PLoS One*. 2013;8(2):e55364. PMID: 23383326

Carella C, Mazziotti G, Amato G, Braverman LE, Roti E. Clinical review 169: interferon-alpha related thyroid disease: pathophysiological, epidemiological, and clinical aspects. *J Clin Endocrinol Metab*. 2004;89(8):3656-3661. PMID: 15292282

13 **ANSWER: C) Expected changes in euthyroid patients on amiodarone**

Amiodarone can have complex effects on the thyroid gland due to both intrinsic drug effects and effects due to its iodine content. Intrinsic drug effects include inhibition of the type 1 and 2 $5'$-deiodinase, decreased T_3 binding to its receptor, and thyroid cytotoxicity leading to thyroiditis. Iodine-related effects include development of hypothyroidism in those with underlying Hashimoto disease and induction of hyperthyroidism in those with autonomous nodules or subclinical Graves disease. Drug-induced hyperthyroidism occurs in approximately 5% of treated patients, while hypothyroidism occurs in approximately 7%.

Amiodarone has dramatic effects on thyroid function tests in clinically euthyroid patients. A large iodine load (74 mg total iodine, 7.4 mg of free iodine per 200-mg tablet) is delivered with each dose. Amiodarone inhibits both peripheral and central (intrapituitary) conversion of T_4 to T_3 through its action on type 1 and type 2 $5'$-monodeiodinase, respectively. Lastly, amiodarone has T_3 antagonistic effects at the nuclear level. The common pattern observed in euthyroid patients is high free T_4 and total T_4, low-normal T_3, high reverse T_3, and high-normal TSH (thus, Answer C is correct). These changes tend to persist over time, although serum TSH values may gradually normalize in some patients. The pattern of these changes is shown (*see figure on the following page*).

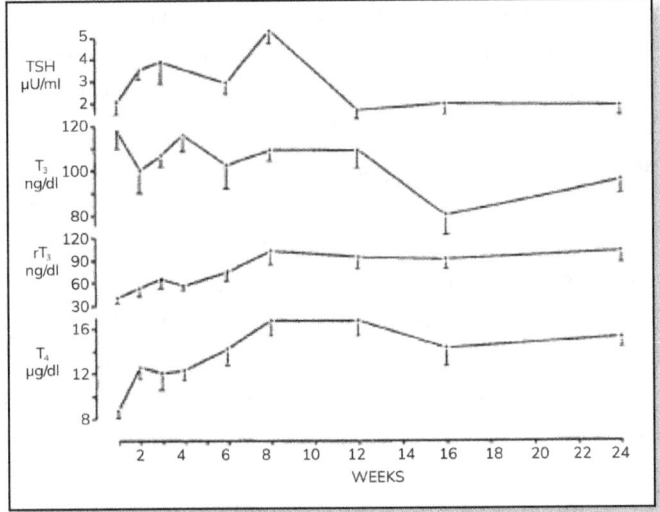

Long-term (6-month) changes in thyroid function in 10 patients on chronic amiodarone treatment. The abscissa indicates the beginning of each week of therapy. By the end of 3 weeks of treatment, each hormone level was significantly different from the pretreatment value, as determined by analysis of variance. Reprinted from Melmed S, Nademanee K, Reed AW, Hendrickson JA, Singh BN, Hershman JM. Hyperthyroxinemia with bradycardia and normal thyrotropin secretion after chronic amiodarone administration. *J Clin Endocrinol Metab.* 1981;53(5):997-1001. © Endocrine Society.

Amiodarone and its metabolites are not known to cause artifactual interference with thyroid function assays (Answer D). This patient's normal TSH and lack of symptoms exclude thyrotoxicosis (Answers A and B). Also, he is not acutely ill, so euthyroid sick syndrome (Answer E) is incorrect.

EDUCATIONAL OBJECTIVE

Distinguish expected changes in thyroid function parameters in patients taking amiodarone from amiodarone-induced thyroid dysfunction.

REFERENCE(S)

Danzi S, Klein I. Amiodarone-induced thyroid dysfunction. *J Intensive Care Med.* 2015;30(4):179-185. PMID: 24067547

Basaria S, Cooper DS. Amiodarone and the thyroid. *Am J Med.* 2005;118(7):706-714. PMID: 15989900

Melmed S, Nademanee K, Reed AW, Hendrickson JA, Singh BN, Hershman JM. Hyperthyroxinemia with bradycardia and normal thyrotropin secretion after chronic amiodarone administration. *J Clin Endocrinol Metab.* 1981;53(5):997-1001. PMID: 7287882

14 ANSWER: D) Levothyroxine, 70 mcg intravenously once daily

When given orally, approximately 62% to 82% of the levothyroxine dose is absorbed and absorption occurs in the jejunum or ileum. Absorption is better in the fasting state (78%-79%) than in the nonfasting state (59%-68%).

Given that 100% of an intravenous dose of levothyroxine reaches the blood stream, when levothyroxine is converted from oral to intravenous dosing, the dose can be reduced to approximately 75%. Therefore, intravenous levothyroxine dosing is generally started at 70% to 75% of the patient's usual oral therapy dosage (Answer D). The remaining choices are either too high (Answers A and B) or inappropriately substitute liothyronine (Answer E). Although case studies have been published describing successful use of intramuscular levothyroxine (Answer C), the US FDA has not approved this route of administration, and the dosage listed is incorrect.

EDUCATIONAL OBJECTIVE

Guide the transition from oral to intravenous levothyroxine in a patient with hypothyroidism.

REFERENCE(S)

Hays MT. Parenteral thyroxine administration. *Thyroid.* 2007;17(2):127-129. PMID: 17316114

Wenzel KW, Kirschsieper HE. Aspects of the absorption of oral L-thyroxine in normal man. *Metabolism.* 1977;26(1):1-8. PMID: 834138

Alexander EK, Pearce EN, Brent GA, et al. 2017 Guidelines of the American Thyroid Association for the diagnosis and management of thyroid disease during pregnancy and the postpartum. *Thyroid.* 2017;27(3):315-389. PMID: 28056690

15 ANSWER: A) Fine-needle aspiration

This patient has a suppressed serum TSH. If she were not in the first trimester of pregnancy, this would suggest the possibility of an autonomous nodule, which would not require FNA. However, in this case, the suppressed TSH is most likely due to the effects of hCG on the thyroid during the first trimester. Therefore, her nodule must be approached as it would be in a nonpregnant patient with a normal TSH level. Based on thyroid ultrasonography, this nodule has a high suspicion pattern according to American Thyroid Association criteria and is moderately suspicious based on ACR-TIRADS (2 points for solid; 2 points for hypoechogenicity, 2 points for irregular margins). Therefore, performing FNA (Answer A) is the best approach.

Nuclear thyroid scanning (Answer B), although appropriate in the workup of thyroid nodules in the setting of low serum TSH outside pregnancy, is not acceptable during pregnancy. Mildly suppressed TSH, which occurs in approximately 20% of pregnancies during the first trimester, does not require treatment with antithyroid drugs (Answers D and E). Thyroid lobectomy (Answer C) is not a reasonable response before performing FNA.

EDUCATIONAL OBJECTIVE

Recommend fine-needle aspiration biopsy of a suspicious nodule despite mildly low TSH in the first trimester of pregnancy.

REFERENCE(S)

Alexander EK, Pearce EN, Brent GA, et al. 2017 guidelines of the American Thyroid Association for the diagnosis and management of thyroid disease during pregnancy and the postpartum. *Thyroid.* 2017;27(3):315-389. PMID: 28056690

Haugen BR, Alexander EK, Bible KC, et al. 2015 American Thyroid Association management guidelines for adult patients with thyroid nodules and differentiated thyroid cancer: the American Thyroid Association Guidelines Task Force on Thyroid Nodules and Differentiated Thyroid Cancer. *Thyroid.* 2016;26(1):1-133. PMID: 26462967

Tessler FN, Middleton WD, Grant EG, et al. ACR thyroid imaging, reporting and data system (TI-RADS): white paper of the ACR TI-RADS Committee. *J Am Coll Radiol.* 2017;14(5):587-595. PMID: 28372962

16   ANSWER: C) Thyroid hormone transporter defect

This patient has a rare defect in thyroid hormone transport involving the monocarboxylate transporter 8 (MCT8) protein (Answer C). Although thyroid hormone was once believed to freely permeate into the intracellular space, it is now known to be actively transported by proteins such as MCT8. Defective MCT8 transport is an X-linked recessive disorder, seen nearly exclusively in males. The patient described has classic features of this disorder. This is known as Allan-Herndon-Dudley syndrome, and treatment with diiodothyroproprionic acid (DIPTA) may help normalize thyroid function and reduce hypermetabolism. When pathogenic variants in the gene encoding MCT8 (*SLC16A2*) are studied in vitro in cell lines, the cells show defective T_4 and T_3 transport.

The correct answer can also be derived by excluding the incorrect options. For example, an activating pathogenic variant in the type 3 deiodinase gene (Answer A) would be expected to result in low levels of both T_4 and T_3 due to enhanced degradation by the activated D_3 enzyme mutant protein. Similarly, a pathogenic variant in the thyroid hormone receptor β gene (Answer B), as occurs in thyroid hormone resistance, would result in high levels of both free T_4 and T_3. An inactivating pathogenic variant in the thyrotropin receptor gene (Answer D) would lead to elevated serum TSH levels. A similar defect in the thyrotropin-releasing hormone receptor gene (Answer E) would lead to a pattern consistent with central hypothyroidism.

EDUCATIONAL OBJECTIVE

Identify the clinical manifestations of a thyroid hormone transporter defect.

REFERENCE(S)

Dumitrescu AM, Refetoff S. The syndromes of reduced sensitivity to thyroid hormone. *Biochim Biophys Acta.* 2013;1830(7):3987-4003. PMID: 22986150

Verge CF, Konrad D, Cohen M, et al. Diiodothyropropionic acid (DITPA) in the treatment of MCT8 deficiency. *J Clin Endocrinol Metab.* 2012;97(12):4515-4523. PMID: 22993035

Kersseboom S, Kremers GJ, Friesema EC, Visser WE, Klootwijk W, Peeters RP, Visser TJ. Mutations in MCT8 in patients with Allan-Herndon-Dudley-syndrome affecting its cellular distribution. *Mol Endocrinol.* 2013;27(5):801-813. PMID: 23550058

17 ANSWER: C) Start a daily prenatal multivitamin containing 150 mcg iodine

Maternal and fetal hypothyroidism due to iodine deficiency has been linked to profound neurocognitive deficits. Even mild maternal iodine deficiency has been linked to lower child IQ. Because of increased thyroid hormone production, iodine transfer to the fetus, and increased renal iodine losses, pregnant women need increased levels of iodine intake. Iodine is transferred into breast milk where it is an important source of infant nutrition. The recommended daily allowance for iodine is 220 mcg in pregnant women and 250 mcg in women who are lactating (compared with 150 mcg in nonpregnant adults). It is currently recommended that women who are pregnant, lactating, or planning a pregnancy should ingest a supplement containing 150 mcg iodine daily (Answer C).

In the United States, and in several other regions of the world, dairy foods are a major source of dietary iodine intake. Therefore, individuals following a vegan diet are at particular risk for iodine deficiency. In a study in Norway, vegan participants who did not take any iodine supplements had lower urinary iodine levels than vegetarians and pescatarians who were also not using iodine supplements. In population studies, iodine sufficiency is generally thought to be indicated by urinary iodine levels above 100 µg/L, whereas the vegan participants in this study had a median urinary iodine concentration of 43 µg/L.

Switching to an animal product–containing diet (Answer A) is unlikely to be acceptable to the patient, and it is not a guarantee of adequate iodine intake. Adding kelp (Answer B) or supersaturated potassium iodide (Answer D) risks excessive iodine exposure, which may lead to detrimental effects, including maternal thyroid dysfunction, fetal hypothyroidism, and fetal goiter. Finally, iodine sublimates during the preparation of salt from seawater, so sea salt (Answer E) is a poor source of iodine.

EDUCATIONAL OBJECTIVE
Recommend iodine supplementation in the preconception period and during pregnancy.

REFERENCE(S)
Leung AM, Lamar A, He X, Braverman LE, Pearce EN. Iodine status and thyroid function of Boston-area vegetarians and vegans. *J Clin Endocrinol Metab.* 2011;96(8):E1303-E1307. PMID: 21613354

Alexander EK, Pearce EN, Brent GA, et al. 2017 guidelines of the American Thyroid Association for the diagnosis and management of thyroid disease during pregnancy and the postpartum. *Thyroid.* 2017;27(3):315-389. PMID: 28056690

Haugen BR, Alexander EK, Bible KC, et al. 2015 American Thyroid Association management guidelines for adult patients with thyroid nodules and differentiated thyroid cancer: the American Thyroid Association Guidelines Task Force on Thyroid Nodules and Differentiated Thyroid Cancer. *Thyroid.* 2016;26(1):1-133. PMID: 26462967

Tessler FN, Middleton WD, Grant EG, et al. ACR thyroid imaging, reporting and data system (TI-RADS): white paper of the ACR TI-RADS Committee. *J Am Coll Radiol.* 2017;14(5):587-595. PMID: 28372962

Verge CF, Konrad D, Cohen M, et al. Diiodothyropropionic acid (DITPA) in the treatment of MCT8 deficiency. *J Clin Endocrinol Metab.* 2012;97(12):4515-4523. PMID: 22993035

Kersseboom S, Kremers GJ, Friesema ECH, et al. Mutations in MCT8 in patients with Allan-Herndon-Dudley-syndrome affecting its cellular distribution. *Mol Endocrinol.* 2013;27(5):801-813. PMID: 23550058

Groufh-Jacobsen S, Hess SY, Aakre I, Folven Gjengedal EL, Blandhoel Pettersen K, Henjum S. Vegans, vegetarians and pescatarians are at risk of iodine deficiency in Norway. *Nutrients.* 2020;12(11):3555. PMID: 33233534

18 ANSWER: C) Thyroid-stimulating immunoglobulin level

Overall, without considering individual risk factors, the chance of remission after 12 to 18 months of antithyroid drug therapy is 30% to 50%. Men, persons older than 40 years, individuals with large goiters, cigarette smokers, and those with higher baseline thyroid hormone levels are less likely to achieve remission (thus, Answers A, D, and E are incorrect). After 12 to 18 months of antithyroid drug treatment, thyroid-stimulating immunoglobulin levels (Answer C) can be used to refine estimates for the likelihood of remission. Patients with negative thyroid receptor antibodies after 18 months of antithyroid drug treatment are more likely to remit than those in whom thyroid receptor antibodies remain detectable. In this patient who is euthyroid on methimazole but whose thyroid-stimulating immunoglobulin level remains high, the likelihood of long-term remission is only approximately 15%. TPO antibody titer (Answer B) is not associated with the probability of remission.

The recommendation from the 2016 American Thyroid Association guidelines for treating hyperthyroidism is as follows: "If MMI is chosen as the primary therapy for GD, the medication should be continued for approximately 12-18 months, then discontinued if the TSH and TRAb levels are normal at that time."

EDUCATIONAL OBJECTIVE
List predictors of remission in Graves hyperthyroidism.

REFERENCE(S)

Franklyn JA, Boelaert K. Thyrotoxicosis. *Lancet.* 2012;379(9821):1155-1166. PMID: 22394559

Barbesino G, Tomer Y. Clinical review: clinical utility of TSH receptor antibodies. *J Clin Endocrinol Metab.* 2013;98(6):2247-2255. PMID: 23539719

Carella C, Mazziotti G, Sorvillo F, et al. Serum thyrotropin receptor antibodies concentrations in patients with Graves' disease before, at the end of methimazole treatment, and after drug withdrawal: evidence that the activity of thyrotropin receptor antibody and/or thyroid response modify during the observation period. *Thyroid.* 2006;16(3):295-302. PMID: 16571093

Ross DS, Burch HB, Cooper DS, et al. 2016 American Thyroid Association guidelines for diagnosis and management of hyperthyroidism and other causes of thyrotoxicosis. *Thyroid.* 2016;26(10):1343-1421. PMID: 27521067

19 ANSWER: B) Screen for occult celiac disease

Celiac disease (Answer B) is a relatively common autoimmune condition that results in intolerance to dietary gluten. Malabsorption is characteristic of overt celiac disease, and refractory hypothyroidism due to levothyroxine malabsorption is well recognized. Recently, a higher-than-expected incidence of occult or previously unrecognized celiac disease has been found in patients with autoimmune thyroid disease. Similarly, unexplained vitamin D deficiency and resultant low bone mass on densitometry can occur in patients with previously unrecognized celiac disease. Several studies have shown the prevalence of celiac disease in patients with autoimmune thyroid disease to be approximately 3% to 5%, compared with approximately 1% in control populations. Similarly, a higher-than-expected prevalence of autoimmune thyroid disease has been described in patients with known celiac disease. Previously unsuspected celiac disease has been described both in patients with malabsorption of levothyroxine and in patients with vitamin D deficiency. Levothyroxine malabsorption in celiac disease is reversed with a gluten-free diet.

Guidelines for treating hypothyroidism recommend excluding causes of malabsorption in patients taking levothyroxine whose dosage requirement has increased or who require unexpectedly higher doses of levothyroxine than would be predicted based on body weight. Based on her body weight and a weight-based dose of

1.4 mcg/kg to 1.6 mcg/kg, this patient would be expected to require approximately 100 mcg levothyroxine. Therefore, evaluating for celiac disease as a cause of malabsorption is reasonable.

The remaining options are not plausible. Four hours of separation of levothyroxine from calcium supplements is generally considered sufficient (thus, Answer A is incorrect). The TSH and free T_4 assays are concordant, making antibody interference with the TSH assay unlikely (thus, Answer C is incorrect). T_3/T_4 combination therapy (Answer D) is preferred by some patients, although randomized controlled trials to date have not provided clear evidence for symptomatic improvement. However, this patient is not complaining of symptoms, and changing to combination therapy will not address the underlying problem. Pernicious anemia may be associated with other autoimmune diseases, but documenting a low vitamin B_{12} level (Answer E) would not provide an explanation for this patient not achieving a normal TSH level while taking 300 mcg levothyroxine, as vitamin B_{12} deficiency would not cause malabsorption.

EDUCATIONAL OBJECTIVE
Diagnose celiac sprue as an etiology of uncontrolled hypothyroidism.

REFERENCE(S)
Virili C, Bassotti G, Santaguida MG, et al. Atypical celiac disease as cause of increased need for thyroxine: a systematic study. *J Clin Endocrinol Metab*. 2012;97(3):E419-E422. PMID: 22238404

Jonklaas J, Bianco AC, Bauer AJ, et al. Guidelines for the treatment of hypothyroidism: prepared by the American Thyroid Association Task Force on Thyroid Hormone Replacement. *Thyroid*. 2014;24(12):1670-1751. PMID: 25266247

20   ANSWER: D) Thyroidectomy from collar incision

The CT shows a substernal goiter with mass effect on the trachea. The patient is symptomatic, with positional dyspnea, most likely due to compression of her trachea by the asymmetrically enlarged thyroid when she lies on her side. She also has dysphagia suggesting an impact of the goiter on her esophagus. More than 90% of substernal goiters can be "delivered" through a collar incision (Answer D).

The remaining therapeutic options listed are less helpful. Specifically, this euthyroid patient's thyroid mass is unlikely to respond significantly to levothyroxine suppressive therapy (Answer A) and she would be at risk for iatrogenic hyperthyroidism. Radioactive iodine therapy with the assistance of recombinant human TSH (Answer B) in a patient with an intact thyroid should be carefully monitored and is potentially dangerous due to a release of thyroid hormone from the gland and to temporary swelling of the thyroid gland under the influence of recombinant human TSH. This might be considered as a potential option in a patient who was not a surgical candidate. This patient is healthy and not in an older age group that would preclude definitive resection of her goiter. Thermal ablation (Answer C) would not prove useful in reducing the size of this very large substernal goiter. No intervention (Answer E) would be inappropriate given her symptomatic disease.

An analysis of studies of goiter treatment either by surgical resection or with use of radioactive iodine therapy showed that both approaches relieved pressure on surrounding structures and improved respiration and swallowing. In a healthy 52-year-old patient, surgery would certainly provide definitive therapy for her compressive symptoms.

EDUCATIONAL OBJECTIVE
Devise a treatment approach to a symptomatic substernal goiter.

REFERENCE(S)
Bahn RS, Castro MR. Approach to the patient with nontoxic multinodular goiter. *J Clin Endocrinol Metab*. 2011;96(5):1202-1212. PMID: 21543434

Fast S, Nielsen VE, Bonnema SJ, Hegedüs L. Dose-dependent acute effects of recombinant human TSH (rhTSH) on thyroid size and function: comparison of 0.1, 0.3 and 0.9 mg of rhTSH. *Clin Endocrinol (Oxf)*. 2010;72(3):411-416. PMID: 19508679

Bonnema SJ, Hegedüs L. Radioiodine therapy in benign thyroid diseases: effects, side effects, and factors affecting therapeutic outcome. *Endocr Rev.* 2012;33(6):920-980. PMID: 22961916

Sorensen JR, Bonnema SJ, Godballe C, Hegedüs L. The impact of goiter and thyroid surgery on goiter related esophageal dysfunction. A systematic review. *Front Endocrinol (Lausanne).* 2018;9:679. PMID: 30524374

21 ANSWER: C) Recombinant human TSH, using 30 mCi ¹³¹I

In 2012, 2 prospective randomized controlled trials comparing remnant ablation using either 30 mCi or 100 mCi, given by either thyroid hormone withdrawal or using recombinant human TSH (rhTSH), documented equivalent rates of successful remnant ablation in the 4 study arms. The 2009 American Thyroid Association guidelines on the management of thyroid cancer recommend that the lowest effective dose of radioiodine be used for remnant ablation, which we now know to be 30 mCi. Given these data and the patient's preference to minimize time away from work, it follows that the best regimen would be recombinant human TSH, using 30 mCi ¹³¹I (Answer C).

The terminology used to describe radioiodine in the management of differentiated thyroid cancer is at times confusing. Radioiodine remnant ablation, which applies to the current case, refers to the destruction of any remaining normal thyroid tissue after radioiodine, when no residual thyroid cancer is known or suspected on the basis of accepted risk factors. The benefit of radioiodine remnant ablation is largely to facilitate patient follow-up. Therapeutic radioiodine applies to the treatment of known persistent disease such as in patients with distant metastases or local invasion that is nonresectable. Higher doses are generally used in this circumstance. Finally, the term adjuvant radioiodine therapy has been recently applied to the use of radioiodine in patients with no definite evidence of residual tumor, but in whom persistent tumor is suspected, as in lymph nodes. An example might be a patient with T₃ or T₄ tumors or those in whom multiple affected lymph nodes are identified at the time of surgery.

EDUCATIONAL OBJECTIVE
List the clinical features that favor the use of recombinant human TSH–stimulated radioiodine remnant ablation in patients with thyroid cancer.

REFERENCE(S)
Schlumberger M, Catargi B, Borget I, et al; Tumeurs de la Thyroïde Refractaires Network for the Essai Stimulation Ablation Equivalence Trial. Strategies of radioiodine ablation in patients with low-risk thyroid cancer. *N Engl J Med.* 2012;366(18):1663-1673. PMID: 22551127

Mallick U, Harmer C, Yap B, et al. Ablation with low-dose radioiodine and thyrotropin alfa in thyroid cancer. *N Engl J Med.* 2012;366(18):1674-1685. PMID: 22551128

Haugen BR, Alexander EK, Bible KC, et al. 2015 American Thyroid Association management guidelines for adult patients with thyroid nodules and differentiated thyroid cancer: the American Thyroid Association Guidelines Task Force on Thyroid Nodules and Differentiated Thyroid Cancer. *Thyroid.* 2016;26(1):1-133. PMID: 26462967

22 ANSWER: A) Primary hypothyroidism

Sunitinib is a tyrosine kinase inhibitor used to treat certain malignancies such as renal cell carcinoma and gastrointestinal stromal tumors. Studies show that sunitinib can induce primary hypothyroidism (Answer A) in up to 85% of patients. Furthermore, sunitinib seems to increase the levothyroxine dosage requirement in hypothyroid patients. Sunitinib therapy would not be expected to result in secondary hypothyroidism (Answer B), primary hyperthyroidism (Answer C), secondary hyperthyroidism (Answer D), or euthyroid sick syndrome (Answer E). Many other tyrosine kinase inhibitors, including sorafenib, cabozantinib, nilotinib, and pazopanib, are also associated with the development of hypothyroidism.

Various mechanisms have been suggested to explain the development of hypothyroidism. In animal studies, hepatic type 3 deiodinase activity increased and thyroid histologic examination showed marked capillary regression. In patients being treated with sunitinib, there is also evidence of altered T_4/T_3 metabolism and some of those who developed hypothyroidism also developed TPO antibody positivity. Interestingly, the development of hypothyroidism appears to be associated with improved overall survival in nonthyroidal cancers.

EDUCATIONAL OBJECTIVE
Predict the most common effect that sunitinib has on thyroid function.

REFERENCE(S)
Illouz F, Braun D, Briet C, Schweizer U, Rodien P. Endocrine side-effects of anti-cancer drugs: thyroid effects of tyrosine kinase inhibitors. *Eur J Endocrinol.* 2014;171(3):R91-R99. PMID: 24833135

Lechner MG, Vyas CM, Hamnvik OR, et al. Hypothyroidism during tyrosine kinase inhibitor therapy is associated with longer survival in patients with advanced nonthyroidal cancers. *Thyroid.* 2018;28(4):445-453. PMID: 29652597

Kappers MHW, van Esch JHM, Smedts FMM, et al. Sunitinib-induced hypothyroidism is due to induction of type 3 deiodinase activity and thyroidal capillary regression. *J Clin Endocrinol Metab.* 2011;96(10):3087-3094. PMID: 21816788

Pani F, Atzori F, Baghino G, et al. Thyroid dysfunction in patients with metastatic carcinoma treated with sunitinib: is thyroid autoimmunity involved? *Thyroid.* 2015;25(11):1255-1261. PMID: 26414109

23 ANSWER: B) Serum thyroglobulin measurement

The differential diagnosis for patients with thyrotoxicosis and low radioactive iodine uptake includes painless and postpartum thyroiditis, subacute thyroiditis, struma ovarii (with low radioactive iodine uptake in the neck, but uptake in the pelvis on whole-body scan), factitious or iatrogenic thyroiditis, amiodarone use, and recent high-dose iodine exposure. In this male patient, struma ovarii and postpartum thyroiditis are not possibilities. He is not taking amiodarone. Subacute thyroiditis is unlikely given the lack of a viral prodrome, fever, or thyroid tenderness, so assessing his erythrocyte sedimentation rate (Answer C) is incorrect. The urinary iodine concentration is not consistent with recent excessive iodine exposure, so repeating the radioactive iodine uptake following a low-iodine diet (Answer A) is unlikely to change results. In this patient, the most likely diagnoses are either factitious thyrotoxicosis or painless thyroiditis. Graves disease has already been ruled out by the low radioactive iodine uptake, so thyroid-stimulating immunoglobulin measurement (Answer E) is incorrect. Thyroid ultrasonography with color Doppler (Answer D) would show absent hypervascularity with both of these entities. However, the serum thyroglobulin concentration (Answer B) in this thyroglobulin antibody–negative patient would be elevated in painless thyroiditis but low in factitious thyrotoxicosis.

Factitious hyperthyroidism can occur when patients take supplements that contain thyroid hormones or when patients take thyroid hormone in order to achieve weight loss. Typically, as in this case, doses of thyroid hormones that are associated with weight loss are also associated with other stigmata of thyrotoxicosis.

EDUCATIONAL OBJECTIVE
Construct the differential diagnosis for low radioiodine uptake thyrotoxicosis.

REFERENCE(S)
De Leo S, Lee SY, Braverman LE. Hyperthyroidism. *Lancet.* 2016;388(10047):906-918. PMID: 27038492

Ross DS, Burch HB, Cooper DS, et al. 2016 American Thyroid Association Guidelines for diagnosis and management of hyperthyroidism and other causes of thyrotoxicosis. *Thyroid.* 2016;26(10):1343-1421. PMID: 27521067

Bernet VJ. Thyroid hormone misuse and abuse. *Endocrine.* 2019;66(1):79-86. PMID: 31617167

Irwig MS, Fleseriu M, Jonklaas J, et al. Off-label use and misuse of testosterone, growth hormone, thyroid hormone, and adrenal supplements: risks and costs of a growing problem. *Endocr Pract.* 2020;26(3):340-353. PMID: 32163313

24

ANSWER: A) Perform FNA biopsy

This patient presents with thyrotoxicosis and neck pain consistent with subacute thyroiditis. She has been treated with prednisone with little improvement. Over a period of only 3 weeks, she has had progressive asymmetric thyroid enlargement, now accompanied by compressive symptoms. The diagnosis in this patient was anaplastic thyroid cancer with thyrotoxicosis due to destructive thyroiditis. There have been reports of this unusual presentation of anaplastic thyroid cancer in the medical literature, and some patients have been treated with prolonged courses of corticosteroids before a correct diagnosis has been made. These patients typically have exceptionally aggressive disease and very limited survival. Although this is an atypical presentation, very rapid thyroid enlargement in an older patient should always prompt concern for anaplastic thyroid cancer. FNA biopsy (Answer A) would determine her underlying diagnosis.

Another malignancy that may present with a rapidly growing goiter is thyroid lymphoma. However, in contrast to this case of thyrotoxicosis due to damage of normal thyroid tissue, thyroid lymphoma typically presents with hypothyroidism due to its association with Hashimoto thyroiditis.

Glucocorticoid therapy may help with the pain from her thyroid inflammation. However, switching to a different corticosteroid (Answer C), starting methimazole (Answer B), or performing contrast CT of the neck (Answer D) would all fail to determine the underlying diagnosis. In addition, methimazole is generally not useful in the management of low iodine uptake inflammatory thyroiditis, since thyroid hormone synthesis is not increased. Thyroidectomy (Answer E) should not be performed in the absence of a definitive diagnosis.

EDUCATIONAL OBJECTIVE

Recognize the rare presentation of anaplastic cancer as thyrotoxicosis and neck pain with rapid thyroid growth and no response to steroids.

REFERENCE(S)

Kumar V, Blanchon B, Gu X, et al. Anaplastic thyroid cancer and hyperthyroidism. *Endocr Pathol.* 2005; 16(3):245-250. PMID: 16299408

Heymann RS, Brent GA, Hershman JM. Anaplastic thyroid carcinoma with thyrotoxicosis and hypoparathyroidism. *Endocr Pract.* 2005;11(4):281-284. PMID: 16006301

Smallridge RC, Ain KB, Asa SL, et al; American Thyroid Association Anaplastic Thyroid Cancer Guidelines Taskforce. American Thyroid Association guidelines for management of patients with anaplastic thyroid cancer. *Thyroid.* 2012;22(11): 1104-1139. PMID: 23130564

Matsuzuka F, Miyauchi A, Katayama S, et al. Clinical aspects of primary thyroid lymphoma: diagnosis and treatment based on our experience of 119 cases. *Thyroid.* 1993;3(2):93-99. PMID: 8369658

25

ANSWER: B) Repeated thyroglobulin and thyroglobulin antibody measurements in 6 weeks using the same radioimmunoassay

This patient has an elevated serum thyroglobulin value shortly after undergoing thyroidectomy for thyroid cancer. Thyroglobulin measurement is a sensitive tool for thyroid cancer surveillance, especially in thyroglobulin antibody–negative patients such as this one, but it is important to be aware of its limitations. In this case, it is simply too soon to measure the serum thyroglobulin postoperatively; values tend to be elevated in the first few days to weeks after surgery given serum thyroglobulin elevations caused by the surgical manipulation of the thyroid gland and the serum half-life of thyroglobulin. It is generally recommended to wait 6 weeks after thyroidectomy or 3 months after radioactive iodine ablation before the initial postoperative thyroglobulin measurement. If the measurements are repeated in 6 weeks (Answer B), the thyroglobulin level will most likely be substantially lower.

Ideally, thyroglobulin should be measured with the same assay over time due to substantial interassay variability (as much as 40%-60%) between methods. Repeating the measurement immediately with a different assay (Answers A and

D) will still most likely result in an uninterpretable value because of timing. Measuring thyroglobulin in serially diluted sera (Answer C) can determine whether thyroglobulin is artifactually elevated (or, less frequently, artifactually decreased) due to the presence of heterophile antibodies. Such antibodies can form a bridge between capture and detection antibody leading to a false thyroglobulin measurement in immunometric assays. However, heterophile antibodies are unlikely to have caused an artifactual thyroglobulin elevation in this patient, since thyroglobulin was measured by radioimmunoassay. The patient has a low-risk tumor based on surgical pathology, so radioactive iodine ablation (Answer E) is not indicated.

EDUCATIONAL OBJECTIVE
Identify common pitfalls with the use of serum thyroglobulin for thyroid cancer surveillance.

REFERENCE(S)
Giovanella L, Clark PM, Chiovato L, et al. Thyroglobulin measurement using highly sensitive assays in patients with differentiated thyroid cancer: a clinical position paper. *Eur J Endocrinol.* 2014;171(2):R33-R46. PMID: 24743400

Haugen BR, Alexander EK, Bible KC, et al. 2015 American Thyroid Association management guidelines for adult patients with thyroid nodules and differentiated thyroid cancer: the American Thyroid Association Guidelines Task Force on Thyroid Nodules and Differentiated Thyroid Cancer. *Thyroid.* 2016;26(1):1-133. PMID: 26462967

26 ANSWER: B) Reduce the methimazole dosage

This patient has a history of thyrotoxicosis and is being treated with methimazole. Her thyroid scan from 2 years ago clearly shows a pattern of toxic multinodular goiter. Unlike Graves disease, which may enter a lasting remission after completion of a 12- to 18-month course of antithyroid drug therapy, toxic multinodular goiter has a natural history of gradual progression. Thus, patients with toxic multinodular goiters usually continue to require either medical therapy with low dosages of antithyroid drugs or definitive therapy with radioactive iodine or thyroidectomy. Because the patient is currently biochemically hypothyroid, her methimazole dosage should be reduced (Answer B) or definitive therapy should be considered. In this patient who has stated that she wishes to avoid therapy with radioactive iodine (Answer E), this avenue should clearly not be pursued.

There is no reason to perform another scan with radioactive iodine uptake (Answer A) because the pattern of uptake and percentage uptake are unlikely to have changed substantially. Discontinuing methimazole (Answers C and D) would result in resurgent thyrotoxicosis. The 2016 American Thyroid Association guidelines for the management of hyperthyroidism state that long-term therapy with low-dosage antithyroid drugs is an acceptable option for patients who prefer to avoid definitive therapy, and a recent meta-analysis concluded that long-term antithyroid drug use is safe.

EDUCATIONAL OBJECTIVE
Recommend continued therapy with a low-dosage antithyroid drug in a patient with toxic multinodular goiter and distinguish this approach from that used to treat Graves disease, which may enter remission.

REFERENCE(S)
Ross DS, Burch HB, Cooper DS, et al. 2016 American Thyroid Association guidelines for diagnosis and management of hyperthyroidism and other causes of thyrotoxicosis. *Thyroid.* 2016;26(10):1343-1421. PMID: 27521067

Azizi F, Malboosbaf R. Long-term antithyroid drug treatment: a systematic review and meta-analysis. *Thyroid.* 2017;27(10):1223-1231. PMID: 28699478

27 ANSWER: B) Iodine

Patients with underlying nodular autonomy are at risk for the development of hyperthyroidism in response to high levels of iodine exposure (Answer B). The tolerable upper limit for daily iodine intake is 1100 mcg, but some supplements contain amounts greatly in excess of this. This patient has all the features of endogenous hyperthyroidism and presumably the high doses of iodine have fueled her previously subclinical hyperthyroidism. In addition to use of iodine supplements, another cause of a similar presentation would be exposure to radiocontrast agents in someone with mild or previously undetected hypothyroidism.

Perchlorate (Answer D) is a competitive inhibitor of thyroidal iodine uptake, and it would be expected to cause hypothyroidism rather than hyperthyroidism.

Thyroid hormone (Answer C) is found illegally in some over-the-counter US supplements, but serum thyroglobulin would be expected to be low, rather than elevated, in a patient taking exogenous thyroid hormone.

Various adrenal extracts (Answer A) have been found in over-the-counter supplements, but they would not be expected to cause hyperthyroidism.

The use of biotin supplements (Answer E) can cause artifactual interference with commonly used biotin-streptavidin immunoassays for TSH, thyroid hormone, and anti–thyrotropin receptor antibodies. A high-dosage biotin supplement could cause assay changes similar to those seen in this patient, but the biotin would not actually be associated with symptomatic hyperthyroidism, or with elevated serum thyroglobulin. High circulating biotin levels cause falsely low measurements in immunometric sandwich assays (such as that for TSH), but falsely high measurements for competitive immunoassays (such as those for free T_4, T_3, and thyroid-stimulating immunoglobulin). Thus, patients taking biotin may have laboratory results identical to those found in Graves hyperthyroidism. However, unlike this patient, the affected individual would not have symptoms of hyperthyroidism. Artifactual thyroid function results have been reported in patients taking at least 1500 mcg of biotin daily, and test results normalize 2 to 7 days after stopping the biotin.

EDUCATIONAL OBJECTIVE
Describe potential effects of iodine excess.

REFERENCE(S)

Leung AM, Braverman LE. Consequences of excess iodine. *Nat Rev Endocrinol.* 2014;10(3):136-142. PMID: 24342882

Kang GY, Parks JR, Fileta B, et al. Thyroxine and triiodothyronine content in commercially available thyroid health supplements. *Thyroid.* 2013;23(10):1233-1237. PMID: 23758055

Kummer S, Hermsen D, Distelmaier F. Biotin treatment mimicking Graves' disease. *N Engl J Med.* 2016;375(7):704-706. PMID: 27532849

Rhee CM, Bhan I, Alexander EK, Brunelli SM. Association between iodinated contrast media exposure and incident hyperthyroidism and hypothyroidism. *Arch Intern Med.* 2012;172(2):153-159. PMID: 22271121

28 ANSWER: B) Refer for immediate total thyroidectomy with neck dissection

Current guidelines for the management of thyroid disease in pregnancy suggest that in general it is safe to wait until after delivery to perform thyroid surgery for thyroid cancer discovered early in pregnancy. The exception, however, is in patients demonstrating a more aggressive course, including growth by 50% of nodule volume (or 20% in 2 dimensions) or aggressive baseline features, such as local invasion. This patient had a doubling of her tumor size and the new appearance of metastatic disease to lymph nodes; therefore, thyroidectomy should not be deferred (thus, Answer B is correct and Answers C and D are incorrect). If thyroid surgery is required during pregnancy, the second trimester is thought to be safest because anesthetic agents may have a teratogenic effect during organogenesis in the first trimester, and surgery in the third trimester has the potential to induce premature labor. Initiating levothyroxine suppressive therapy (Answer A) might be helpful, but it would not be an acceptable substitute for thyroidectomy. Ethanol ablation of the lymph node (Answer E) is incorrect, as it only addresses the known metastatic node and not the primary tumor, which could continue to progress.

EDUCATIONAL OBJECTIVE
Recommend options for thyroid cancer treatment in pregnant women.

REFERENCE(S)

Alexander EK, Pearce EN, Brent GA, et al. 2017 Guidelines of the American Thyroid Association for the diagnosis and management of thyroid disease during pregnancy and the postpartum. *Thyroid.* 2017;27(3):315-389. PMID: 28056690

Gibelli B, Zamperini P, Proh M, Giugliano G. Management and follow-up of thyroid cancer in pregnant women. *Acta Otorhinolaryngol Ital.* 2011;31(6):358-365. PMID: 22323846